IMPROVING WITH AGE

HOW TO LIVE TO 101 AND STILL HAVE FUN

By

Bernard Singer, Ed.D.

D1416163

IMPROVING WITH AGE: How to Live to 101 and Still Have Fun

ISBN 978-0-9709859-1-0

1. Longevity. 2. Nutrition. 3. Spirituality. 4. Vegetarian Diet.
5. Alternatives to Drugs. 6. Weight Loss. 7. Tai Chi. 8. Meditation

Published by the Society of Faithists, a Non Profit Corporation

Notice:

The author of this book shares his experiences and opinions. The knowledge and information contained in this book is based on the author's life experiences, education and research. The author and publisher are not offering medical advice, or other professional advice, and are not liable for any damage or any claims made by the reader due to reading or following any information in this book. This book is intended as a reference volume only, not as a medical manual. The information given here is designed to help you make informed decisions about your health. It is not intended as a substitute for any treatment that may have been prescribed by your doctor. If you suspect that you have a medical problem, we urge you to seek competent medical help.

Bernard Singer is the author of an earlier book, *Life Beyond Earth: The Evidence and Its Implications,* which was published by the Society of Faithists in 2001.

For further information you may contact the Society of Faithists on their website, fathistsociety.com

Cover design, photography and typesetting by Charles LaPadula
of CMS Consulting Group, Inc. - http://www.cmsconsulting.com

Acknowledgements

I would like to dedicate this book to my wife, Ruth, who although departed from Earth, gave me the love and support that enabled me to achieve three degrees at Rutgers University, and write a book while I worked at a full-time job. Although she is very active in the spiritual realm, she did take the time to visit me on two occasions after her demise to confirm the fact that life does go on after so-called death.

I would also like to thank my two sons, Barry and David for their love and support and for their magnificent accomplishments in their fields of endeavor which help to make this a better world to live in; David as a physician and consultant, and Barry as a producer of musical shows.

My nephew Arnie Holtz and his wonderful wife Mary, who both heal people with natural methods, have supported me in many ways in my endeavors to write books that heal.

Dianne Denenberg has been of great help in editing this book as well as my previous book, *Life Beyond Earth: The Evidence and Its Implications.* Her skills of healing with such techniques as color therapy and Reiki brought my attention to those healing modalities.

I would like to express my appreciation to my granddaughter, Kimberly and to her husband David Reynolds for their valuable assistance in helping solve my computer problems whenever the need occurred.

My illustrator, Tania Singer-Cergnul, deserves special mention for the vivid cartoons she created for this book.

My heartfelt thanks to my friend, Charles LaPadula, for his many hours of help in bringing the book to completion with his software, photographs, cover design and editing.

Many thanks to Paige Edwards, librarian at the Omega Institute Ram Dass library, for her help with my research.

Table of Contents

Part One: Longevity

Part Two: Alternative Health Care

FOREWORD

When Awareness Runs Over Your Dogma

I am Carlos Garcia, a Medical Doctor by profession. Although I started my career in corporate allopathic medicine, my fate directed me into the misunderstood, often feared, through ignorance and all too maligned, *'alternative, integrative or natural medicine'* specialty. I grew my practice into the largest in the United States. In December 2005, the United States government raided my offices for the heinous crime of helping people get healthy without the need of drugs. It seems that correctly done, natural medicine can remedy most illnesses and get people off of FDA approved medications and their predictable and reliable side effects.

Today in 2009, our country is torn by *'health care reform'*. But wait, who ever claimed that we have *health*care is clearly delusional, I think. Yes, corporate traditional allopathic medicine is great but only when used in treating trauma, i.e. gunshots, auto accidents, cuts etc. In just about every other medical application, corporate traditional medicine feeds our American fantasy that some magic pill will make everything better. What America has in 2009 is *sick* care, I think. Americans, in general, will gladly subscribe to any pill that allows us to eat like pigs, drink like fish and smoke like chimneys, while neglecting exercise, and providing an abdominal six pack as a side effect. Being stewards of your body and responsibility for your health is American heresy.

It is an American rarity, in these times, to find anyone with a true zeal for life anymore. Today's society lives just for the moment with little regard, if any, for the future. Ignorance is bliss appears to be the motto for today's generation. Heck, today's generation make the hippies of the 60's appear intellectual and physically active by comparison.

About a year ago, while consulting with a good friend of mine, David Singer, D.C., he informed me that his father was on his way to meet with him at my office. I braced myself for what I knew was going to be another *'meet my dad, please tell him that he is doing well'*. I think some misunderstand my sensitivity. I asked David his father's age – he stated 92. I was now prepared, so I thought …

I got a call from my receptionist stating that Bernard Singer had arrived, looking to meet with his son, Dr. Singer. So I took a deep breath and prepared for the inevitable, the 'meet and greet'. In spite, of David's good health, I was anticipating a relatively frail older man. There was a knock at the door. He entered, and I said to myself: *"Wow"*. If I had never spoken with David, I would have guessed Bernard's age somewhere mid- to late- sixties. He walks erect, with a spring in his walk, and a firm handshake. He is educated and articulate, quick as a whip, intellectually. No Alzheimer's here. He is a fascinating human enigma.

He could see a perplexity about my face. Thinking that I had misheard David, or that he was joking, I asked Bernard his age: he stated with pride: *'92'*. He then proceeded to show off his physical dexterity and coordination. I sat back onto my black leather chair in amazement. We began having a most delightful and insightful conversation, one that I will remember for quite some time.

We discussed a plethora of different topics. He is clearly well read and spoken, but more overly, he had integrated his knowledge. All too frequently, I meet and converse with those who understand one or two areas of medicine. Some understand energy, while others understand nutrition, others exercise etc. But they are unable to see the entire mind-body integration. Yet Bernard's greatest achievement is, not that he integrated his knowledge, but that he applied what he learned. Unlike many well read people, Bernard executed a plan that works. He is a living proof of what he writes about in his book.

Whereas this book may not be the holy grail of integrated medicine, or an exhaustive encyclopedic marvel, it is full of practical and insightful information. Suffice to say, that most of you will benefit from the sage wisdom found within this volume.

For those of you who want to start your journey of health and wellness, this book is a great beginning. For those on your journey, this book may facilitate your integration of your knowledge. For those naysayers who believe in corporate traditional allopathic care, I recommend that you look around and see how many relatives and friends depend on drugs. If bypass surgery is curative, why is it all patients need drugs *after* their surgery?

Hook or crook, deliberately planned and executed or just by happenstance; I can honestly state: *'I want to be like Bernie when I get old(er)'* –

Remember only you can cure you. The only person any doctor can cure is himself or herself.

Wishing all a safe and healthy journey through life,

-- Carlos Manuel Garcia, Medical Doctor
Founder and Director of the Utopia Wellness Institute
www.utopiaawaits.com

Preface

The present healthcare system is in a state of disaster. It should more aptly be called a sick care system. New evidence keeps piling up about the terrible side-effects of drugs. In spite of the fact that Americans spend much more than any other country on healthcare, the United States ranks 23rd in the world in longevity. Healthcare costs have continued to increase to the point where many major corporations have had to declare bankruptcy. There is an urgent need for a change away from the present failed medical system to a system based on natural alternative methods that work without any harmful side-effects and at a fraction of the cost.

Dr. Bernard Singer, in his new book, *Improving with Age: How to Live to 101 and Still Have Fun,* not only offers alternatives to the medical system, he offers a wealth of practical knowledge that can be used to maintain optimum health and joy of living. At his present age of 93, he is a living proof of what he writes about. He will be 94 on March 18, 2010.

The twelve chapters of the book are filled with a vast amount of factual knowledge based on Singer's personal experiences together with over 60 years of research into nutrition, exercise and spiritual knowledge which empowers the reader with the ability to apply holistic methods to improve their health and quality of life. He is a retired teacher, having taught children with learning disabilities for 25 years. Chapter Six in the book on ADD and ADHD is filled with practical knowledge that can be put to use by parents, prospective parents and anyone else who is interested in the prevention and cure for these ailments.

Due to the life-threatening illness of his infant son, sixty years ago, which required a strict diet to overcome; Singer began to study everything he could about nutrition which he has pursued up to the present time. His excellent health and longevity are a testament to his making use of the knowledge he acquired. Chapter One titled Nutrition contains a wealth of knowledge which the reader will find to be of great practical value.

Singer is a master Tai Chi instructor with over 20 years of experience. He still actively practices Tai Chi every morning and teaches classes all year round. During the past three summers he has taught Tai Chi at the famous Omega Institute. One of the reasons for his longevity, he believes, is Tai Chi. He describes the many health benefits of Tai Chi in Chapter Two of his book.

Dr. Singer holds three degrees from Rutgers University in the fields of social sciences and education. He is the author of an earlier book, *Life Beyond Earth: The Evidence and its Implications.* He is available for talks and book signings on his books. He is an excellent speaker and has been interviewed on radio and television shows and featured in many newspaper articles.

INTRODUCTION

This book was written largely because of the many people who were bombarding me with questions about how I was able to arrive at my present age of 93 in such excellent health and youthful vigor. As you read this book, it is my hope that you will acquire new insights and practical knowledge that will enable you to have a healthier and happier life. The book is based on my personal experiences and knowledge which I obtained during my long life plus my intensive studies into all aspects of health. I believe my longevity is largely due to my beliefs, diet and lifestyle.

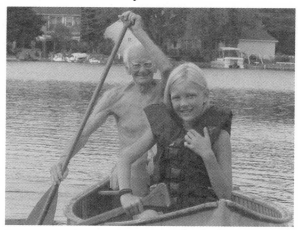

Dr. Singer at age 93 canoeing with his Great-Grand-Daughter, Jade

Information issued by the medical and pharmaceutical industries has led to the assumption that people are now living longer because of improvements in the medical system. This may be based on the simple fact that there are large numbers of baby-boomers who are now reaching the age of 60. We actually rank lower in life expectancy than **28 other countries.** Another very important factor to consider is how many of these elderly people are still enjoying good health. It is one thing to reach an older age but what good is it if you are unable to enjoy it because of physical and mental illnesses? In this regard the statistics show an alarming increase in the number of people dying from cancer and heart disease together with an increase of people coming down with other diseases such as obesity, Alzheimer's disease, lupus, Parkinson's, multiple sclerosis, and diabetes.

New equipment and techniques used in hospital intensive care units prolong life, and new surgery procedures used for cancer and diseases of the heart do appear to prolong life but do these procedures produce a healthier person? Are the underlying causes of these diseases being corrected or eliminated so that it prevents their reoccurrence? For the most part conventional medicine places its emphasis on the suppressing of symptoms, not on healing the body. Prescription drugs are used for this purpose and are being used in ever greater amounts in spite of the fact that they all have serious side-effects.. This problem has become even more dangerous because of the fact that there is a serious over dosing of patients due to the over-prescribing of drugs. This practice has become so common that there is a new word for it, **polypharma,** which appears in *Webster's Revised Unabridged Dictionary* as "the act or practice of prescribing too many medicines." Most people rely on medical doctors to take care of their health needs but are unaware of the connection between the doctors and the pharmaceutical industry which is primarily interested in selling drugs. The extent of this problem is revealed in an article appearing in the *AARP Bulletin*, Jan./Feb.,2008, as follows:

"The results of a national survey were published in 2008 in the *New England Journal of Medicine,* in which 94 percent of the doctors polled said they had 'direct ties' to the drug industry …Whether they know it or not, 'many doctors have been prescribing according to industry profits rather than the patient's needs. Each day more than 101,000 drug company reps call on the nation's doctors. Primary care physicians, on average, have 28 interactions per week with drug reps, according to a 2005 report by the Health Strategies Group, a consulting firm for manufacturers of health care products."

The drug problem is discussed at length in this book. Evidence is provided showing the link between the increased use of drugs and the increased incidence of deadly diseases. Many people have become aware of this problem and are turning to alternative health care methods that have been proven to be helpful without any of the harmful effects of drugs. Non-invasive health care methods that heal without side-effects are described in detail together with preventative measures to insure health and longevity.

Although there are larger numbers of older people at the present time, the fact remains that elderly people now have more diseases than ever before. The increase of known cancer cases is particularly alarming as shown by the results of scientific studies: "From 1950 to 2001 the incidence for all types of cancer in the United States increased by 85 percent, and that was the age-adjusted rate, which means the increase has nothing to do with people living longer. The fastest growing rate of cancer for any age group has been among children, who cannot be accused of having smoked or partied or worked or stressed themselves into a diseased state. Dr. Samuel Epstein, an internationally recognized expert in toxicology, laid the blame squarely on the synthetics chemical revolution which made use of new technology in 1940 to produce chemicals from petroleum for every purpose imaginable."[1]

Such things as auto exhaust emissions, chemical fertilizers, pesticides, weed killers, and additives to food and water came into widespread use resulting in the pollution of our air, food and water. Many of the chemicals that are added to our food and water are poisonous by-products of industrial wastes. The full extent of this problem and the things that can be done to protect our planet, ourselves and our loved ones are presented throughout this book. The main causes of disease and what can be done about it are found in chapters three and five.

You might think that my longevity is due to my genetic background but that is not the case. My father died of cancer at age fifty-four and my mother died of cancer at the age of 80. If genes have anything to do with it, I should have died from cancer a while ago. Research studies actually show that genes play only a minor role in determining longevity. Based on numerous studies, it appears that the most important factors in determining longevity are diet, exercise and stress. Mental attitudes and the realization that a loving God does exist are also important factors in maintaining a peaceful state of mind and buoyant health. Increased energy and the reduction of stress by such activities as deep breathing, yoga, Tai Chi and meditation can also be of great benefit. All of these aspects of longevity are

---

[1] Diamond, Harvey. *Fit for Life*. NY: Kensington Books, pp.36-37.

covered in great detail in this book. I was fortunate to learn of these aspects of health and apply them early on in my life, which I believe was the reason for my health and longevity. As I mentioned above, I do not believe that my genetic background had anything to do with my longevity.

Not only did I not enjoy the benefits of a healthy genetic background, but I started life as a sickly child. I suffered from frequent infections of my respiratory tract such as colds, la grippe, and the flu. I vividly remember being brought to a hospital to have my tonsils removed. It seemed like there was an epidemic of tonsillitis going on since almost every child was having their tonsils removed at that time .I was saved from this trauma by the fact that my parents requested financial aid since they couldn't afford to pay for an operation. The doctor told my parents that my tonsils were not so badly enlarged that they needed to be removed at that time and sent me home. Thank God, I still have my tonsils.

When I entered Junior High School, I experienced another traumatic incident. I was given a physical examination and shortly afterward, a nurse came to visit my mother. She expressed concern that I appeared thin and undernourished. She asked me to drop my pants and pointed out to my mother that I had bowed legs. Then she started to whisper to my mother suggestions as to what could be done to improve my health. Suffice it to say that I became very aware of what appeared to me to be a terrible handicap. From that point on, I had a very poor self-image and feared exposing myself naked or in shorts before anyone. It resulted in my developing an inferiority complex.

This state of affairs lasted for many years and was magnified when my teen-age friends poked fun at my legs. One day while I was in Weequahic Park in Newark, New Jersey, I had an experience which, I now believe, led to an epiphany that cured my feelings of inferiority. I was lying on my back basking in the sunshine when the pleasant feeling I was experiencing was interrupted by my feelings of inferiority. It was so annoying to me that I put my ego aside and asked for help. Help came in a totally unexpected way. I started to think about what the real cause of my misery could be. There was certainly more to life than my mere physical appearance. I began to think about my strengths and weaknesses and what was really important in my life. I knew that my strong dedication to work for peace in the world was very important to me and I knew that the most important people in my life loved me just as I was. It then dawned on me that I should only be concerned about what the important people in my life thought about me and should not be concerned at all about what other people thought. The most important thing that I really wanted was to be loved. I then expressed my thanks for the insight I had received.

A short time later I had an unusual experience while hiking in the Ramapo Mountains in New York State which not only resulted in my achieving freedom from my fears but in giving me a totally new perspective on life. Whether it was an epiphany or the grace of God, it had the most profound effect on me. It changed me from a self-conscious, fearful person, with a poor self-image, into a new person with self-confidence and a profound feeling of inner peace. The incident occurred as follows: I was hiking with friends on a mountain trail through a dense forest when I came to an opening in the forest. My friends were a distance behind me as I stood alone on top of a huge boulder. I was no longer hemmed in by the darkness of the forest. I was in bright sunshine facing a hillside in a gorgeous array of fall colors. As I stood there taking in the beautiful scene, I started to feel as though all of the tensions in my mind and body were being drained away. An unusual light surrounded me. I experienced sensations of loving acceptance, inner peace, ecstasy and extreme joy. Words cannot express adequately the tremendous feelings I had at that time.

Suddenly, I felt that I was out of my body and moving rapidly through the air until I was hovering over a large city. As I looked down I could see what appeared to be a large number of people scurrying about busily engaged in such activities as earning a living and of shopping for various things. They appeared to be so involved with their everyday activities that they were not at all aware of the happiness and joy that could be theirs if their minds were free and open.

It occurred to me that "letting go" of the usual concerns about getting more money and more things was a prerequisite to a peaceful state of mind which could lead to a state of bliss. I realized that what I was experiencing was so unusual that it had to come from a higher source. From that moment on I have believed in the existence of God. My faith in God has been a deep conviction of mine that has never wavered through all the vicissitudes of my life. I thank God for all of my blessings every day. When I am faced with what appears to be an impossible problem for me to solve, I ask for help and "let go" of the problem in complete faith that God will resolve the problem and invariably the problem is resolved.

To get on with my story, I became aware that I was back on the mountainside, still surrounded by bright light and still in a state of bliss, when a thought entered my mind that I could not remain in that state much longer without permanently leaving my body. I, also, became aware that I could make a choice as to whether I wished to remain in a blissful state of existence or return to 'earth'. It was pointed out to me that I should continue my efforts to work for peace and to be with my family and friends. I then found myself back to 'normal' as my hiking friends joined me on the mountainside and we then continued hiking back to where the car had been parked.

My state of mind continued to improve, especially after I met and started to date a lovely girl, Ruth, who was later to become my wife. We had two sons. My younger son David had a serious condition. He could not digest the milk formula that was prescribed by our pediatric doctor since my wife could not breast feed him. He was constantly crying and had to be held to quiet him down. The doctor said that he probably had a condition called colic. We became alarmed when he started to lose weight when he was eight months old. At that point, our doctor told us that he could not understand what was causing the weight loss and that it was imperative that the cause be determined as soon as possible. He immediately arranged for our son to be admitted to the New York University Hospital where they would be able to diagnose our son's condition. We entered our son in the hospital. He was kept there for thirty days before we could bring him home. He was subjected to all kinds of tests including spinal taps.

We had to go to our doctor to learn the results of the tests. He told us that the tests showed that our son David could not digest fats, starches or sugars. He told us that we should go to a specialist who was familiar with that kind of problem. We were fortunate to find a specialist who knew just what had to be done. He told us that our son had a condition known as celiac and that he should be kept away from all foods that had fats, starches and white sugar. For the next six months we fed our child a diet consisting of dried banana flakes that came in a can called "Kanana Banana Flakes" plus no-fat cottage cheese. David thrived on this diet which also included a multi-vitamin supplement plus sublingual vitamin B-12. Other kinds of food were gradually added to the diet over a period of time and David finally was able to eat a normal diet. This incident got me started on what was to become an intensive interest in the role of nutrition and health.

Shortly after my son David was on his road to recovery, I came into possession of a book which was to have a profound effect on me for the rest of my life. The title of the book is *Oahspe*. Oahspe means earth, sky and spirit. It was channeled to earth by angels from higher realms in the spirit worlds. It contains a wealth of knowledge of the origins of all religions; the influence of angels on humans; how the solar systems and galaxies are created; and much more. It is written in the biblical style as in the Holy Bible. A detailed description of the origin of *Oahspe* can be found in Appendix A.

I became a vegetarian after reading *Oahspe* because of the frequent references to the importance of being a vegetarian as an important preparation for spiritual development, and also as the way that human beings can become more peaceful and less aggressive. As you can see, I became a vegetarian for spiritual reasons. The health benefits of being a vegetarian were an added benefit. Chapter Three in this book provides substantial evidence for the value of a vegetarian diet.

The unusual way in which I obtained copies of the books of revelation, plus the occurrence of many other unusual experiences in my life, made me become aware of the fact that many important incidents in our lives are probably brought about by spirit influence rather than by what appear to be, at the time, isolated events or coincidences. It turned out that my strong belief in God plus my vegetarian diet, together with my active life style among other things, contributed to my long life and general well-being. The importance of diet, beliefs, attitudes, exercise, plus alternative health care in relation to longevity, are gone into in great detail in later chapters in this book.

My deep interest in the study of the *Oahspe* book led me to seek for other readers of the book to share my thoughts with. I learned of a group in Duxbury, Massachusetts who held daily prayer services during which portions of *Oahspe* were read. I contacted this group and started to travel to their meetings whenever I could. I learned that they were vegetarians and also that they grew most of the food they consumed in their large organic garden. My wife and my son, David, who was now in college, joined me on these trips.

On one occasion, we were traveling home from Massachusetts when we ran into a heavy snow storm. The snow started to come down so thick and fast that it was almost impossible to see. The driver, a friend of my son, steered the car into the right lane and slowed the car down. Suddenly a car appeared to be stopped in the lane we were in. The driver turned the car sharply to the left to avoid a collision. We wound up in the fast lane and everyone sighed with relief for avoiding the collision and then we were hit in the rear by a car coming quite fast with a violent impact. Our car was spun around so it was now facing on-coming traffic. As we sat there wondering what to do, we saw a truck heading straight for us. The driver didn't see my car because of the heavy snowstorm and plowed into the front of my car with full force. As a result of that accident, my wife, my son and I suffered many injuries. After we returned home, my son decided to go to a chiropractor in New York City. Within two months he was fully recovered from his injuries. My wife and I went to an orthopedic doctor because we felt that medical doctors were superior to any other kind of physician. He placed us on pain killer drugs and sent us to a physical therapist for treatments. We suffered with much pain for two years without much relief. My son had entered a chiropractic college and was urging us to go to a chiropractor. When we were told that the only way to get rid of our pains was to have surgery we finally decided to go to a chiropractor. The results from chiropractic treatments were excellent. Within a short period of time both my wife and I were free from almost all of our pains and we gradually recovered from all of our injuries. From that time on, up to the present, I have not used a medical doctor for any ailments. For an occasional back pain, I go to my chiropractor. I never take any medications, not even aspirin, antibiotics or flu shots. My health has been excellent since that time. I have been a vegetarian and eat organically grown foods as often as possible. I was fortunate in learning about the organic method of growing foods shortly after the facts were published in the magazines published by the *Rodale Press* in the 1940's such as *Organic Gardening* and *Prevention.* I made an intensive study about the people involved with the pioneering research which led to the organic farming methods of growing crops. I found the books about the Hunza people of India very fascinating and enlightening. They were among the first people to raise their own crops with compost that they prepared themselves. It was the only fertilizer they used. They had none of the diseases that are prevalent throughout the world and many of them lived to over a hundred years of age. A more extensive description of the Hunza people and the basic research which led to the organic food movement is presented in Chapter One of this book which deals with the role of nutrition and health.

There are so many books and magazines devoted to the role of nutrition and health that it has resulted in a great deal of confusion because of the various aspects of the subject. The knowledge presented in this book is based on the best available information that covers all aspects of the subject distilled from the hundreds of books and health publications that were read by the author plus the insights gained from the many experiences acquired over a long lifetime.

The need for exercise, as an essential for good health, is widely accepted but not always practiced, or if practiced may not be done in the most effective way. Chapter Two describes the benefits of exercise, plus detailed information about the practices of Chi Gong, Tai Chi and Yoga. Chapter Three contains a wealth of knowledge about the "Power of Thoughts," plus practical methods of achieving and maintaining peace of mind freed of all blocks that obstruct a joyful, healthy life.

Chapter Four, titled "Power of Beliefs," presents a wealth of evidence about the benefits of knowledge about spiritual realities such as "life after death," and contacts with angels. Chapters Five to Twelve are devoted to the important aspects of alternative health care. There is a crisis in the health care system due to the fact that it has been dominated by the medical approach that depends largely on prescription drugs, surgery, radiation and chemotherapy to treat the major diseases that are destroying the lives of ever increasing numbers of people in spite of these medical treatments. The historical reasons for the present crisis in health care are presented in detail. Alternative health care treatments and methods are described in great detail such as kinesiology, chiropractic, NAET, acupuncture, and acupressure; plus the use of curative foods and herbs that can both prevent and cure most diseases, without the dangerous side-effects of medical treatments.

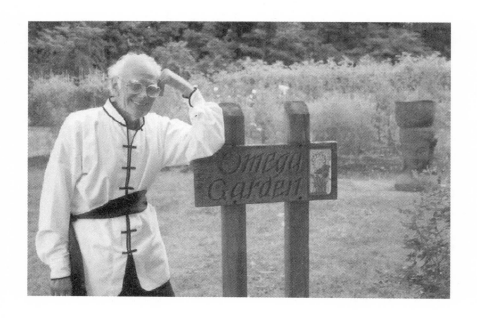

Dr. Singer at the Omega Holistic Institute where he teaches Tai Chi

PART ONE

LONGEVITY

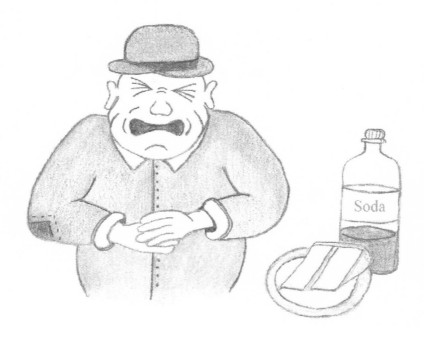

You can avoid digestive problems without resorting to medicine which only treats the symptoms and usually has dangerous side effects by making use of the knowledge contained in this chapter.

CHAPTER ONE

NUTRITION

There are so many books and magazines devoted to the relation of nutrition to health that it has led to much confusion and misunderstanding about the role of nutrition. For example, proper nutrition for optimum well-being should not be based on one goal alone such as weight loss. There is obviously a great need for a solution to the problem of obesity. Recent surveys indicate that obesity is on the increase throughout the general population in spite of all the weight-loss programs and books that have been published on how to lose weight. This book furnishes the reader with information that will help anyone who applies the knowledge presented with the things that can be done to achieve a state of well-being. In the state of well-being the body will usually reach the ideal weight for the particular individual. Because of the fact that there are no two persons identical in every respect, there cannot be one program that will address every person's goal for the weight that each person wants to achieve. That is the reason why every popular weight program designed to help a person lose weight cannot satisfy everyone. Most weight-loss programs, in fact, can result in some loss of weight, but there can also be serious side-effects by following these programs. This book does not get into dieting for the purpose of weight-loss but it does furnish the reader with the tools for a nutritious diet that promotes health and may bring about either a reduction or increase of weight, if that is what your body requires for a state of overall well-being.

The best approach to maintaining your health and well-being is to make use of the knowledge of lifestyles that have been proven by demonstration and research to be most effective. This chapter contains a wealth of practical knowledge that you can put to use to improve your health and longevity and avoid obesity at the same time.

A very recent study into the value of consuming dark green, leafy vegetables that are liquefied together with sweet fruits showed that chronic ailments could be cured by this program as well as controlling weight. All that is needed is a powerful blender to mix the ingredients into a liquefied drink that is called a green smoothie. After learning about this program, I decided to give it a try. I can tell you that I have never felt better since being on the program for just three months. I intend to continue with this program for the rest of my life. The program is described in great detail by the woman who created the method, Victoria Boutenko, in her book, *Green for Life*. A thorough description of this program including recipes is presented later in this chapter in the section on vegetable protein.

Many recent studies have shown that there is a direct relationship between the quality of the food we eat and our health. Unfortunately, most of the foods available in food stores and restaurants are derived from large-scale farms that use chemical fertilizers and dangerous pesticides in growing their crops. On top of that there are many chemical additives used by the food industry to preserve and increase the shelf life of foods. Basic foods such as sugar and flour are refined to the point that they lack the nutrients essential to health such as fiber, vitamins and minerals that are found in the whole food before being processed. Sugar substitutes are even more dangerous than the processed sugar. The subject of sugar is presented in more detail in Part Two of this book. In order to avoid the highly dangerous chemicals that are present in most foods it is necessary to grow or buy foods that are grown organically. At one time organic foods were very difficult to obtain unless you grew your own foods or found a health store that carried such foods. At the present time it is possible to obtain such foods in large supermarkets because of popular demand which shows that it is possible to bring about change when enough people become aware of the dangers that face them. In order to fully understand the importance of this situation the background of organic agriculture is described on the next page.

Organic Food Movement

The knowledge about organically-grown foods is based on the research conducted by two Englishmen who were knighted for their discoveries which culminated in the basis for the organic food movement. One of the men was Sir Albert Howard and the other one was Sir Robert McCarrison. Howard was a bio-chemist who had developed a theory about the importance of organic topsoil in sustaining life on our planet. He had observed that trees and plants in a forest grew abundantly without human intervention. He found that the main factor in sustaining life in the forest was the topsoil. Upon analyzing samples of the topsoil he discovered that there was a certain amount of decayed vegetation from fallen leaves and dead plants and a certain amount of animal waste from animal droppings and from dead animals and dead insects. He also found that there was a ratio of three parts of decayed vegetation to one part of decayed animal wastes. He called the end product of this decomposition humus.

Howard was also very concerned about the large increase of plant diseases at that time. His studies led him to believe that the increase of plant diseases was directly related to the increased use of chemical fertilizers which had become popular with farmers. The reason farmers turned to the use of chemical fertilizer was largely due to the theories of a famous German chemist, Justus Von Liebig, who analyzed the composition of plants to find out what the chief ingredients were. He identified three minerals in the plants: nitrogen, phosphorous and potash. This was hailed as a great discovery because it was assumed that all that was needed to stimulate plant growth was the replacement of these minerals to the soil. He wasn't aware of the importance of the many other components of soil, such as trace minerals and humus. He believed that organic matter, humus, was not essential to the growth of plants. Liebig was so highly respected that his ideas were accepted throughout the world. He became known as the father of chemical fertilizers.

At the end of World War I, there were huge stockpiles of nitrates left over from the manufacture of dynamite. Since nitrogen is the chief ingredient in stimulating plant growth, chemical companies started a campaign to sell their nitrates to farmers and to lawn companies as the best kind of fertilizer to use. The chemical fertilizers did produce rapid growth and led to the widespread use of chemical fertilizers which continues to this day. Anyone who applies fertilizer to their lawns knows about the formula NPK which stands for Nitrogen, Phosphorous and Potash. Gardeners also know about the use of highly toxic chemicals to kill weeds and to protect their lawns and plants from disease. The minerals sold for fertilizer are not in their natural organic form as supplied by nature. They are highly toxic to the living organisms in the soil killing off beneficial enzymes, bacteria and earthworms. The crops and grasses grown with these fertilizers are sickly and require additional chemicals to offset diseases and insect pests which gave rise to the need for pesticides.

Howard's concern about chemical fertilizers led him to visit farms in different parts of the world to compare the results of farming which made use of chemical fertilizers with farming which made use of natural manures or humus. In the early twenties, he went to India to investigate a large farm that was known to use humus that was composed of the 3 to 1 ratio of natural topsoil. While there he found out how they made the humus and that they referred to the humus as compost. He made a very important discovery about the relationship of disease to the quality of food. He observed on several occasions that cattle raised on a farm which used organic fertilizer did not contract foot-and mouth disease even when the cattle rubbed noses with diseased cattle on an adjoining farm which used chemical fertilizers. In his book *The Soil and Health,* Howard had the following to say about the relationship of disease to the way that foods are produced:

"Foot-and-mouth is considered to be a virus disease. It could perhaps be more correctly described as a simple consequence of malnutrition ...One of the most likely aggravations of the trouble is certain to be traced to the use of artificial manures instead of good old-fashioned muck or compost." [2] Howard also wrote another book titled *An Agricultural Testament* which provided the basis for the organic farming movement.

Another Englishman, Robert McCarrison became famous for his discovery of the health secrets of the Hunzakut people who lived in the northern part of India known as Hunza country. He was sent there by the British government to provide medical treatment for the Hunzas since there were no doctors in that remote area. He found to his

---

[2] Sir Albert Howard. *Soil and Health.* NY: Devin Adair, p.19

surprise that the Hunzakuts had only one ailment. They suffered from an eye irritation during the winter months because the huts they lived in had no ventilation and were heated by burning wood or goat dung. McCarrison stayed with the Hunza people for ten years in an effort to find out what the reasons were for their excellent health and longevity. Many of them lived to well over 100 years and were in excellent health until they died. They had none of the diseases of modern societies. He found that the chief reason for their health and virility was the way they grew and fertilized their crops making use of every bit of organic matter to add to their gardens. They saved all animal wastes including human and mixed it with any dead vegetation they could find. The result was a rich organic fertilizer that they applied to their soil. The crops were free of insect pests and free of all plant diseases requiring no additional fertilizers or chemical sprays. They ate only the foods that they grew by themselves except for a clarified butter called ghee that they purchased at the closest store. The store was about ten miles away from their village at the bottom of the mountain and they would walk the round-trip in one day. One of their main foods during the long winter months was apricots. They ate the kernels as well as the fruit. McCarrison made the following observations about the Hunza people:

"During the period of my association with these people I never saw a case of asthenic dyspepsia, of gastric or duodenal ulcer, of appendicitis, of mucous colitis of cancer....Among these people the abdomen over-sensitive to fatigue, anxiety, or cold was unknown. Indeed their buoyant abdominal health has, since my return to the West, provided a remarkable contrast with the dyspeptic and colonic lamentations of our highly civilized communities." [3]

When McCarrison and Howard finally met, they were pleased to find out that they had both reached the same conclusion as to the importance of using only organic fertilizer together with certain minerals obtained from natural rocks that were needed for different soil conditions. Other scientists, such as Selma Waksman and Ehrenfried Pfeiffer, added to our knowledge of how to make compost quicker by the use of different types of anaerobic and aerobic bacteria. They found that compost piles made with these added forms of bacteria

---

[3] Ibid. p.177

decomposed more rapidly and produced superior humus. This method has come to be known as bio-dynamic agriculture and is one of the popular methods of producing organic crops on large farms.

Dr. McCarrison made another great contribution to our knowledge of nutrition. After he was appointed in 1927, as Director of Nutrition Research in India, he began to conduct a series of experiments comparing the effects of different diets on the health of experimental albino rats. Different diets typical of the diets of various population groups of humans were fed to the rats for an extended period of time. Everything was the same for each group except the food. The rats that were fed the organic diet which the Hunza people ate were all alive and had no illnesses at the end of the experiment. They were vigorous and appeared to be in excellent health. Rats that were fed the diets of most Englishmen or that of typical Indian people came down with the diseases common to those groups of people. When the results of these experiments were applied to various groups of people, the results were amazing. People who were ill became better and well people became healthier. The results of the rat experiments were described by the British Medical Testament as follows: "In every case the average standard of health of a given human group was faithfully mirrored in the rats, including the percentage incidence of specific diseases. Nor was this reflection confined to bodily ailments, for neurasthenia, and bad temper showed themselves in the rats fed on the common English diet. During the course of this series of experiments, McCarrison found, and listed, diseases of every organ of the body among the 2243 rats fed on faulty Indian diets…All these conditions," said McCarrison, "these states of ill-health had a common causation; faulty nutrition with or without infection." [4]

We can thank J. L. Rodale for spreading the knowledge of the benefits of organic foods through his publications such as *Organic Farming and Organic Gardening*. He also wrote several books on the subject and thus made this knowledge available to people all over America. In his book *The Healthy Hunzas* he has this to say about the Hunza people: "The causative relationship that exists between methods of growing food and their ultimate effect on the physical condition of the consumer is impressively exemplified in the pheno-

---

[4] E. B. Balfour. *The Living Soil.* London: Faber and Faber, 1944, p. 35.

menally unique good health of the Hunzas.....They are a group of 20,000 people, *none* of whom die of cancer or drop dead with heart disease. In fact, heart trouble is completely unknown in that country! Feeble-mindedness and mental debilitations which are dangerously rampant in the United States are likewise alien to the vigorous Hunzas." [5]

Additional information about the Hunza people was provided by Dr. Allen Banik who was sent to Hunza by the Art Linkletter TV show to learn all that he could about the health and lifestyle of the Hunzakuts. Dr. Banik wrote a book describing his trip titled *Hunza Land.* An excerpt from the book follows:

"In Hunza, I seemed to be in another world; a world of friendliness and good nature. Envy, covetousness, and jealousy were nonexistent; no police force was needed to keep order; unlocked doors were not a temptation. But I was most strongly impressed by the evidences of good health I witnessed among the Hunzakuts of all ages. Their freedom from a variety of diseases and physical ailments was remarkable. Cancer, heart attacks vascular complaints and many of the common childhood diseases such as mumps, measles and chickenpox are unknown among them. I am convinced that the diet upon which these people have lived for centuries is responsible for the enviable good health they enjoy. It cannot be matched in our civilization with its depleted soils, processed foods that robbed of life-giving elements, and cooking methods that effectively destroy a substantial percentage of the vitamins and trace elements that are essential to sound bodies. My attitude toward eating changed radically after I observed the Hunza way of life. I realized that it is time for the Western world to awaken to facts and do something about changing its 'civilized' food habits." [6]

It is one thing to know about the many benefits of organically-grown foods but it is important to know that not all foods sold in stores as organic are truly organic. The powerful food conglomerates such as Dole, Kraft, ConAgra, Archer Daniels Midland and Gerber have come out with products that are labeled organic but do not necessarily have 100% organically-grown foods in their products.

---

[5] J. I. Rodale. *The Healthy Hunzas.* Emmaus, PA: Rodale, 1949, p. 34.
[6] Dr. Allen Banik. *Hunza Land.* Long Beach, CA: Whitchorn Publishing, 1995, pp. 174-175.

Fitzgerald has this to say about the situation:

"Much like what happened when the vitamin industry came to be dominated by pharmaceutical companies, this takeover of organic foods by the makers of chemical foods threatens a redefining of what organic means, until the word itself becomes just another meaningless marketing term.

This does not necessarily mean that produce labeled as organic is the same as produce farmed with chemical methods." Fitzgerald goes on to say, "Despite this general lack of purity in organic foods, research has shown that organic fruits and vegetables contain only about one-third of the chemical residues found on conventionally grown foods. What continues to set organic foods clearly apart from foods intentionally doused with chemicals are the nutritional advantages.

A study in the *Journal of Applied Nutrition* analyzed and contrasted the mineral content of conventionally grown versus organically grown vegetables over a two-year period. Organic proved far higher in mineral content.

Other studies showed that organic foods contained higher levels of antioxidants than conventional foods and research studies have shown that soup made from organic vegetables contained significantly higher levels of salicylic acid than non-organic soup. Salicylic acid is the active anti-inflammatory ingredient in aspirin, and evidence suggests that it can reduce the risk for heart disease and bowel cancer." [7]

We can benefit from the research described above by including organically grown foods in our diet and avoiding the commercially prepared foods found in most food stores and restaurants. Fortunately organic whole-foods are presently available in health food stores and are even being found in many large food supermarkets. Other sources of organic produce are farmer's markets and local farmers; or better yet learn to grow your own foods organically if you want to obtain fresh produce and know exactly how your food is grown. A list of books about the Hunza way of life and helpful suggestions on how to grow foods organically can be found in the Selected Bibliography. It

---

[7] Randall Fitzgerald. *The Hundred Year Lie.* NY: Dutton, 2006, pp.193-194.

is strongly recommended that organic foods be included in the diet in addition to other important aspects of nutrition and health presented below:

The China Study of Foods and Health

A massive study was conducted in China to determine the number of people who had cancer in each of the provinces of China. Teams of researchers were sent to every province in China to find out how many people died from cancer in each province. The results of the study showed that people who lived in remote parts of China had little or no deaths from cancer while people who lived near industrial areas or in large cities had a very high incidence of cancer. Follow-up studies showed that the people who ate the diet of rural Chinese people, which consisted largely of whole grain rice together with some fruits and vegetables, had little or none of the common degenerative diseases such as diabetes, multiple sclerosis, cancer, Alzheimer's, and cardiovascular diseases. Obesity was rarely found among the rural population.

A follow-up study was conducted in China by a team of researchers from the United States and China in the 1980s to find out what the causes were of these diseases. The study was led by a distinguished nutritional researcher, Dr. T. Colin Campbell. The results of the study together with the results of other large-scale studies were published in a book titled *The China Study.* The findings showed a direct relationship between diet and disease. The message was clear: if you want to be healthy, change your diet. The need for changing the diets of people in the Western World, commonly referred to as the western diet, is of paramount importance. Dr. Campbell describes the background and scope of the study as follows:

> I decided to start an in-depth laboratory program that would investigate the role of nutrition, especially protein in the development of cancer...By carefully following the rules of good science, I was able to study a provocative topic without provoking knee-jerk responses that arise with radical ideas. Eventually, this research became handsomely funded for twenty-seven years by the best reviewed and most competitive funding sources...Then our results were reviewed (a second time) for publication in many of the best scientific journals.

What we found was shocking. Low-protein diets inhibited the initiation of cancer by aflatoxin, regardless of how much of this carcinogen was administered to these animals. After cancer initiation was completed, low-protein diets also dramatically blocked subsequent cancer growth. In other words, the cancer producing effects of this highly carcinogenic chemical were rendered insignificant by a low-protein diet. In fact, **dietary protein proved to be so powerful in its effect that we could turn on and off cancer growth simply by changing the level consumed**.

We found that not all proteins had this effect. What protein consistently and strongly promoted cancer? Casein, which makes up 87% of cow's milk protein, promoted all stages of the cancer process. What type of protein did not promote cancer, even at high levels of intake? The safe proteins were from plants, including wheat and soy. As this picture came into view, it began to challenge and then to shatter some of my most cherished assumptions.

These experimental studies didn't end there. I went on to direct the most comprehensive study of diet, lifestyle and disease ever done with humans in the history of biomedical research. It was a massive undertaking, jointly arranged through Cornell University, Oxford University and the Chinese Academy of Preventative Medicine. This project surveyed a vast range of diseases and diet and lifestyle factors in rural China, and more recently in Taiwan. More commonly known as the China Study, this project eventually produced more than 8,000 statistically significant associations between various dietary factors and disease.

What made this project especially remarkable is that, among the many associations that are relevant to diet and disease, so many pointed to the same finding: **people who ate the most animal-based foods got the most chronic disease. Even relatively small intakes of animal-based food were associated with adverse effects. People who ate the most plant-based foods were the healthiest and tended to avoid chronic disease. These results could not be ignored. From the initial experimental animal studies on animal-protein effects to this massive human study on dietary patterns,**

the findings proved to be consistent. The health implications of consuming either animal or plant-based nutrients were remarkably different.

I could not, and did not, rest on the findings of our animal studies and the massive human study in China, however impressive they may have been. I sought out the findings of other researchers and clinicians. The findings of these individuals have proved to be some of the most exciting findings of the past fifty years.

These findings show that heart disease, diabetes, and obesity can be reversed by a healthy diet. Other research shows that various cancers, autoimmune diseases, bone health, kidney health, vision and brain disorders in old age (like cognitive dysfunction and Alzheimer's} are convincingly influenced by diet. Most importantly, the diet that has time and again been shown to reverse and/or prevent these diseases is the same whole foods, plant-based diet that I had found to promote optimal health in my laboratory research and in the China Study. The findings are consistent. [8]

Among the findings were the following items which can be applied to the daily diet in order to maintain optimum health:

The protein in cow's milk, called casein, was found to have a direct relationship to the onset of breast cancer and to childhood diabetes. The message is clear, avoid cow's milk.

The total amount of animal protein consumed on a daily basis is of the utmost importance. A high consumption of protein, 15% or higher, is associated with a high incidence of the common diseases of western societies. A low protein diet, 10% or less, results in a low incidence of the common western diseases.

A diet high in fat, especially animal fats, was found to be closely associated with the incidence of breast cancer, large bowel cancer and heart disease. [9]

Dietary fiber is also an important factor. The China Study

---

[8] Colin Campbell. *The China Study.* Dallas: Benbella Books, pp. 6-7.
[9] Ibid., p. 84

provided evidence indicating the fact that high-fiber intake was consistently associated with lower rates of cancer of the rectum and colon. High fiber intakes were also associated with lower levels of cholesterol. Of course, high fiber consumption reflected high plant based food consumption; foods such as beans, leafy vegetables and whole grains are all high in fiber. [10]

The China Study sheds light on the weight loss debate. 'Understanding that diet can cause small shifts in calorie metabolism that leads to big shifts in body weight is an important and useful concept. It means that there is an orderly process of controlling body weight over time that does work, as opposed to the disorderly process of crash diets that don't work. It also accounts for the frequent observations that people who consume low protein, low fat diets composed of whole plant foods have far less difficulty with weight problems, even if they consume the same, or even slightly more, total calories. ..We now know that eating a low-fat, low-protein diet high in complex carbohydrates from fruits and vegetables will help you lose weight.' [11]

Dr. Campbell sums up his findings with this statement: 'The strength and consistency of the majority of the evidence is enough to draw valid conclusions. Namely, whole, plant-based foods are beneficial, and animal-based foods are not. Few other dietary choices, if any can offer the incredible benefits of looking good, growing tall and avoiding the vast majority of premature diseases in our culture.' [12]

Excellent Reasons to Eat a Vegetarian Diet

I became a vegetarian about 60 years ago for spiritual reasons as I mentioned in the Introduction to this book. My vegetarian diet, no doubt, is one of the reasons that I am enjoying excellent health at my present age of 93.

The China Study mentioned above provides enough scientific evidence to prove the value of a vegetable diet. The problem most

---

[10] Ibid., p. 92.
[11] Ibid. p. 102.
[12] Ibid., p. 107.

people in America face is the constant barrage of misinformation publicized about the importance of eating a high protein diet. This encourages the eating of meat and the consumption of high protein foods and drinks.

When we eat meat we're feeding ourselves the poisonous adrenaline that was secreted by the terrified animal before it was slaughtered.

Lions and tigers and other carnivores are provided with a very short intestinal tract. They process flesh very quickly and eliminate it before it putrefies and becomes toxic while humans have a very long intestinal tract which is not geared to the proper digestion of animal protein. If you're worried about being weak without eating meat, think about the elephant. This great and powerful beast who feeds only on plants –lives very long, and is extremely intelligent.

Meat will leave a residue of uric acid in the bloodstream. Uric acid is considered by some to be a carcinogen (cause of cancer). Uric acid is a toxin that makes it harder to reach a higher, clearer meditative state of mind since it is an irritant in the bloodstream. Uric acid also causes the PH of body cells to become too acidic. Undigested protein and saturated fat may accumulate in the large intestine and over time clog the colon resulting in poor assimilation of food and elimination of waste from the body.

Vegetable protein

The results of the China Study mentioned above showed that the consumption of a diet high in animal proteins is a major cause of many illnesses including cancer. Unfortunately, most Americans think that they must have a high protein diet due to their ethnic cultural backgrounds and also largely due to a massive promotion in recent years stressing the need for a high protein diet. High protein bars and drinks can be found in every food store including health food stores. Casein, the protein found in the whey of milk is a major cause of cancer, as determined by the China Study, and yet it is one of the most popular forms of protein used in these products.

Green Smoothies

In the book *Green for Life* by Victoria Boutenko there is a wealth of information presented showing the superiority of the protein in the leaves of green leafy vegetables as compared to the protein in foods from animals. Boutenko analyzed the diet of humans compared to that of chimpanzees and pointed out the importance of changing our diet to include a much higher percentage of green vegetables and fruits and a much lower percentage of animal-based foods. She was interested in finding a cure for a chronic ailment that she had plus a program that would help her lose weight. She had tried all of the popular weight-loss programs and was unable to lose weight and keep it off. She tried a vegetarian diet and found it helpful but not completely effective. After studying the diet of the chimpanzees, she decided to eat only dark, green, uncooked, leafy vegetables.

Boutenko compared the diet of humans to the diet of chimpanzees in order to find out how chimpanzees were able to grow so strong on a diet which consisted mostly of green, leafy plants and fruits. She had dark, green leafy vegetables analyzed and found that the proteins in plants are superior to animal proteins. Here's what she has to say about proteins:

"Every protein molecule consists of a chain of amino acids. An essential amino acid is one that cannot be synthesized by the body, and therefore must be supplied as part of the diet. The U.S. RDA for protein is greatly overestimated according to the results of the China Study. Studies of the diets of chimpanzees compared to that of humans confirm the same truth: Chimpanzees maintain a fairly low and constant protein intake. The amount of protein found in green leafy vegetables like kale actually exceeds the amount of protein recommended by the USDA. The popular assumption that greens are a poor source of protein is inaccurate. The lack of research on the nutritional content of greens has led to a great confusion among the majority of people, including many professionals. Dr. Joel Fuhrman wrote in his book *Eat to Live:* 'Even physicians and dieticians are surprised to learn that when you eat large quantities of green vegetables you receive a considerable amount of protein.'

Since most people were not aware that greens have an abundance of readily available essential amino acids, they were trying to eat foods from the other food groups known for their rich protein content. However, let me explain the difference between complex proteins fond in meat, dairy, fish, etc. and individual amino acids found in fruits, vegetables, and especially in greens. It is clear that the body has to work a lot less when creating protein from the assortment of amino acids from greens, rather than the already combined, long molecules of protein, assembled according to the foreign pattern of a totally different creature such as a cow or chicken....Your body has a hard time trying to make perfect molecules of protein out of an animal's molecules, which consist of a different combination of amino acids. Plus, your body would most likely receive a lot of unnecessary pieces that are hard to digest. These pieces would be floating around in your blood like garbage for a long time, causing allergies and other health problems. Professor W. A. Walker from the department of Nutrition at the Harvard School of Public Health, states that, 'Incompletely digested protein fragments may be absorbed into the bloodstream. The absorption of these large molecules contributes to the development of food allergies and immunological disorders.

The ironic result of consuming this imperfect source of protein (animal protein), is that many people develop deficiencies in essential amino acids. Such deficiencies are not only dangerous to health, but they can drastically change people's perceptions of life and the way people feel and behave. ..According to the research of Julia Ross, a specialist in nutritional psychology, if your body lacks certain amino acids, you may develop strong symptoms of mental and psychological imbalance and severe cravings for unwanted substances. For example, let us consider the symptoms of a deficiency in tyrosine and phenylalanine. The symptoms of a deficiency in these amino acids can cause: Depression, lack of focus and concentration, lack of energy, and ADD (Attention deficit disorder). In addition, the symptoms of a deficiency in these amino acids may lead to cravings for: Sweets such as Sugar and Aspartame found in most commercial foods plus Caffeine, Starch, Alcohol, Cocaine, Chocolate, Marijuana, and Tobacco.

Using data from official sources I have calculated the amounts of these two essential amino acids that we can receive from either chicken or dark green endive:

CHICKEN (One serving)	ENDIVE (one head)
222 mg tyrosine	200 mg tyrosine
272 mg phenyalanine	261 mg phenyalanine

As you can see, contrary to the popular opinion, there are plenty of high quality proteins in greens. According to the explanation of Professor T. Colin Campbell, 'There is a mountain of compelling evidence showing that so called 'low-quality' plant protein, which allows for slow but steady synthesis of new proteins, is the healthiest type of protein'. For example, the protein from greens doesn't have cancer as a side effect. Yet, in many books, greens are not even listed as a protein source because greens have not been researched enough. In summary, greens provide protein in the form of individual amino acids. These amino acids are easier for the body to utilize than complex proteins. A variety of greens can supply all the protein we need to sustain each of our unique bodies." [13]

Boutenko was interested in finding a cure for a chronic ailment that she had plus a program that would help her lose weight. She had tried all of the popular weight-loss programs and was unable to lose weight and keep it off. She tried a vegetarian diet and found it helpful but not completely effective. After studying the diet of the chimpanzees, she decided to eat only dark, green, uncooked, leafy vegetables such as kale and collard greens. She found that it was impossible to eat enough of the greens by chewing them, so she tried liquefying them. This did not work well because most of the fiber was expelled by the liquefier. She finally found a high-speed blender that liquefied the greens when she added a glass of water and was able to drink the mixture. After a few weeks on the drink, she found that her physical ailments were improving and that she was losing weight. After several months the improvements were so noticeable that her family and friends wanted to know what she was doing to bring about such a dramatic change.

Her husband, who had several chronic ailments that had not responded to conventional medical treatments, decided to try the Green Drink. After a month on the drink, he started to feel much better. Before long about 20 people were on the Green Drink. Her two daughters tried the drink but found the strong chlorophyll taste unpleasant. She then tried adding fruit to the mixture, such as a banana plus one other fruit. That made the drink quite pleasant to the taste. Her daughters found certain fruits to their liking and then became

---

[13] Victoria Boutenko. *Green for Life*. www.rawfamily.com: Raw Family Publishing, 2005, pp. 41-47.

very fond of the drink. They called the drink 'Green Smoothies.' Her older daughter had asthma that she had from early childhood which hampered her ability to participate in vigorous sports. She loved soccer but could only play for a short time in a game. After being on the Green Smoothies for several months she was able to play a full game and over time, the asthma no longer was a problem.

A doctor, Dr. Paul Feiber, came to her home to find out about the Green Smoothies. He became convinced of its benefits and asked Boutenko if she would be interested in conducting a scientific study of the drink in order to establish a scientific basis for its benefits. He helped her set up the study which came to be known as the Roseburg Study. Thirty people agreed to participate as subjects in the study which consisted of the following procedures:

The subjects had to agree to consume one quart of the Green Drink each day. One pint had to be taken for breakfast and the other pint for dinner. Lunch could be any food that each subject wanted to eat, preferably without meat. Each subject had to be given a physical test just before and at the end of the study which was to last for 30 days. They were tested for their stomach acidity and for the pH of their blood. Each one had to complete a questionnaire about their lifestyle, state of health and other pertinent data.

Boutenko describes the importance of stomach acid in regards to our health as follows: "There is a need for an adequate amount of stomach acid (HCL) in order to properly digest our foods. Without stomach acid, nutritional deficiencies inevitably develop leading to disease. If stomach acid is insufficient, there is no barrier against parasites. The natural level of stomach acid helps to digest large protein molecules. If stomach acid is low, then incompletely digested protein fragments get absorbed into the bloodstream and cause allergies and immunological disorders. HCL decreases as we age, especially after the age of forty. Over eating, especially over consumption of fats and proteins, wears out the parietal cells of the stomach that secret HCL." [14]

Dr. Fieber, who participated in the study, made the following comments about the results of the experiment:

After 30 days of drinking one quart of green smoothie

[14] Ibid, pp. 62-63.

each day, we then completed another HCL challenge test to see what improvement occurred over the month. **It was remarkable to me that 66.7% of the participants showed such vast improvement.** The fiber content and nutrient value of the green smoothies made for an incredible success. All the participants also noted many other improvements in their health, some of which were dramatic changes.

I would like to give my own personal testimonial as my wife and I had been drinking the green smoothies about two months before the study was conducted. My blood pressure, pulse rate, and cholesterol readings all improved substantially. We lost all cravings for cooked food. The most significant change for me concerned a small growth that had appeared on my nose. After one month on the green smoothies, the growth fell off. This proved to me the tremendous healing properties of the green smoothie. The Roseburg experiment demonstrated that regular consumption of green smoothies greatly benefits the health of people through improving the level of hydrochloric acid. Therefore the consumers of green smoothies should expect:

1. To have better absorption of valuable nutrients
2. To lessen the possibility of infection and parasites
3. To heal allergies
4. To improve overall health

As a result of regular consumption of the green smoothies for just one month, people reported the following health benefits: increase in energy, depression lifted and suicidal thoughts gone, less blood sugar fluctuations, more regular bowel movements, dandruff healed, insomnia gone, asthma attacks stopped completely, none of usual 'PMS' symptoms any more, fingernails became stronger, less coffee needed, sex life was improved, skin cleared up, cataracts improved, and many more. It was interesting to see that most of the participants who wanted to lose weight lost anywhere from five to ten pounds, and a couple of people who wanted to gain weight, were able to gain one or two pounds. [15]

---

[15] Ibid, pp. 72-76.

According to Boutenko, "Food is not the only factor that affects our pH balance. Any stress can potentially leave an acid residue in our body; conversely any activities that are calming and relaxing can make us more alkaline.

Factors that make us more acidic include hearing or saying harsh or bitter words, loud music and noise, being in a traffic jam, feeling jealousy or wanting revenge, hearing a baby crying, over-working and over-exercising, beginning or finishing school, going on vaccination, watching scary or stressful movies, watching and listening to TV, talking on the phone for a long time, taking on a mortgage, paying bills and credit cards, etc.

Factors that make us more alkaline are: giving or receiving a smile or a hug, laughter and jokes, classical or quiet music, seeing a puppy, hearing a compliment or blessing, receiving a soft massage, being in nature, watching children laugh and play, walking and sleeping under the stars and moonlight, working in the garden, observing flowers, singing or playing a musical instrument sincere friendly conversation, and many others. Boutenko came to the following conclusions based on her experiences and research:

"It is impossible to maintain a good alkaline pH balance without consuming large quantities of dark leafy greens. Some people try to keep a normal pH balance by taking supplements containing dried greens. While this certainly is better than eating junk foods, I strongly believe that to consume fresh greens is thousands of times better because supplements are processed food and their nutritional content is altered, as a result of which some qualities of the nutrients disappear so that the value of the nutrients changes greatly. Also, when consumed in the form of capsules and tablets, they enter our body in huge, concentrated doses creating extra work for the elimination system.....

For this reason, out of all the choices that we have to consuming greens, the green smoothie is a winner because it is a complete food, it is fresh, and it takes less than a minute to prepare." [16]

---

[16] Ibid, 82-85.

Some of the green smoothie recipes presented in this book are shown below: (They all must be blended well: liquefied). [17]

Raw Family Wild Banango
    2 cups of lambquarters (or other weed like plantain, chickweed or purslane)
    1 banana
    2 cups water

Blueberry Pudding
    1 stalk of celery
    2 cups fresh blueberries
    1 banana
    2 cups water

Aloe Live
    1 cup apple juice
    1 banana
    1 mango
    1 small piece of aloe
    5 leaves of kale
    2 cups water

Summer Delight
    6 peaches
    2 handfuls of spinach leaves
    2 cups of water

Freshness
    6 to 8 leaves of Romaine lettuce
    ½ medium honeydew
    2 cups water

Kiwi Enjoyment
    4 very ripe kiwis
    1 ripe banana
    3 stalks of celery
    2 cups water

Raspberry Dream
    2 Bosc pears
    1 handful of raspberries
    4-5 leaves of kale
    2 cups water

Green Delicious
    5 leaves of kale (purple)
    ¼ avocado
    3 cloves garlic
    Juice of ½ lime
    2 cups water
    2 Roma tomatoes
    ½ tsp. Salt

Boutenko points out that the green drink should not be made in a liquefier but in a blender that spins at a very rapid rate in order to make a drink that is liquefied but also contains all of the fiber.

---

[17] Ibid., pp.101-102.

Longevity and Nutrients

From the above presentation, it is apparent that a diet consisting mostly of fruits, vegetables and whole grains will provide the foods necessary for a long, healthy life.

In order to assist the reader in making use of some of the most beneficial foods that have come to my attention the following items are listed below:

A Synergistic Trio of Foods (potent when taken together)

Garlic is considered a sacred herb by the ancients for its powerful therapeutic effects. It has also been found to be effective against certain cancers when taken raw with olive oil. Garlic oil has been known to battle effectively against many types of viruses and bacteria....In fact, garlic was known in the former Soviet Union as 'Russian penicillin'! Best eaten raw, garlic can also be taken in capsule form.

Onions are known for being a universal healing food. It not only attacks harmful bacteria and purifies the blood, but it helps build new blood. It has been said 'An onion a day keeps the doctor away.' Onions will help you avoid dysentery.

Ginger The root is both soothing and strengthening to the nerves when the body is under stress. Ginger tea is very useful for women to drink during menstruation. It strengthens the nerves instead of harming them as caffeine does.

Alpha Lipoic Acid

Lipoic acid is a powerful antioxidant that has numerous health benefits. It not only protects the body from free radical damage, it has a unique ability to neutralize toxins, chelate heavy metals, and protect against DNA damage. This makes lipoic acid potent against diabetes, liver damage, cancer, cardiovascular disease, AIDS, vision problems, Parkinson's and Alzheimer's - it even slows down aging.

The suggested dose for anti-aging purposes is 400 mg per day.

Apple cider vinegar

In the book, *Folk Medicine,* written by Dr. Jarvis, the importance of apple cider vinegar in relation to health is presented in great detail. He learned from his patients and from extensive research that the daily use of cider vinegar was beneficial in preventing and in many cases curing many ailments such as the common cold and the flu. He found that the combination of one or two teaspoons of the vinegar together with one teaspoon of honey in a glass of water was the ideal way to reap the benefits. It is a pleasant tasting drink tasting something like apple cider. It can be sipped slowly several times during the day. Taken the first thing in the morning, it helps to restore the acid/alkaline balance in the body, thus strengthening the immune system. It can also be used as a gargle to relieve sore throats and coughs.

Vinegar may also help fight diabetes. "In a recent study, healthy patients and patients with a pre-diabetic condition known as insulin resistance drank a vinegar drink (1/8 cup of vinegar, diluted with cup of water and sweetened to taste) or a placebo drink before a high carbohydrate meal. The vinegar drinks improved insulin sensitivity in both groups by up to 40%." [18]

Vinegar can also be used for several skin disorders such as jock itch, impetigo and cuts since it's an anti-bacterial agent.

Bee Pollen

Raw honey, that is honey which has not been heated, is widely known for its health benefits. The pollen, which is not changed to liquid form by the bees in the hive, settles to the bottom of the hives where it can be collected. It has been discovered that the bee pollen has extraordinary health benefits. A scientist, William Fischer, made a study of bee pollen and reported the following:

"A Russian botanist and biologist, Dr. Nikolai Tsitsin found that the centenarians living in the Caucasus Mountains who were 125 years of age or older all ate bee pollen as a basic food. After intensive research, he determined that including bee pollen in their regular diet was responsible in a large part for the incredible age these people attained. He was also impressed with the quality of their lives in that all of these people were actively working and in singularly good health in spite of their advanced age.

Working independently, other Russian scientists reached the same conclusions. Dr. Naum Yoirich of the Soviet Academy summa-

---

18 *The Top Lifesaving Secrets of the World's Greatest Doctors.* Bottom Line Books, Boardroom, 2007, p.48.

rizes his research in these words:

'Bee pollen is one of the original treasure houses of nutrition and medicine. *Long lives are attained by bee-pollen users.* It contains every important substance necessary to life.'" [19]

Bee Pollen can be obtained as tiny granules or in capsules at any health food store. Granules should be fresh as possible and not so hard that they can't be chewed without discomfort.

Human Growth Hormone (hGH)

Human Growth Hormone (hGH) is one of the many endocrine hormones such as estrogen, progesterone, testosterone, melatonin and DHEA that all decline in production with age. Of all the hormones, hGH is the most important in its overall effects on the health and longevity of the mind and body. Not only can it prevent biological aging, it can also reverse a broad range of signs and symptoms associated with the aging process. Thousands of studies have been conducted to determine the effects of hGH. The results confirm the tremendous benefits of hGH. Some of the benefits of an adequate supply of hGH are:

- Strengthens the immune system providing resistance to common illness.
- Reduces risk of heart attack and stroke
- Emphysema patients find their oxygen intake improves.
- Osteoporosis is prevented.
- Wrinkled skin is restored to youthfulness.
- Hair color is restored.
- Brain shrinkage is stopped.
- Metabolism is increased resulting in weight loss and increasing muscle mass at the same time.
- Reduces blood pressure.
- Increases energy

There are supplements available that when taken orally, stimulate the release of the body's own anti-aging hormone hGH. This product can be obtained in health food stores and from mail order health product companies such as Purity Products and Swansons.

---

[19] William L. Fischer. *How to Fight Cancer and Win.* Baltimore: Agora Health Books, 2001, p. 189.

Since hormones have such a profound effect on the body, it is advisable to consult your health care provider before taking any product that stimulates your hormones.

Maca

Maca is a root vegetable that grows in many parts of South America. It is famous for many medical miracles, but this is only true for the plants that grow in the highest parts of the Peruvian Andes. Among its reputed benefits are the following:

A Healthy Prostate. Maca has been shown to reduce prostate size significantly. This is due in part to its rich supply of plant sterols, including *beta sitosterol* - a powerful treatment for benign prostatic hyperplasia. Maca has another well-known prostate shrinker, compounds called *glucosinates* - which protect against cancer as well.

Improved Sexual Performance. Maca is helpful for men with erectile dysfunction (ED) by gently and gradually reversing the underlying circulatory problem without any of the dangerous side-effects of drugs like Viagra.

Improved Fertility. With a daily dose of 1500 mg benefits in women include increased fetal growth and reduced miscarriage rates. Men enjoy an average 200 percent increase in semen volume as well as significantly increased sperm counts and increased conception rates. All of these benefits occur without meddling into sex hormone levels. It appears that maca activates an anabolic (tissue-building) gene pathway known as insulin-like growth factor (IGF), which is a critical determinant of fertility and fetal development, and which is known to decline with age.

A Clearer Mind. Maca is rich in phytoestrogens and flavonoids such as quercetin, one of the most powerful food-sourced antioxidants and anti-inflammatories known—with proven protective effects on cognitive performance, particularly learning and memory. Maca also contains anthocyanins (of blueberry fame) which have been shown to enhance memory, problem-solving skills, and equilibrium/balance in the elderly.

Healthier Joints. Joint replacement has become commonplace. You joints are at risk of needing this radical solution mainly because joint cartilage is naturally subject to breaking down and not too good at building itself back up. If you lose enough cartilage to have bone against bone, you're in serious trouble and serious pain. Maca can prevent that. A recent study using human cartilage found that maca almost triples cartilage's anabolic activity, even if there's current inflammation. When combined with another Peruvian herb: **Cat's claw**, the anabolic stimulation in the cartilage almost quadruples.

A Healthy Liver. Although Maca is a medicinal herb, it does not damage the liver as does a drug such as Vioxx. Lab studies show that not only does it not hurt your liver. It actually appears to have liver-protective effects.

Adaptogen, Menopausal Relief. Maca is an adaptogen because it promotes the body's ability to shrug off the imbalances caused by stress. The body's weakening ability to compensate for stress, as we age, is at the root of just about every health problem. Maca has been shown to reverse stress-induced ulcers, bring stress-elevated cortisol levels back to normal, and reduce the glucose levels and weight gain that result from chronic stress. Maca's adaptogen properties make it ideal for relieving the stressed-out systems of menstruating and menopausal women. Most importantly, maca achieves menopausal relief not by adding hormones or targeting symptoms but rather by helping your body restore its own balance. There's been a wealth of research done with maca over the past several years, beyond the red-hot marketable stuff about its aphrodisiac effects. The truth is that when you're healthy and balanced and stress rolls off your back, everything works better, including your libido, and that's what a good adaptogen can do for you. [20]

Melatonin

According to Gary Null, melatonin has many benefits: in addition to its well-known role in promoting sleep as presented below:

"Data indicate that melatonin can be a potent scavenger hence; melatonin can slow aging and even postpone the onset of age-related diseases including cancer. Results of animal studies also indicate that melatonin has cardioprotective, anti-diabetic,

---

[20] Dr. Marcus Laux. *Naturally Well Today,* Feb., 2008.

anti-glucocorticoid, anticonvulsant, and immune-enhancing effects. It improves adrenal function and can reduce the severity of colitis, seizures, brain injury, and gastric lesions. It can delay disease onset and death due to viral encephalitis.

Jet lag is a common problem for which melatonin can provide an answer. A double-blind placebo-controlled study found that 5mg of melatonin taken once a day for three days prior to a flight, once during the flight, and once a day for three days after the flight alleviates jet lag and fatigue in healthy travelers.

"The ideal daily dose varies according to each individual, but experts believe 1 to 3 mg taken at night will produce positive effects in most people." [21]

Another nutrition expert, Dr. Marcus Laux, points out additional information about the benefits of melatonin as follows:

Researchers consider melatonin to be one of the most promising 'new' cancer therapy agents. The incidence of breast cancer is about five times higher in people who live in industrialized countries where excess light interferes with the natural day-night rhythms, and where working the night shift is common. People with low levels of melatonin are at significantly higher risk of many different kinds of cancer, including breast, endometrial, and colorectal. Cells from these and other kinds of cancers slow down or even stop growing in response to melatonin alone.

Melatonin strengthens your immune system through a number of different avenues. It does all this as a modulator, not a stimulator—it helps you launch a stronger defense against any challenge, including cancer, while also fighting excessive inflammation, to keep your immune system from becoming overreactive and self-defeating.

There's a strong link between depressive disorders and the loss of synchronization of your body's natural rhythms. Sleep disturbances are common in just about every form of clinical depression and anxiety. Recent studies show that melatonin's antidepressant properties are at least partly related to its ability to restore your natural circadian rhythm (your body's 24 hour clock

---

[21] Gary Null, Ph.D. *Power Aging*. New York: New American Library, Division of Penguin Group, 2003, p.84.

that regulates body temperatures and hormone levels, among many others). *There's also a direct link between melatonin and another major mood-mediating neurohormone, serotonin.*

With all these health-protective effects, it makes sense that melatonin is being recognized as a major player in the fight against aging. [22]

Mushrooms

You don't have to be sick to benefit from them. They help maintain optimal health and wellness. They have no side-effects or drug reactions and don't cost much. Some of the most potent ones are listed below:

Shitake is considered to be a potent weapon against tumors. Research also shows shitakes to be good for lowering blood pressure, reducing cholesterol, cleansing the liver and kidneys, and boosting energy.

Reishi is a member of the polypore family of mushrooms, the shelf or bracket fungi that grow on living and dead trees and help recycle organic matter in forests. It is recommended for its anti-inflammatory effects without any of the side effects of anti-inflammatory drugs. Known in China as an 'elixir of immortality,' researchers have found this mushroom to enhance immunity, fight viruses, reduce cholesterol, and help prevent fatigue. Like shitakes, reishis are also known to combat cancer by boosting the body's killer agents. They may be used to treat arthritis and possibly the brain swelling associated with Alzheimer's disease.

Maitaki mushrooms may be the most potent immune-booster because of their ability to reach and activate more immune cells. They also contain many nutrients.

Enoki has been found to be a very potent immune booster. It is popular in Japan for its delicate flavor. Researchers found that families of enoki mushroom growers had nearly one-third less death from cancer than the rest of the community. [23]

---

[22] Dr. Marcus Laux. *Naturally Well Today*, June 2, 2000, p.5.
[23] *More Ultimate Healing.* Pp.190-191.

Nuts

Nuts are an excellent source of protein. They are richer in protein than meat with none of the harmful effects of eating meat. Certain nuts also have curative powers such as almonds, walnuts and apricot pits. Almonds and apricot pits contain anti-carcinogenic properties which help prevent and may help cure certain cancers. Walnuts, especially black walnuts, help destroy parasites in the intestinal tract. Nuts are also loaded with Omega 3 fatty acids which help reduce inflammation.

Peroxide

One of the most powerful weapons against infectious diseases is hydrogen peroxide, an inexpensive product that can be obtained at any pharmacy or health food store. It is not necessary to take antibiotics with their many side-effects. Hydrogen peroxide is available as a food grade product. It can be added to bath water or to water and food. Use it according to the directions provided.

According to Dr. Douglas, "It's safe, backed by decades of solid research. Did you know that your own white blood cells produce hydrogen peroxide? Yes they do. Lots of it. Know why? Because that's how they kill invading germs. It's your body's first and best defense against any infection. Kills bacteria, viruses, yeast and parasites—all the bad guys. But how? The hydrogen peroxide molecule (H_2O_2) is basically water (H_2O) with an extra oxygen atom attached. When that oxygen gets released against germs, it oxidizes them. Poof, they're goners." [24]

Pregnenolone

Much like DHEA, pregnenolone is a completely natural hormone, manufactured in the body from cholesterol. Indeed, pregnenolone is the grand precursor from which almost all of the other steroid hormones are made, including DHEA, progesterone, testosterone, the estrogens, and cortisol. It is frequently referred to as the 'mother hormone.' Among its benefits are:

Improves memory, focus and concentration. Tests showed pregnenolone to be the most potent memory enhancer yet found.

Reduces allergic reactions, lessens inflammation and produces a

---

[24] Douglas Report, Summer, 2009, p. 19.

relaxing mild euphoric, 'stress buffer effect,' without any of the negative side-effects of cortisol.

Unlike synthetic steroid hormones, which can have terrifying side effects, pregnenolone is completely natural (it is made from an extract of Dioscorea yam), and clinical studies have shown it to be virtually free of side effects. It can be obtained from vitamin supplement companies in tablet or capsule form.

Policosanol (54% Better Than Statins)

"Supplements containing Policosanol have been found to work well to balance cholesterol counts. Biochemically speaking, policosanol is made up of a series of what is known as fatty alcohols. Policosanol supplements are usually made from either sugar cane or beeswax. Citrus peels, wheat germ and caviar are other rich sources of policosanol. Recent studies have shown policosanol to be up to 54% more effective for cholesterol than statin drugs such as Pravasatin, and causes none of the adverse effects statins can cause. As a matter of fact, in a study of nearly 28,000 people who used policosanol for two to four years, less than half of one percent of the subjects experienced notable adverse effects from their daily dose." [25]

Wheat Germ Oil

There are many health benefits associated with such oils as olive oil, sesame oil, and flaxseed oil which are described elsewhere in this book. Wheat germ oil is included here because of its importance to longevity. It is an excellent natural source of vitamin E which is absorbed readily by the body unlike the synthetic vitamin E found in the typical multivitamin pill. It can be obtained as a liquid or in capsules at health food stores and from the Standard Process Company which uses organically-grown foods as the base for its vitamins and herbal products.

It is best taken sublingually in the liquid form or by crushing capsules in your mouth until you can feel the oil coming out of the capsule. You can feel the effects quickly as the oil is absorbed through your mouth. Some of the benefits are an increase in energy and in endurance; lubrication of the joints and vertebrae, healing skin disorders from the inside and also when applied externally for itching due to jock itch or acne.

---

[25] Bottom Line Editors. *The Top 50 Lifesaving Secrets of the Worlds Greatest Doctors.* Stamford, CT: Bottom Line Books, 2007, p.6.

Tea Tree Oil

Tea tree oil has become very popular for its antiseptic and healing properties to the skin, according to Dr. Mark Stengler: "This oil comes from the leaves of the Australian *Melaleuca alternifolia* tree. There are approximately 100 chemicals in tea tree oil. The oil has natural anti-inflammatory, analgesic, antiseptic and healing properties. It destroys bacteria, fungus and viruses. It can be used topically for almost any skin condition. Examples include acne, athlete's foot, and fungal infections of the skin, boils, bruises, buns, cold sores, cuts, dandruff, insect bites, rashes, lice and warts. It can also be used for gingivitis and vaginitis.

Tea tree oil is very safe for topical use. It is generally nonirritating and nontoxic. As with any substance, some people may be sensitive to this oil. Pure undiluted tea tree oil should not be applied to the skin of children or pregnant or lactating women. These people should use a commercial cream or gel. The oil is excellent for the topical treatment of skin infections. It has been shown to be effective against many types of bacteria and fungus including *staphylococcus, candida albicans,* and many others. Tea tree oil can be applied topically to warts as it has antiviral properties. It is **especially useful for plantar warts.**" [26]

Longevity and Toxins

Although many of the beneficial foods with detoxifying properties are mentioned in other parts of this book, a list of special foods that have been proven to detoxify the body are described in this section in more detail. At the present time it is next to impossible to live anywhere in the world without being subject to extremely dangerous chemical toxins. Dr. Thomas Slaga, an eminent health scientist, provides us with a wealth of practical knowledge on how to best protect ourselves from these dangerous toxins. Excerpts from his book, *The Detox Revolution,* follow below:

"The toxins and carcinogens found in the air we breathe, the water we drink, and the foods we eat can overload our systems and endanger good health. By now, the health benefits of such foods as green tea and soy have been well touted. But what you

---

[26] Mark Stengler. *Natural Healing Supplement.* Bottom Line, Boardroom, 2007, pp. 75-79.

may not know is through a carefully structured diet, which balances the 'right super foods' with supplements, and lifestyle strategies you can help your body perform at optimum levels of health and energy, while greatly reducing the risk of disease.

Results of more than two hundred epidemiological studies and literally thousands of human and experimental animal studies support the scientific view: a diet based on plant foods leads to a decrease in cancer and other degenerative diseases.

Of all the botanical families, none has greater scientific association with the prevention of cancer, especially breast and prostate cancer, than *cruciferous* vegetables, including broccoli, cabbage, and cauliflower. These hardy plants also provide protection against ischemic stroke, the most common type of stroke. Chief among the members of the cruciferous family, watercress contains certain phytochemicals that work incredibly well together to increase the overall activity of the xenobiotic detoxification system. The odor that we commonly associate with cruciferous vegetables is actually caused by a class of nitrogen, sulfur, and glucose-containing chemicals called glucosinolates.

Garlic, onions, leeks, chives, asparagus, and scallions are members of the allium botanical family and are also characterized by their strong odor. This odor results from the activity of certain sulfur compounds that are known to be effective in both the anti-oxidant and xenobiotic detoxification systems. The compounds in onion and garlic extracts are protective against cancer and cardiovascular disease. Garlic extracts are also effective in lowering cholesterol and triglycerides. In addition, garlic and onions have been found to increase glutathione, a powerful anti-oxidant that helps support the detoxification systems.

The leguminous family, or legumes, which include many kinds of beans and peas, is a good source of protein, fats, carbohydrates, vitamins, minerals, fiber, and phytochemicals. Among the different types of legumes, the soybean stands out as one of the most widely consumed food sources. Not surprisingly, it is also one of the most studied for the health benefits it possesses. It is high in protein and protective phytochemicals. Studies have shown that soy protein helps to prevent heart disease by lowering total cholesterol. Soybeans also have cancer-fighting isoflavones, which help prevent hormone-dependent cancers such as those of the breast and prostate. In addition, soy isoflavones help to prevent osteoporosis. The observed low rates of these diseases among Asian populations are due to the large consumption of soybeans, according to many scientists.

All colorful fruits and vegetables contain flavonoids, caretenoids, or other beneficial phytochemicals. They inhibit inflammation; lower cholesterol, and prevent cancer, heart disease, and other illnesses. Studies have shown that blueberries contain the highest antioxidant strength, followed by strawberries, prunes, black currants, and boysenberries. Other flavonoids fruits and vegetables include blackberries, raspberries, red grapes, and alfalfa sprouts.

Not only fruits and vegetables but also spices contain important classes of phytochemicals that make unique contributions to all aspects of our detoxification systems. Spices contain potent ingredients that are effective inhibitors of cancer, especially skin, breast, and colon cancer. Curcumins are phenolic compounds, present in turmeric and mustard which have strong antioxidant and anti-inflammatory properties which inhibit cell proliferation and reduce inflammation. To help detoxify dangerous forms of estrogen associated with breast cancer and to inhibit the formation of skin and colon cancer, be sure to cook with rosemary, sage, oregano, and thyme.

Water and Health

Drinking enough *pure* water each day is essential to maintaining health. Water makes up more than 60 percent of your body weight, and if you don't get enough, any other nutrients you take in will not be utilized efficiently or not at all. Drinking sodas of any kind will deplete the water in your body and should be avoided. A lack of enough water affects everything from your digestion to your immune system. In the book, *Super life, Super Health,* there is a list of 9 ways that water fights aging, as follows:

1. *Feeds and cleans your cells.* Water constantly moves in and out of your cells—dissolving nutrients, delivering them where they need to go and carrying waste out of your body.

2. *Improves your digestion.* Like oil in a machine, water helps your digestive system run the way it is supposed to.

   Suffer from constipation? Water helps soften your stools so you can pass them more easily. Ever get that painful burning in your chest? Heartburn is an uncomfortable fact of life for many people. You get it when acid in your stomach backs up into your esophagus and irritates it. Water helps wash the acid out. Try drinking water about an hour before or after meals to keep your stomach from bloating.

3. *Keeps your body temperature even.* When exercise or fever makes you sweat, the water evaporating off your skin actually helps cool you down. Your body has a hard time handling extreme heat or cold, so during a summer heat wave or winter freeze, you need to drink even more water. If you don't, your body may shut down altogether, leading to serious problems such as heatstroke or frostbite. Drinking lots of water will keep you from getting dehydrated and help prevent heat stroke.

4. *Helps your body heal itself.* If you're sick or having surgery, drinking water is an easy way to put yourself back on the road to recovery. Water is also one of your best bets to prevent urinary or bladder infections. Six to eight glasses o water a day will also help you beat a cold or the flu.

5. *Lubricates and cushions your joints.* Water molecules don't like to be crowded together. This aversion actually protects your joints. By spreading out, water forms a cushion that helps lubricate your joints, which make them easier to bend and move around. When arthritis makes you stiff and achy, your first thought should be, 'I need some water.' If you're bothered by gout, you especially need to drink a lot of water. It dilutes and carries away the uric acid that causes your discomfort. Along with cushioning your joints, water acts like a shock absorber inside your eyes and spinal cord.

6. *Moisturizes your skin and lips.* Water is absolutely critical to healthy skin. It makes your skin elastic and supple

instead of dried up and shriveled like a prune. If you take long, hot showers or linger in a hot bath, you are doing your skin more harm than good. It can strip your skin of natural oils, which help keep moisture in. Use a humidifier in your home. Moist air means moist skin. And don't forget what it does for your lips. Water keeps them supple, and kissably soft.

7. *Stops stones before they start.* Water helps flush out the building blocks that form kidney stones before they can join forces to make you suffer. If your problem is gallstones, make water your lifelong friend. Bile, a fluid secreted by the liver and stored in the gall bladder, helps in digestion, especially of fats. When your bile has enough water, it can easily dissolve the cholesterol that forms gall stones.

8. *Watches your weight.* Guess what's at the center of your weight-loss program? That's right, good old-fashioned H_2O. Drink a glass before eating. Water fills you up, making it easier to resist that mound of food on your plate. It helps you eat more slowly. Drink more whenever you're active. It helps you exercise longer and harder.

9. *Rinses away germs.* Water can do just as much good from the outside as the inside. Soap and water is the number one way to stop germs from spreading. Fewer germs mean fewer illnesses. And that means a healthier you." [27]

Drinking an adequate amount of water each day is very important. However it must be from a source that is not only free of the usual contaminants such as chlorine but is also free of the fluoride additive which supposedly protects the teeth. See section of this book on the dangers of fluoride which include damage to the brain resulting in Alzheimer's disease among other things.

---

[27] Thomas Slaga. *The Detox Revolution.* New York: McGraw-Hill, pp.179-182.

Vitamins, Natural vs. Synthetic

The importance of vitamins is well recognized and supplements should be used as needed but there is a very important factor to be aware of: Synthetic vitamins are not the same as natural vitamins, as described below:

A pioneer in drawing such distinctions was Royal Lee, who pointed out that a natural vitamin is a working process consisting of nutrients, enzymes, coenzymes, antioxidants, and trace mineral activators. Since then chemists have noted that at the molecular level there is a difference between natural molecules and the synthetic ones designed to mimic them.

Synthetic vitamins are made from coal tars and use artificial colorings, preservatives, coating materials, and other additives. Although we have been led to believe that ascorbic acid, a synthesized form of vitamin C, is really vitamin C, it is not. Alpha tocopherol is not vitamin E. Retinoic acid is not vitamin A. And so on through the other vitamins. Vast energy and resources have been expended to make these myths part of conventional wisdom. However, the truth is that vitamins are not individual molecular compounds. Vitamins are biological complexes. In addition to ascorbic acid, real vitamin C must include bioflavonoids like hesperidin, rutin, quercetin, tannins, along with other naturally occurring compounds. Mineral cofactors must be available in proper amounts. If any of these parts are missing, there is no vitamin activity.

Dr. Bruce West states: "Synthetic B vitamins are useless against heart disease. Trying to fulfill vitamin deficiencies with synthetic B vitamins (no matter how 'potent') is a waste of time and money. They will not help, and may even hurt. When treated properly with the correct nutritional complexes (including the natural vitamin B complex), the heart is easier to repair than any other organ in the body." [28]

What the chemical industry foists upon us as vitamins essential to our health are actually more of the synthetic 'magic bullet' drugs that our bodies treat as toxins, and that have weakened our immune systems, and contaminated our foods.

---

[28] Dr. Bruce West. *Health Alert Newsletter,* Sept., 2006, Vol.23, No. 9, p. 4.

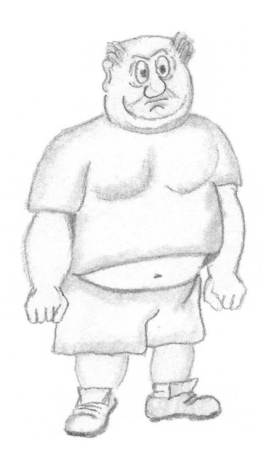

You don't have to look like this.
This chapter will show you how to improve your physique
and health simultaneously.

CHAPTER TWO

EXERCISE

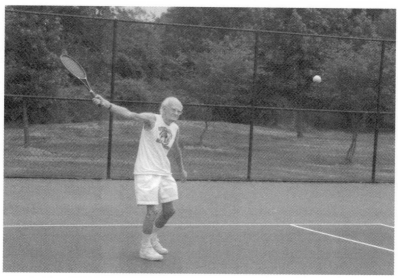

Dr. Singer playing tennis at age 93

Although proper nutrition is of primary importance in achieving an optimum state of health and longevity, we must also include exercise as part of a complete program for well being. Exercise is essential for maintaining your strength, vitality and flexibility. All major illnesses can be improved by exercise. It is a must in the prevention and cure of candida, osteoporosis, obesity, arthritis, and cardiovascular diseases. The best nutrition will not be sufficient as it will not be properly assimilated when there are blockages in the circulatory system. The colon must be cleansed and a slightly acidic pH maintained in order for acidophilus flora to flourish. This is a major factor in the overall health of the body, and particularly in the prevention of candida. The proper functioning of the lymph system is of great importance since it bathes the tissues and acts as a filter for the body. It is only through exercise the lymph can be kept circulating and continue to cleanse the system of toxins and thus help maintain the proper pH in the colon. Exercises that are helpful for the lymph system are swimming and jumping on a trampoline. A small home trampoline requires only about 10 minutes each day which will help circulate the lymph.

One of the most important things to keep in mind when doing any kind of exercise is to be aware of what you are capable of doing without injuring yourself. If you have any doubts about a particular exercise program consult your physician. Another thing to be aware of is the importance of warming up before getting started. Warm ups should include stretching, deep-breathing and focusing on each movement. Muscles that are tight can be loosened by certain movements. An excellent way to loosen-up is to use the progressive relaxation method. This involves focusing your mind on one part of your body at a time. Then deliberately tense the muscles and hold the tension for a while and then let go. If you have a problem doing this by yourself, find someone who can help you such as a Yoga or Tai Chi teacher. Very beneficial exercise programs that can improve health and longevity are described below:

Walking, Jogging and Running

Walking is the most frequently used method of exercise but has to be done with a purpose in mind in order to get the full benefits. Just walking casually and slowly does not confer the benefits that walking with intention does. To improve your health keep in mind the following things as you start a walking program:

- Walk as if you want to get somewhere in a hurry (stay within your comfort zone)
- Swing your arms with shoulders hanging loose, matching the rhythm of your stride.
- Pick an area which has trees and open areas so that you can enjoy the peace and beauty of nature.
- Let go of any thoughts which could keep you from enjoying the experience.

- Breathe deeply.

Have a schedule of when and how often you will walk. This is very important since doing it on a regular basis will insure that you stay with it; Walking for about one hour a day is ideal.

Start walking for a distance that is in your comfort zone and then gradually increase the distance until you can do at least two miles on a regular basis. If you cannot reach that goal do the best you can.

Running requires more strength and dedication than walking. Here again, you should start out slowly; building up your endurance by adding a little longer distance over a period of time until you reach the maximum that you wish to achieve. Warm up stretching exercises should be part of your routine before starting each session of running. A cool down period after running should also be part of your program.

Jogging is a good introduction to running for distance. It is done for shorter periods of time and for shorter distances. Running on natural turf is the ideal as it places less stress on the knees than does running on concrete or other hard surfaces. There are special types of sneakers which are supposed to cushion the shock of running. There are mixed reactions as to the value of some of the more expensive types.

For those who are able to achieve the level of long distance running, there are many benefits to look forward to as listed below:

- Increased strength
- Increased endurance
- Increased confidence
- Feelings of exhilaration

Dr. William Glasser wrote an entire book on what he called the *Positive Addiction* that is experienced by many long distance runners. A unique state of mind occurs after running for a long period of time that results in feelings of euphoria. On the basis of extensive research Dr. Glasser presents evidence that explains why this unique experience occurs:

"Almost all runners emphasize the pleasure of motion, the gliding or floating feeling that frequently occurs. I believe that running creates the optimal condition for PA because it is our most ancient and still most effective survival mechanism. We are descended from those who ran to stay alive, and this need to run is programmed genetically into our brains. When we have gained the endurance to run long distance easily, then a good run reactivates the ancient neural program. As this occurs we reach a state of mental preparedness that leads to a basic feeling of satisfaction *that is less critical than any other activity that we can do alone.* If you wish confirmation of the genetic need to run, watch a child. See the parents of a two or three year-old constantly nagging at their child to slow down. Urged to run by a neural program written millions of years ago, the child like a puppy, runs naturally.

It is because this activity is so non-self-critical and so completely programmed in the ancient pathways of our brains that when we run without fatigue we are able to free most of the brain for other activity. When this happens it is easy to slip into the euphoric, unique PA state.

These feelings are best described by runners; a few samples follow:

'I enjoy physical and mental satisfaction, feeling that everything is alright, elimination of worries. I can't carry a personal or job problem all the way through a run. They fade into inconsequence; thoughts become long, slow motion, drawn out. I often kick my mind out of gear resulting in a heightened awareness of light, temperature, and odors, sometimes an inexpressible joy, I want to stick my arms out and float.

In terms of psychological benefit, John says: 'I have never had any seriously bad habits but running has been responsible for reducing frenetic nervous drive, compulsive overwork, and impatient demand for immediate social change. I am much less serious, far more easygoing, less committed to abolishing all the evils overnight, easier to live with, have greater ability to ignore and eschew peripheral issues and that jazz...

'Everybody should run. It would down hates, aggression, and make people happier; create a greater sense of self-worth....To run you have got to build yourself up around a half-hour, hour, whatever, in which you run and say that absolutely nothing else is to interfere with this.

Jim describes his state of mind as he runs: "I simply perceive as I run. I react instinctively to obstacles which suddenly appear. I float. I run like a deer. I feel good. I feel high. I don't think at all. My awareness is only of the present. Even that cannot be called awareness. Brain chatter is gone....I am a less uptight person since running. I believe I have seen goodness by virtue of my runs. This awareness of the goodness in the world allows me to see it in people. I am more open with people and it seems to make them more open to me, thus my inter-personal habits or skills have improved." [29]

Chi Gong (Qigong)

One of the recognized masters of Qigong and Tai Chi, Dr. Yang, Jwing-Ming has this to say about the benefits of these practices:

Qi is the foundation of all Chinese medical theory and Qigong. It corresponds to the Sanskrit 'prana' and is considered to be the vital force and energy that flows in all living things. According to the experience of Qigong practitioners, Qi can best be explained as a type of energy very much like electricity, which flows through the body. When this circulation becomes stagnant or stops you become ill or die.

It was discovered in recent years to be a form of bioelectricity – which circulates in all living things...In Qigong training the mind controls the flow of Qi, just as it controls other body functions. Thinking of a tense situation can cause you to tighten your muscles so much that your muscles become sore. Your mind can also relax your body just by thinking about it. Many people use this approach to control their pulse or blood pressure without drugs.

In Qigong training, concentration is the key to success. By concentrating attention on the abdomen and doing certain exercises, Qi is generated and circulated throughout the body. This leads to the development of extra energy and its more efficient use.

Another way of increasing Qi circulation is called Nei Dan. In this method Qi is accumulated at the Dan Tian, a spot an inch and a half below the navel. Once sufficient Qi has accumulated, then you use your mind to guide the Qi to circulate throughout the vessels or channels in your body.

---

[29] Dr. William Glasser. *Running: Positive Addiction.* Pp.104-114.

Wai Dan is the practice of increasing Qi circulation by stimulating one area of the body until a large energy potential builds up and flows through the Qi channel system.

There are two types of Wai Dan exercises, moving and still. In moving Wai Dan, a specific muscle or part of the body is repeatedly tensed and relaxed as you concentrate on that muscle. Use as little tension as possible because great tension will constrict the Qi channels and prevent the flow of energy. When you exercise a part of your body in this way for several minutes, the Qi accumulates in that area which usually results in a local feeling of warmth. Both energy and blood are collected in this high potential area. When the muscles relax, the highly charged Qi and blood will spread to nearby areas with a lower energy state and so increase the Qi circulation.

In moving Wai Dan exercises, the mind concentrates on the breath and at the same time imagines guiding energy to a specific area. S was mentioned earlier, the Qi channel system and the brain are closely related, so that when you concentrate, you can control the circulation of Qi more efficiently. This in turn results in the muscles being able to exert maximum power. This is what is known as Wai Dan internal power. For example, in order to guide the Qi you have generated to the center of your palm, imagine an obstacle in front of your palm and try to push it, if you relax, calm down, and imagine pushing the object, you will find the object will now move. Therefore, in practicing the moving Wai Dan exercises, you should be calm, relaxed and natural. The muscles should never be strongly tensed, because this tension will narrow the Qi channels. Concentrate on breathing with the Dan Tien and on guiding the Qi.

There is a disadvantage to Wai Dan moving exercises. Because of the repeated tensing and relaxing of the muscles during training, the muscle itself will be built up, as in weight lifting, and can become overdeveloped. This over development will slow you down, and at the same time will constrict the channels. When these overdeveloped muscles are not regularly exercised, they accumulate fat, which will further narrow the channels, and the Qi and the blood will become stagnant. Common symptoms of this phenomenon are high blood pressure, local nerve pain, and poor muscle control. As long as you avoid over-developing your muscles this will not happen.

In still Wai Dan, specific muscle groups are also stressed, but they are not tensed. For example, in one type of still Wai Dan practice you extend both arms level in front of your body and hold the posture. After several minutes the nerves in the arms and shoulder become excited, and reach a higher energy state. When you drop your arms and relax, the generated Qi will circulate to areas of lower potential, much like an electric battery circulates electricity when a circuit is made. In still Wai Dan, there is no danger of overdevelopment because the muscle is not being exercised as it is in moving Wai Dan. Although the muscle is not built up in still Wai Dan training, its endurance is increased. If you practice Nei Dan meditation after you do the Wai Dan exercises, you can avoid the harmful effects of overdeveloped muscles.

Another powerful set of Qigong exercises is called Da Mo after the Shaolin monk who developed them during the sixth century. These exercises are easy and their benefits are experienced in a short time. When practicing the Da Mo exercises, find a place with clean air, stand facing the east with your back relaxed and naturally straight, and your feet shoulder –width apart and parallel. Facing the east takes advantage of the earth's rotation and the energy flow from the sun. Keeping the legs apart will relax the legs and thighs during practice. Keep your mouth closed and touch your palate with the tip of the tongue without strain. In Chinese meditation, this touch is called Da Qiao or Building the Bridge because it connects the Yin and Yang circulation. Saliva will accumulate in your mouth; swallow it to keep your throat from getting dry. The key to successful practice of this exercise is concentrating on the area being exercised, and concentrating on your breath. Without this concentration the original goal of Qi circulation will be lost and the exercise will be in vain. [30] (A complete description of these exercises can be found in the book by Dr. Yang)

It is one thing to understand the theory and benefits of Chi Gong, but it is also necessary to do the exercises in order to get the benefits. The best way to get started is to find a chi gong or Tai Chi instructor in the area where you live. If that is impossible you can get books and DVDs on the subject and follow the directions as best you can.

---

[30] Dr. Jwing Ming Yang. *ChiGong for Health and Martial Arts.* Boston: YMMA Publication, 1998, pp. 9-24.

You can also find some of the exercises on the internet on the Google website. An example of the tremendous benefits of Qigong is shown below:

According to Qi theory, cancers are caused by the stagnation of Qi and blood, which results in changes to the structure of the cell. Several types of cancer that may be cured by swinging the arms are cancer of the lungs, esophagus, and lymph. Other kinds of disorders that can be helped by swinging the arms are hardening of the liver, paralysis caused by high blood pressure, high blood pressure itself, heart trouble, and nervous disorders.

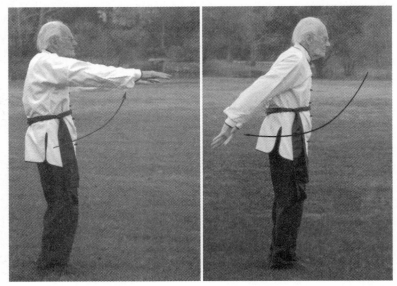

Figure 1   *Figure 2*

The method is very simple. Stand with your feet shoulder width apart, with the tip of your tongue touching the roof of your mouth. Swing your arms forward until they are horizontal with the palms facing down (demonstrated in Figure 1 above), then swing them backwards as far as possible with the palms facing up (Figure 2 above). Keep your entire body relaxed. Start with two hundred to three hundred repetitions, then gradually increase to one or two thousand, or up to half an hour.

Many Qi channels terminate in the feet and pass through the hip joints. Walking in place has many of the health benefits of swinging the arms for similar reasons. As a matter of fact, you can do both at the same time. [31]

According to acupuncture theory the Qi channels are connected to the internal organs. If Qi is circulating smoothly, then the organs will function normally. If an organ is not functioning normally, then increasing the Qi flow in the corresponding channel will help to restore its normal function. Acupuncture also increases Qi circulation by the insertion of fine needles at certain points in the channels or meridians of your body. Other ways of increasing circulation are: Tai Chi, massage, slapping the skin, and acupressure.

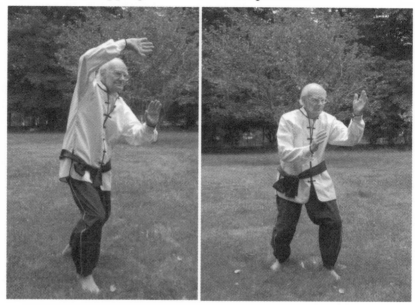

Dr. Singer Practicing Tai Chi in 2009 at age 93

Tai Chi

One of the best exercises you can do to improve your balance and overall health is Tai Chi. Research shows that practicing Tai Chi improves flexibility and coordination and also helps reduce stress. The basis of Tai Chi was Chi Gong which was introduced in China about six thousand years ago. Chi Gong made use of stretching movements and deep breathing to help prevent illnesses and develop overall strength. This gradually led to the development of Tai Chi as a martial art. In addition to the physical movements, Tai Chi includes

---

[31] Ibid, p. 139.

deep breathing to increase the amount of energy, "Chi," that your body will absorb as you do the movements.

Tai Chi, in the Chuan style, calms and relaxes the emotions focusing the mind, thus making an outstanding contribution to one's overall health and well-being. Movements are practiced at a slow and even speed, making this form of exercise appropriate for all ages and abilities. Tai Chi promotes relaxation, straight posture and balance, in addition to improving all bodily functions. It helps to prevent aging and disease

The most potent energies in the universe are invisible. We are all familiar with oxygen which is essential for life. Chi is also an invisible source of energy which is available to all living entities. It helps sustain life and when absorbed into the body by deep breathing it increases the vitality and general well-being of humans. In India it is called prana and in Japan ki. An expert on the subject of Tai Chi, Bruce Frantzis, has this to say:

"Energy can be increased in a human being. Consequently, the development of chi can make an ill person robust or a weak person vibrant; it can enhance mental capacity too. The concept of chi also extends beyond the body, to the subtle energies that activate all human functions, including emotions and thought. From the perspective of thought, when your mental chi becomes more refined it enhances your creativity at all levels.

When we are under stress we experience various levels of tension which can lead to serious diseases. Tai Chi helps to alleviate stress and thus performs a very valuable function in the protection from disease and also in the cure of disease.

In our fast-paced, high-pressure society, people are constantly bombarded with stress on a daily basis that can continuously activate the 'fight or flight' response.

This can lead to persistently high circulating levels of stress hormones and subsequent pathological consequences. For these reasons stress is often considered to be the leading cause of disease in the West today....Tai Chi conditions you to decrease your stress through the subtle learning process of how to do this art and through regularly doing the movements....For Tai Chi to work, you must practice a reasonable amount every week. To gain Tai Chi's benefits, you must do the form, not just think about it....Doing the Tai Chi form cools down and relaxes your nervous system and replenishes the chi that stress drains from your reserves....Tai Chi consistently trains you to recognize what is possible within your capability to be productive at the present moment without being stressed out, as it allows you to achieve physical, emotional, mental, and spiritual relaxation. *Tai Chi helps you to profoundly relax - physically, emotionally, mentally, and spiritually - so that joy and compassion can flourish."*

Many of the benefits of Tai Chi result from the frequent turning at the waist as you do the movements. This results in all of the important organs in the abdomen being massaged in a gentle and effective way restoring the organs to health and vitality. As you do the constant shifts of weight back and forth from one leg to the other it results in stretching all of the muscles of the lower back, legs, and feet resulting in stronger muscles and releasing tension which eliminates pains caused by tension. The synovial fluid which provides lubrication for the joints is also increased by these Tai Chi movements. Achieving a state of complete relaxation is another one of the many benefits of Tai Chi.

Acupuncture also increases Qi circulation by the insertion of fine needles at certain points in the channels or meridians of your body. When the channel is stimulated, Qi builds up and circulates in that channel. Other ways of increasing circulation are: massage, slapping the skin, and acupressure. [32]

The following description of what actually takes place physiologically was prepared for the Taoist Tai Chi Society by a physiotherapist Anne Carper, as described below:

Anatomy and Tai Chi

The Joints - Tai Chi is often promoted by referring to the beneficial effects it has on joints. For those who practice Tai Chi it would be useful and interesting to understand exactly what is being affected and benefited from the slow, continuous movements. There are many aspects of the joints which could be considered, but this article will restrict itself to the role of cartilage in the joint.

---

[32] Bruce Frantzis. *Tai Chi: Health for Life.* Berkley, CA: Blue Snakes Books, 2006, pp.7-12.

A joint is defined as a place where two or more bones are held together. There are two basic kinds of joints: those with little or no movement and those where the bones move freely. The most common, and most important functionally, is the second group, the Synovial joints, which normally provide movement.

There are four distinguishing features of a synovial joint. These are 1) a joint cavity; 2) articular cartilage; 3) synovial membrane; and 4) articular capsule. As the function of this kind of joint is movement, it is structured to reduce friction between the bones. The articular (adjoining) surfaces are covered with a thin layer of cartilage which is lubricated by synovial fluid produced by the synovial membrane. This is all encased by the articular capsule.

Cartilage is a soft, flexible material (tissue) found throughout the body. The ear and nose are formed from one type of cartilage, and parts of the skull, vertebrae and pubis consist of a second type. By far the most common type of cartilage, however, is that found on the ends of bones which are, therefore, the articular surfaces of joints. This cartilage is a translucent, bluish-white material (e.g., the shinny surface at the ends of chicken bones) and before birth formed the entire skeletal system before it was replaced by bone. By the time adulthood is reached the only cartilage that remains in the structure of the bones is at their ends, providing a smooth surface for movement.

Cartilage does not have a nerve supply and functions as a cushion of elastic material, kind of shock absorber. At age 20, cartilage is 70-80% water. Under load it compresses like a sponge losing water, and when it isn't bearing it re-expands by absorbing water. Cartilage also does not have a blood supply. For nutrition it relies on synovial fluid, a very thin, viscous layer of lubricating material that occupies the tiny space between the cartilage surfaces in the joint. The compression and release occurring in movement pumps the synovial fluid into the cartilage keeping it viable.

Tai Chi movements are very effective in lubricating the cartilaginous joint surfaces in two ways: rotation and compression. The rotational component of the movement brings all parts of the cartilage into contact with the opposing cartilage by putting the joint through a full range of motion. In addition, the movement is done with alternating compression and release; and slow, sustained pressure has been shown to be most affected for the transfer of nutrients, as opposed to the sudden impacting movement in many forms of exercise.

As people age, they tend to move less, and there are areas of cartilage which are never under compression. These areas loose water, become brittle, and the cartilage degenerate; the smooth surfaces becoming rough and uneven. This results in the loss of flexibility associated with aging, and is so common it is considered normal. By medical standards, supposedly, everyone over thirty has osteoarthritis, meaning that by this age there is evidence of the beginning of degeneration in the joints. Tai Chi, however, by requiring movements in all parts of the joints can retard or prevent this degeneration (depending on how many Tor Yus you do).

Evidence for the beneficial effect of full range of movement with compression can be seen in the comparative infrequency of arthritis in the ankle. Walking even a small amount puts the ankle through a full range under load and consequently the cartilage at the ankle stays viable in many people. In the same way, Tai Chi ensures that all joints are used maximally, and the cartilage is kept nourished and intact. A joint with healthy cartilage is able to move freely, and the movement in turn keeps the cartilage healthy – a non-vicious circle. Above all, a person with full pain-free movement in all joints is physically young regardless of their chronological age.

The Muscles and Tai Chi

Tai Chi as an exercise system has specific effects on the muscles of the body. Any exercise will improve strength in the muscles required to perform that exercise. Tai Chi is distinct from many exercise systems because it requires the use of almost all of the over 600 muscles that you have. In addition, Tai Chi does not produce the same alternation of muscle contour as other exercises produced because it is a balanced exercise.

In order to understand the changes Tai Chi cause, it helps to consider the structure of the muscles. A skeletal muscle is made up of smaller units called motor units. A motor unit is defined as a group of muscled fibers and the single neuron innervating these fibers. There are three types of muscle fiber that make up muscle, and each motor unit has only one type of fiber. These fibers differ in how quickly they react, how easily they tire, and whether or not they require oxygen as an energy source. The number of fibers-per muscle does not change but the diameter of each can increase with exercise, and with consistent neural input fibers of one type can be converted into another type. Exercises for endurance increase blood circulation and favor the development of non-fatigable fibers which use oxygen. Exercises for strength favor the development of fibers that contract quickly, do not require oxygen and fatigue quickly. Certain exercises or sports predispose the development of one type of fiber, and this is why a person who lifts weights has a different musculature than a person who jogs or dances. Tai Chi is considered an endurance exercise.

Muscles grouped together are wired in the spinal cord together, so that in the nervous system any movement prepares the muscle of the body for its opposite movement. The Tai Chi set utilize this relationship. Stretching, which is the distinguishing feature of Taoist style Tai Chi, is a very important component of building balanced muscle strength. Because of the way muscles are innervated, a muscle contraction in strongest following maximum stretch. The converse is also true. A muscle can relax and lengthen maximally following a maximum contraction. The alternating contraction and expansion that Tai Chi moves require can be thought of as preprogrammed in the reflex wiring of the spinal cord. Tai Chi improves your reflexes because it uses the spinal reflexes to maximize efficiency.

In addition to stretching and contracting, Tai Chi movements are also circular, having diagonal and rotational components. This means more muscles are called into play to execute the movement, and no muscle is developed more than others. For example, if you put weight on your ankle, sit on a chair, and repeatedly straighten your knee, the quadriceps muscle on the front of your thigh will be strengthened. If you do enough of this, you will be able to see the outline of the muscle which will harden and enlarge. The kind of muscle fiber required to perform maximum work of short duration will be produced: quickly reacting, easily fatigable fibers. In Tai Chi, however, you use the quadriceps to control the sitting and standing motions, but you use it in conjunction with the hamstring muscles on the back of the thigh. This will not produce a hard, defined quadriceps muscle, but since you are supporting the weight of your body on the leg, you will still be building strength. By strengthening and balancing the muscles in both groups, you will develop fast reacting, non-fatigable muscle fibers which are effective for endurance. Because these types of fibers have a high oxygen requirement, the circulation to the muscle is automatically increased. Tai Chi is therefore an endurance exercise which increases circulation to the muscles.

Strength in Tai Chi is developed slowly and is a process of learning to relax the muscles and allowing them to contract. Many people come to Tai Chi with a high level of muscle tension created by poor physical habits, bad postures or emotional states. Their nervous systems are signaling the muscles to contract in the absence of a reason for the tension. Tense muscles are brittle, not strong, and an excess of tension not only makes movement stiff, it decreases the blood circulation. By practicing Tai Chi, you learn to use the body efficiently, posture is improved and a foundation of using the naturally strong muscles of the legs, thighs, pelvis and back is laid. Tai Chi is a total exercise: it develops the muscles in all of the major muscle groups; it improves strength, includes stretch and develops endurance. Few other forms of exercise offer this.

The Lower Back and Tai Chi

When you begin the practice of Tai Chi, the legs and pelvis are consciously moved by the large muscles used in standing, sitting and walking. As you progress in Tai Chi, initiation and control of the movement of the legs and pelvis shifts to the spine. When you can "sit", you do not actively rotate the pelvis, nor contract the stomach muscles, nor flex the hips to strengthen your back...you simply relax and the spine straightens automatically.

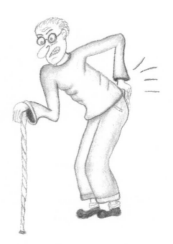

The term "spiral turning" is often used by Mr. Moy. One aspect of this principle is to stretch the muscles, ligaments and joints in the lower back and this, in turn, carries through into the entire spine. "Spiral turning" is difficult to achieve in the lumbar spine because the structure of these five vertebrae mechanically resists rotation. The plane of the facets (boney projections) which make up the joints between successive vertebrae is vertical so that the joints normally allow movement backward and <u>forward</u> only. Therefore, rotation in the lumbar spine can only occur when the spine is straightened. Flattening the lower back combined with turning and stretching the entire spine opens these joints so that rotation can occur. The "tor yu" exercise in Tai Chi works precisely on turning and stretching combined with the sitting motion.

Opening the joints has many <u>connotations</u> in Tai Chi, but anatomically this means separating the joint surfaces to allow play or movement in the joint. The deepest spinal muscles are very small and join one vertebra to the next; the action of these muscles is rotation. Advancing in Tai Chi can be considered a progress from gross movement of the superficial muscles which turn the hips and upper body, to small movements of deep muscles which turn the individual units of the spine.[33]

---

[33] Anne Carper. Taoist Society of Florida pamphlet, 2007.

Yoga

The practice of Yoga has many health benefits over and beyond the usual benefits of physical exercise. There are a number of separate forms such as Hatha Yoga which involves the various postures (asanas) and movements; Pranayama which focuses on techniques of controlled breathing in order to increase the benefits of meditation; and Raja Yoga, which among other things trains the mind to focus on one thing such as the flame of a candle or on one thought or sound in order to free the mind of one's usual thoughts resulting in a heightened sense of awareness and peace of mind.

The physical movements involved with the various postures result in increased lubrication of the joints and strengthening of the ligaments and tendons. Yoga massages all of the internal organs and glands in the body in a thorough manner even involving organs such as the prostate which hardly ever gets externally stimulated.

Among the various postures of Hatha Yoga are the inverted postures which have many health benefits. When the legs are raised above the head it increases the flow of blood to every organ of the body. Inverted postures cleanse and boost the health of the immune system and also benefit the glands of the endocrine system that produces vital hormones such as adrenalin, estrogen and testosterone. A simple standing forward bend inverts the body and brings the head below the heart. In this position the pituitary gland is stimulated. This gland is involved in the regulation of blood sugar levels and body temperature. The forward bend also gently stretches the spine and lengthens the entire back of the body.

Although each form of Yoga has its particular focus many of the features of each one are utilized by the others resulting in the total power of Yoga to increase mental, physical and spiritual benefits. For example, sitting in the lotus posture with legs crossed is a part of every form of Yoga, especially when meditating. The focus on Yogic breathing is also a part of each form as is the concentration of the mind in Raja Yoga. You will experience the benefits of Yoga shortly after you begin to practice the techniques on a regular basis. Yoga delays aging, increases energy, and results in a remarkable zest for life.

Learning to concentrate and control the mind leads to freedom from fears and anxieties which results in peace of mind. Using techniques of meditation advanced students, after many years of strict efforts, may reach the state of enlightenment (Samadhi.) In this state one can connect the conscious mind with the Universal mind. A state of transcendental powers can be achieved, enabling one to transcend our known laws of physics and make use of metaphysical energy. We can experience heavenly bliss which words cannot describe. In this transcendental state you can extend your lifespan as advanced yogis do.

There is another form of Yoga which involves advanced poses and special breathing exercises that is known as Kundalini Yoga. One of the most powerful remedies for many ailments is called the *Breath of Fire.* It consists of seven long breaths, holding each inhalation to the maximum. You can reach a state of euphoria doing this exercise because of the increased volume of oxygen and prana that enters your body. A skilled teacher is needed in order to acquire the necessary techniques and to monitor your progress.

A special full care drugless 3 HO Drug Rehabilitation Facility in Tucson, Arizona makes use of Kundalini Yoga as the main feature of the program.

Some of the basic techniques and benefits of Pranayama Yoga are described in the chapter on breathing which follows below. There are many books on Yoga containing specific instructions and illustrations providing a wealth of information on how to make use of the various techniques. Space does not allow for the inclusion of the wealth of available information in this book. Actually, the best and quickest way to learn Yoga is to find an experienced teacher or class where you can receive personal guidance.

CHAPTER THREE

THE POWER OF THOUGHTS

In addition to the physical needs of our bodies, an extremely important factor in achieving longevity is the state of our minds as demonstrated by our attitudes and thoughts. We actually bring about what we focus our thoughts on. There are several factors that greatly influence our state of mind such as early childhood experiences and beliefs inculcated by parents and the society one lives in. For example, a dislike or hatred for people who have different racial, ethnic or religious backgrounds than our own. Feelings of fear and guilt are also inculcated into young minds by certain religious creeds.

Painful experiences may become lodged in our reactive mind and lead to illness and aberrative behavior. It is important to free ourselves from these negative and destructive thought patterns. This chapter provides a number of powerful methods that can help you achieve freedom from negative influences and achieve a joyful positive state of mind.

I have been fortunate during my long lifetime to have had a number of personal experiences which have provided me with insights into the power of our thoughts and which, I believe, have had a profound effect on my achieving and maintaining the state of vibrant health that I now have at age 93. I described some of the experiences that I had in the Introduction to this book, which convinced me of the reality of God and the fact that we are not just human beings; that we are also spirit beings as well. This led me to a conviction that life continued on after death.

My research into the subject of life after death led me to write a book on the subject titled *Life Beyond Earth: The Evidence and Its Implications.* In that book I present the evidence that supports the reality of life after death. Further confirmation of this fact was provided by my wife after she passed on in March, 2005. She appeared to me and to six other people after she passed on. First-hand personal accounts of my wife's visitations are presented later in this chapter.

Although that knowledge provided me with such benefits as peace of mind and the inner strength to handle adversities, there were times when I needed additional help. In my search for answers, I learned about *A Course in Miracles, The Power of Attraction,* and the *Power of Intention* which further enriched my life. Each of these topics is presented later in this chapter.

Earlier in my life, I was introduced to two programs: EST and Dianetics by my son, David. Both of these programs helped to clear my mind of negative thought patterns which had limited my abilities and restricted my joy of life. Dianetics proved to be the most effective program and brought about positive improvements in both my mental and physical health.

Dianetics

Dianetics provides a technique which brings suppressed painful memories to your conscious awareness and then proceeds to permanently erase the reactive, negative influence of these memories. For example, I was enabled to clear my mind of debilitating thoughts of painful childhood experiences that were suppressed at a subconscious level called the reactive mind in Dianetics. This was accomplished by my participating in a series of courses given by a trained auditor.

The courses were based on the teachings of Ron Hubbard, the author of *Dianetics: The Modern Science of the Mind* and the founder of Scientology. The underlying power of Ron Hubbard's theories is presented in his many books and lectures. His chief contribution to the field of mental health was his discovery that memories of very painful experiences that occur on a subconscious level while a person is unconscious or in a very weakened state of health are stored in a memory bank, below our conscious level, in what he called the reactive mind. His unique discovery was the fact that the initial painful experience usually involved a short period of unconsciousness during which comments by people who were present were stored in the memory. This in itself does not usually cause a problem. However, when another similar experience occurs or when someone makes a comment similar to one associated with the original experience, then the memory becomes 'keyed in' and becomes magnified with powerful emotional reactions called engrams which are stored in the reactive mind without any conscious awareness that this has taken place. This then became a memory associated with the innate need for survival.

Any future incidents which are perceived to be associated with the engram tend to 'restimulate' the emotional charge and cause the person to act or say things with great emotion out of all proportion to the current situation. A person may react in many different ways such as running away; committing violent or destructive acts; and/or becoming ill without any apparent reason for such behavior. The basic reason for this problem is the need for survival which doesn't allow time for conscious evaluation of a perceived threat. While engrams remain in the reactive mind they drain the body of energy and curtail the ability of the individual to function at an optimum level.

After identifying this problem, Hubbard proceeded to study how to eliminate the destructive power of engrams which led to his discovery of the principles and techniques of Dianetics. After applying the techniques to thousands of patients whom he classified as 'pre-clears', Hubbard learned that the technique was universal. It worked in every case regardless of the person's background or severity of the case. The methods employed, known as auditing, were found to eliminate the engrams and restore the pre-clears to a state of heightened well-being which he called *clear*. Eventually Dianetics became part of an organization known as Scientology. A simplified version of how auditing works is described below:

The pre-clear sits facing the auditor. It is a very relaxed atmosphere, in a private room free of any distractions. You are given two small cans, similar to the juice cans on airplanes, to hold in each hand. The cans are attached by wires to an instrument called an e-meter which faces the auditor. The e-meter registers the amount of emotional charge coming from the person being audited as different memories are brought to a conscious level. This enables the auditor to identify when a person being audited is experiencing an emotionally charged memory and this is followed by the technique that results in eliminating the engrams, once and for all. The technique has been refined and made more and more effective by the lessons learned through the years following its discovery in 1950. On the surface it appears to be a very simple process of having the pre-clear repeat the details, which were associated with the original painful memory, over and over again, until the memory is restored to the conscious level and thereby eliminated permanently from the reactive mind.

There is actually more to it than that. The skillful auditor makes use of the basic methods which include questioning the pre-clear in a way that enables the pre-clear to recall all of the details of the engram, no matter how painful they may have been. This includes making use of all of the senses in the recall process such as colors, sounds, odors, etc. associated with the engram. The auditor also knows the importance of getting the pre-clear to go back in his memory to the origin of the engram in order to clear it completely.

Most of our memories are stored in a memory bank at our conscious level and can be recalled easily most of the time. Our very painful memories that are associated with survival are kept in a memory bank called the reactive mind. By the process called auditing they can only be brought to conscious awareness through the processes described in Dianetics. The auditor does not become involved with the person being audited. He or she makes no comments about the pre-clear's memories assuring the pre-clear that no one will ever be told about the incidents being divulged by the pre-clear. An indication of how it works was my personal experience with being audited as described below:

I had been subject to three unexplainable fears that I believed were part of an inferiority complex that I had somehow acquired. I had a fear of drowning, a fear of authoritarian persons and a fear of speaking to a group of people. I went into a panic when I was in deep water and when I had to speak with a high school debating team and I went into an even greater panic when I was selected to be in a high school play. Encouraged by my son, David, my wife and I enrolled in a series of courses at a Dianetics Mission in Clearwater Florida. A review of what took place follows:

When I was audited I found it to be a very pleasant experience. The auditor kept asking me to recall memories at different stages of my life such as what was happening when I first entered school; or what did I feel about the first girl I got interested in; and what did I feel or see when I was born. This is called going up and down the time-line. It appears that every single detail of every incident in our lives is stored somewhere in our memory banks. The safe environment and the skill of the auditor enable the pre-clear to freely express the most personal and emotionally charged memories so that the actual facts are revealed.

In my case, an incident occurred while I was in kindergarten that was the seat of most of my mental problems. By careful questioning, the auditor zeroed in on an incident that caused me to store an extremely painful memory in my reactive mind. I remembered being pulled by the hand by the teacher, who was very angry at me and dragged into a small bathroom near the entrance to the kindergarten room. She then proceeded to force me to keep my mouth open while she put a bar of soap in my mouth that gagged me while she kept scolding me severely. She then left me there and went back to the classroom. After a while, I started to go back in the classroom and I heard the children giggling and staring at me. I felt so embarrassed and ashamed that I went into the cloakroom adjoining the classroom and knelt in a corner and remained there hidden behind some jackets. It seemed like a very long time passed by and then my mother came and brought me home.

I felt like I must have done something terribly wrong to be punished so severely. The auditor kept asking me to remember more details. I then remembered being in the center of a circle and the children in the circle were throwing a heavy ball at me, while playing a game of dodge ball. The teacher suddenly started screaming at me and dragging me to the bathroom. I still had no idea of why the teacher was so angry. After repeated questions by the auditor, asking me to repeat the incident over and over; starting at the very beginning, it suddenly dawned on me as to what had provoked the teacher. One of the children had thrown the ball at me very hard and struck me in a painful part of my body causing me to utter some kind of a curse word. When I realized what had caused me to be so severely punished, I felt completely relieved. I realized that I had done nothing terribly wrong. After reviewing the details again a number of more times, the auditor said to me: "The needle is swaying freely." This indicator on the E-meter showed that there no longer was any emotional charge associated with the engram and the memory was now part of my standard memory bank where it no longer had any harmful effects on me.

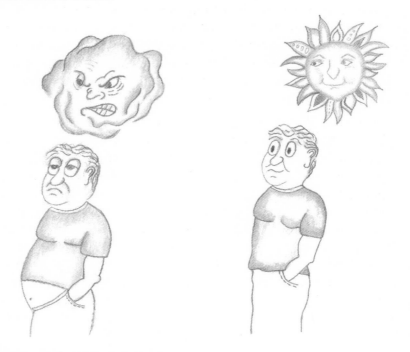

Thoughts Create Our Reality

In her book, *The Healing Power of Light,* Primrose Cooper presents evidence showing how thoughts can initiate healing energies that bring about miraculous cures. Excerpts from the book follow below:

It is absolutely necessary first, to understand that we exist as consciousness; and secondly, to become conscious of this reality of existence. Physical or mental healing is based on the belief that we are somewhere between our feet and our head, and it attempts to do something about a physical existence. Spiritual healing has an entirely different basis. Spiritual healing is dependent on the individual's becoming consciously aware of the truth that we do not exist in the body or as the body, but that we exist as infinite, divine consciousness.

Perhaps the first thing we should be aware of is the energy of thought. It is, in fact, faster than the speed of light (Bell's Theorem mentioned this) and a fourth dimensional tool not bound by our third dimensional limitations of time and space. As we have indicated, at this level prayer and radionics (the projecting of the energy of number and form for healing) and the sending of healing thoughts in whatever form – color, sound pattern, number – are effective. I never cease to be amazed that it is so and yet it is not really amazing. It is simply in accordance with the laws that operate at that level and are as yet not fully understood by contemporary science.

It is well known, however, that energy follows thought. The ideas in the mind, the desire of the heart have their energy which follows on to bring about a manifestation on the physical level of the idea or desire. Intention is of major importance at this level. So, even if a method of or performance in healing is less than brilliant, the good intention will always be honored and, where necessary, corrections made and inadequacies compensated for. There is a divine economy in which we are part of a far greater scenario than we can imagine and where angels, guides, friends and saints support our healing work.

At this level our perceptions also change. Good and evil may impact on our systems as warmth or cold or light and darkness. A friend of mine who has a gift for clearing people and places of bad or evil influences speaks of 'seeing the darkness turn to light' when she has prayed and cleared a room. I have been with her when she has done this and I have not seen this change visually, as she has, but I have sensed the lifting of the oppressiveness and a coming in of a new purity.

Sometimes a spirit or an entity may get into a place or a person's auric field. The spirit may be lost, not able to go to the Divine Light and may be living parasitically off the energies of the person to whom it has attached itself, unwilling to go anywhere else. It is important that such a spirit be helped to find the Light of God and it's fulfillment there. Those trained in releasement therapy know something of this important aspect of healing. Negative and destructive influences do need to be cleared and a blessing and protection given to the place or person concerned. To call upon the Divine Light and to put on the Armor of Light is a very important protection for each person every day. Evil cannot penetrate such protective Light. [34]

In the book, *Spontaneous Healing,* Dr. Andrew Weil tells us about his real life experiences with patients who were healed of debilitating illnesses by the use of psychosomatic techniques, which enabled the patient to heal themselves by guiding their thoughts in the healing process. This healing power is available to us as described in the following true story about his wife's pregnancy:

In August 1991, when my wife, Sabine was seven months pregnant with her fourth child, we were in British Columbia, where I was teaching a workshop on health and healing. One of the participants was a friend and colleague, Marilyn Ream, a family practice doctor from Spokane, Washington, who works in a woman's health clinic. Marilyn was completing training in interactive guided imagery therapy. I wanted her to give a demonstration of the method, and Marilyn asked Sabine if she would consent to be a volunteer subject in front of the group. Sabine agreed.

My wife has a history of back trouble associated with pregnancy. Usually around the seventh month her lower back goes out and she is in the habit of getting weekly chiropractic adjustments to help. On this occasion we had been traveling for several weeks, no one was available to adjust her, and she was living with steady pain. Marilyn asked her if she wanted her back to be worked on in a guided imagery session. Sabine said no; she thought it was a mechanical problem needing a mechanical solution. Instead she wanted to work on issues around her birth. She wanted the baby to come on time, because I was scheduled to leave shortly and she had had long and difficult labors with her previous pregnancies.

Marilyn asked Sabine to lie on the floor, loosen her clothing, and take a series of deep breaths. Interactive guided imagery uses the forms of hypnotherapy to induce a state of light trance and openness to the unconscious mind. It assumes

---

[34] Primrose Cooper. *The Healing Power of Light.* NY: Agora, 2006, pp. 104-106.

that the unconscious mind comprehends the nature of disease processes and how to resolve them. Marilyn began the process by asking Sabine to picture herself in a familiar place where she felt completely secure, then to describe it. Sabine described a site in the canyon country of southern Utah. Marilyn told her to focus on small details, to try to hear sounds and smell scents, as well as see the place. Sabine warmed to the task and quickly became very relaxed.

Marilyn then asked her to shift her focus to her uterus and to the baby inside it. Sabine was soon in contact with the baby. Marilyn guided her through a dialogue with the baby, in which Sabine asked her to come on time (she agreed to do so) and to help make the labor quick and uneventful. In this dialogue, Sabine would speak the words she 'heard' the baby use in reply to her questions. After a time, Sabine felt she had completed this work, and Marilyn told her to return to her spot in southern Utah.

'How do you feel?' Marilyn asked.

'Great, very peaceful.'

'Is there anything else you'd like to work on? How about your back?'

'Mmmm. Okay.'

'Good. Then put your attention on the part of your back that hurts and tell me what you find there.'

Sabine gave a little gasp.

'What is it?' Marilyn asked.

'It's all black.'

'Go to the blackness and see if it has anything to say.' Marilyn suggested.

'It says it's really angry, 'Sabine answered, sounding surprised. 'It's angry at me.'

Sabine was quite unprepared for the intensity of her back's anger at her. With Marilyn's guidance she entered into a tentative conversation with it and discovered that it was angry at her for being angry at it, and for not taking care of it.

'Ask it what it wants.' Marilyn directed.

'It says it wants me to put warm towels on it.'

'Will you do that?'

'Yes, but I've been putting cold on it, I thought cold was better for it.'

'Tell it you'll put warm towels on it and ask if it will stop hurting.'

'I did. It says it will stop.'

'How does it feel now?' Marilyn asked.

'Better,' Sabine replied. She moved around on the floor. 'Definitely better. That's the first time in weeks it's been any better.'

'Is it completely gone?'

'No.'

'Ask it if it can go away entirely.'

'It says it can.'

'Ask it to please do so.'

'Okay. I did. And I think it did.'

'Now how does it feel?'

'My God, I think it's gone.'

'Is it gone?'

Sabine moved this way and that. 'Yes, it's really gone.'

When Sabine returned to normal consciousness, the pain was still gone. It remained absent that night and the next day. (Nonetheless, Sabine kept her promise to keep warm towels on her back.) In fact the pain did not return for the remainder of her pregnancy, even though Sabine got no further chiropractic work. She had never before been free of back pain in the last two months of a pregnancy.

Three weeks before Sabine's due date I asked a friend and colleague, Dr. Steve Gurgevich, who practices hypnotherapy, to do a session with her, again in the interest of a timely, quick, uncomplicated birth. The baby was in a posterior presentation at that time, which worried us. Sabine's last baby had been posterior, causing long painful labor. Steve did an hour-long session with her, encouraging Sabine to talk with the baby, asking her to turn around before the beginning of labor and help make the labor quick. When he brought Sabine out of her reverie, she looked supremely relaxed. After Steve left, Sabine and I went to the kitchen to start dinner. Suddenly, she clutched her belly and bent over.

'What is it?'' I asked

'I think the baby's turning,' she said, amazed.

It happened that our midwife was coming for dinner that night. She examined Sabine and reported that the baby was now in anterior presentation, having turned within twenty minutes of being asked to do so. The baby came right on her due date, October 4. Labor lasted a mere two hours and six minutes, which was, if anything, a little too brief in that we barely had time to prepare. Needless to say, Sabine and I are both true believers in the effectiveness of mind and body approaches, and when we hear doctors and researchers dismiss the role of the mind in health and healing, we exchange knowing smiles. [35]

A number of real life experiences which support the reality of mind over matter and the power of visualizations were described by the famous actress and author Shirley MacLaine in two of her books, *Out on a Limb,* and *It's All in the Playing.* In the latter book, she describes how the weather was changed by a combination of factors including focusing of her thoughts, use of visualization and prayer. She was in the Andes Mountains in Peru taking part in a film about her book *Out on a Limb.* There was an urgent need to finish filming the last scene on the top of a mountain peak before the film would be scrapped due to cost overruns caused by inclement weather conditions. By concentrating her thoughts on the need for clear weather, she was led to consulting a Peruvian psychic named Benito. She describes what took place:

'Benito earnestly conducted his ceremony and talked to me of my life. By now he had spread a gigantic bag of coca leaves across the daybed. I had been to enough psychics to know that tarot cards or tea leaves or palm reading or *I-ching* were only tools that enabled the psychic to attune to a higher level of awareness. That awareness is available to all of us because it is only contact with the higher self, which is all-knowing and directly connected to the Divine Universal Energy Source. But psychics have had more training in attuning to that energy level, so they are able to trust it more readily than the rest of us are.

---

[35] Dr. Andrew Weill. *Spontaneous Healing.* pp. 93-97.

'You must do ceremony for good weather at Mt. Picchu. The high priest of Inca agrees to help if you will do your part. Everything stems from within. You will manifest what you sincerely believe. Do not doubt. Be not afraid. Do not be mistrustful. What you believe is what will occur.'

Then he piled all the natural objects together and made a package out of them. He tied the package tightly, blessed it, and handed it to me.

'You must take this,' he said, 'to the highest point of Mt. Picchu, face the East, and burn the packet. While burning you will think only of your vision of good weather and your wish will come to pass. Do not doubt what you wish to happen.'

Simo woke me the next morning at 4:00. This was the big day. Crew members were all over Cuzco were rising and wondering if the arduous train trip would be worth it this time. The drive to the train for Machu Picchu would take several hours. The fog was so thick that a snail would have beaten us. I wondered how the camera truck with all our equipment was going to make it in time to load onto the train. With prayers in our hearts we scanned the skies as the train pulled into the station just below the Machu Picchu monument. We piled into the buses and with uncertain emotions made our way up the winding road to the mountain top.

Fifteen minute later our worst fears were confirmed. A solid thicket of fog accompanied by a cold drizzle enveloped the Lost City. Machu Picchu wasn't even visible. Four of us started to climb to the top of the mountain to perform the ceremony which would help control the weather, according to Benito.

The climbing entailed in getting to the top of Machu Picchu is no joke. Even if the sun did come out I wondered how the guys would lift the equipment to the top. No matter. That's show business. We stopped took a look below us. Nothing was visible. It was as though we had ascended into a sprinkly fog heaven and left the earth below us forever. When we reached the top, we proceeded to follow Benito's instructions. We faced East, lit a fire under the packet and started to visualize.

'Picture the weather you would like to have, Benito had said.' Your mind's picture will manifest if you trust it.'

About half an hour went by. Then, as though on cue, the four of us broke our meditation. The 'element' package was ashes now. There was only a thin waft of smoke left from the ashes. There was nothing left to do or say—except for something I felt very strongly. So I said it out loud.

'It will be sunny in about an hour,' I announced, absolutely sure of my words. The others nodded and shrugged. I went to change and get ready for the shoot. I looked out of the window to check on the weather. The drizzle had stopped. The crew was carrying the equipment to the top of the mountain.

When we reached the top of the mountain, the sun had broken through the clouds completely. The sun's rays cast an aura around the ruins as well as the trees. The third dimensional mystical quality was even more pronounced than I had visualized. It was a poetic painting…perfect. We got the scene.

The camera guys set up quickly in another location. For two and a half hours we shot. We shot every conceivable angle of the Machu Picchu ruins so we'd have plenty to choose from in the editing room. Finally we got the last shot. We looked up. As God is my judge, a cloud drifted in front of the sun. Clouds seemed to materialize out of the thin air. Yudi yelled, 'Let's get a crew picture. And then something happened which I will never forget as long as I live. The photographer took about five shots of the entire crew. Then, as though by direct cue from an unseen director, the photographer said, 'That's it—I'm out of film.' And immediately the skies literally *dumped* sheets of rain on us. Our small band of movie makers was drenched within one minute. It actually made us laugh; it was so 'coincidental.'

When we returned to Cuzco it wasn't long before the word spread that I had controlled the weather and made sunshine happen in Machu Picchu on a day that was intrinsically gloomy. [36]

---

[36] Shirley MacLaine. *It's All in the Playing*. New York: pp. 283-294.

On the way back to the United States, Shirley focused on the psychic aspects of her experiences while in Peru and came up with the following insights:

The levels of both our psychic and our mental capacities are far greater now than they ever were in the far past. This is a testament to the spiritual and mental progress of the human race. Our minds are more capable today of accepting unusual, unfamiliar, more complex ideas.

In the past, death belonged in the province of an exterior, unknowable 'God'; the mythological garden of paradisiacal afterlife, untouchable and unrealized by mortals who longed to know its promise, its secrets, and, indeed, whether it existed at all.

Lately, more and more people are claiming to have seen the actual 'light,' the blinding, indescribably loving light that they are certain is 'Heaven.' 'God is light,' they say after having had an out-of-body experience. 'I died and lived to tell about it,' they say. The reports are increasing; almost as though the numbers of people experiencing the light are increasing as a testament to the level of receptivity and openness to higher and higher consciousness.

The *light* is expected now. It had always been there, but more and more we are beginning to recognize that in fact we are the *light,* if only we can bring ourselves to hold that evolved and sophisticated concept. The light is not outside of us. And whenever we recognize that light inside of us, we know we have found the secret to life well kept. We have been a secret to ourselves. That is what has been missing. We have been missing the light from ourselves. [37]

The above story by Shirley MacLaine may seem too unusual to believe but based on my own experiences during a long lifetime, it is my personal belief that many incidents in my life that can be dismissed as 'coincidences', were actually interventions by some higher power beyond the physical realm.

---

[37] Ibid, pp. 334-335.

Guardian Angels

One of the unseen powers beyond our own mental visualizations is the power of spirit entities, such as angels to intervene on our behalf in many ways without our being aware of their presence. In the book, *Ask Your Angels,* many real-life experiences are described providing evidence that angels do take an active part in the lives of humans, as illustrated by the following excerpt from the book:

Angels are intelligent beings, capable of feelings, yet a different species, which have their existence on a slightly finer vibrational frequency from the one to which our physical senses are tuned. This means we can't perceive them ordinarily with our eyes or ears, but they can perceive us. Our realities interpenetrate one another – with their reality encompassing and enfolding ours.

The word *angel* is a generic name for the collective group of beings - citizens of 'inner space' - whose responsibilities include the harmonious organization of the inhabited universe. A relatively small number of this vast multitude is immediately concerned with humanity and our planet. Among these are our closest companions—our guardian angels—and also the many millions of angels who watch over virtually every aspect of human activity. For example, we were given an angel by the name of Joy to help us in the creation and writing of this book.

In the autumn of 1988 I was going altogether too fast—an occupational hazard of New York living—and as can happen when I am blundering along not giving myself the time to listen, I found myself laid low with a bout of flu that stopped me in my tracks for five days. Once I got over the raw pain in all my joints, I fell again into contact with my guardian angel, Joy. I was completely unprepared for what Joy told me.

JOY: Beloved, welcome. I should indicate to you, that this process of dictation falls under the aegis of another. One you might call a close colleague, but an entity who, in many ways, is more adequately equipped for such work...Let me introduce you to Abrigrael who is a recording angel who has been entrusted with the thought patterns that many have centered on for this work. We trust you will find it valuable to have one particular terminal who is prepared to make this document of general and real application to the widest possible audience.

ABIGRAEL: The first and most important fact is, Dearest One, as it always must be, love. Our contact and communication is made possible through love. If there's little love, there can be little contact. And if there is no love in a person's heart, then it is well-nigh impossible for us to make any inroads...

Let it first be said that the conditions you live under on your planet are rather exceptional ones. On more regular planets which are inhabited by beings much as yourselves, we aren't hidden, neither are we unknown. The mortal and angelic worlds have a full and cooperative aspect. The mystery and disbelief surrounding our order of beings on your world is by far the greatest exception to the natural rhythms of ordinary planetary existence. Another way to express this might be to say that under more normal circumstances, we'd be evident as your planetary helpers and ministers, without whom it would be considered extremely difficult to live out your full term as a human being.

If I understood Abigrael correctly, all mortal beings, regardless of whatever physical form they may take on due to local planetary conditions, have angels! What a wonderful feeling! What a splendid communality! Yet it occurred to me how few of us even start to really understand how our universe really works. We are almost completely unaware of the presence of angels.

The utter necessity of this understanding that you are surrounded with intelligent life is of paramount importance at this point in the development of your species, for reasons that must be growing more obvious to you by the year.

You are awakening from your nightmare, from your dream of fear. But have no fear. All this is changing. You will behold a reality of such love and joy as you have never been able to conceive possible. This, Dearest One, is the reason why we of the angelic realm are making ourselves known to you. This is why we greet you with such enthusiasm as each one of you individually awakens. This is the true meaning of the New Reality that is arriving for us all. [38]

---

[38] Alma Daniel, et al. *Ask Your Angels. New York: Ballantine Books, pp* 84-89

Letting Go

There is great value in 'letting go' of all attachments in order to achieve and maintain a peaceful state of mind. The teachings of Zen Buddhism point out the value of letting go of all desires. However, it appears to be very difficult to give up all desires unless you are a Buddhist monk in a monastery in the Himalaya Mountains. What is the way out of this dilemma?

The concept of Yin and Yang, which is illustrated by a circle with two halves separated by an S shaped line, represents the law of opposites. Yin represents the female aspect of life with the characteristics of yielding and gentleness while Yang represents the male aspect with the characteristics of strength and aggressiveness. The two aspects are the two sides of the whole. Pairs of opposites are a part of life, such as night and day; black and white; sweet and sour, etc. When we think of the opposites, we think of duality. When we put aside discrimination and think of everything as part of the whole, we can accept the oneness of the universe. The challenge we face is how to maintain a balance between the two opposites in our daily lives. The desire to acquire things comes naturally to us but the letting go of desires requires much effort.

The goal should be: how to satisfy our desires within the limitations of what is beneficial for everyone, and to let go of all desires which are not actually good for us and for others. This requires us to become aware constantly of how our desires can be controlled so as to benefit everyone. This is not an easy thing to do, but we can make use of the philosophy and techniques developed over a great many years by Zen Buddhists. An excellent source of this knowledge is contained in the book *Nothing To Do Nowhere To Go*. The author of the book Thich Nhat Hanh draws upon the teachings of Master Linji, one of the founders of Zen Buddhism. One of the key bits of knowledge found in the book is the emphasis on 'living in the moment.' By focusing our attention on each moment in our daily lives, we not only learn to appreciate each moment, but we also obtain release from stressful thoughts. Since we can only think about one thing at a time, focusing on the moment frees the mind of all other thoughts including the stress of fulfilling all of our desires.

The following excerpts from the book contain many insights into how to let go of desires and the great benefits to be derived from freeing ourselves from most of our desires:

What's important is not the goal we're seeking - even if that goal is our enlightenment - but living each moment in our daily lives truly and fully...Master Linji invented the term 'business-less person', the person who has nothing to do and nowhere to go. This was his example of what an ideal person could be. The ideal person was the bodhavistattva, a compassionate being who, on the path of enlightenment, helped others. [39]

The purpose of Master Linji's work is to help us cease all our seeking and come back to ourselves in the present moment. That's where we can find everything we're looking for whether it's Buddha, perfect understanding, peace, or liberation ....Master Linji would shout: 'Don't come to me seeking something. The enlightenment, happiness, stability and freedom you seek are already inside you.' [40]

Friends, do not go in search of things described in words. It will only make your mind more agitated and your intellect more weary. ...In the past, when I had not yet seen the way of practice clearly, I was still in dark obscurity. I did not dare waste any time in idleness; a quantity of hot blood in me was always pushing me to wander around looking for someone to learn about the Path from. Thanks to the power of understanding that I received later on, I am now able to sit here and talk to you. I advise you not to waste your time over food, clothes, and honors." [41]

Another aspect of letting go has to do with the release of problems which one cannot resolve by oneself. This was already mentioned above but bears repeating since it affects so many people and can help to eliminate burdens which can result in illness due to stress. What I am referring to is the fact that there are sources of help in the spirit realm which are

---

[39] Thich Nhat Hanh. *Nothing to do Nowhere to Go*. Berkley: Parallax Press, 2007, p.10.
[40] Ibid, pp.15-16.
[41] Ibid, p.57.

available to everyone by simply asking for help to solve any kind of problem with complete faith in it being handled and then 'letting go.' The request can be in the form of an earnest plea or prayer with the complete faith that it will be answered. And then it is very important that you 'let go' of the problem completely, making no further efforts to handle it yourself. It is an amazing experience when you discover how well it works. I know from my own experience and that of many other people who have told me how it worked for them. Give it a try; you have nothing to lose.

Perhaps the first thing we should be aware of is the energy of thought. It is in fact, faster than the speed of light. At this level prayer and radionics (the projecting of the energy of number and form for healing) and the sending of healing thoughts in whatever form—color, sound pattern, number— are effective. I never cease to be amazed that it is so and yet it is not really amazing. It is simply in accordance with the laws that operate at that level and are not as yet fully understood by contemporary science.

It is well known, however that energy follows thought. The idea is in the mind, the desire of the heart have their energy which follows on to bring about a manifestation at the physical level of the idea or the desire. Intention is of major importance at this level. So, even if a method of or performance in healing is less than brilliant, the good intention will always be honored and, where necessary, corrections made and inadequacies will be compensated for. There is a divine economy in which we are part of a far greater scenario than we can imagine and where angels, guides, friends and saints support our healing work.

At this level our perceptions also change. Good and evil may impact on our systems as warmth or cold or light and darkness. A friend of mine who has a gift for clearing people and places of bad or evil influences speaks of seeing the darkness turn to light when she has prayed and cleared a room. I have been with her when she has done this and I have not seen this change visually, as she has, but I have sensed the lifting of the oppressiveness and a coming in of a new purity.

Sometimes a spirit or an entity may get into a place or a person's auric field. The spirit may be lost, not able to go to the divine light. And may be living parasitically off the energies of the person to whom it has attached itself, unwilling to go anywhere else. It is important that such a spirit be helped to find the Light of God and its fulfillment there. Those trained in releasement therapy know something of this important aspect of healing. Negative and destructive influences do need to be cleared and a blessing and protection given to the place or person concerned. [42]

In the book, *Power Versus Force: An Anatomy of Consciousness,* Dr. David Hawkins presents an in-depth presentation of the power of being aware of the fact that our consciousness should not be identified with our ego since that limits our ability to be receptive to the unlimited power of the universe. The following excerpt from his book provides an insight into how we can achieve unlimited blessings by becoming aware of whom and what we are:

The mind identifies with its content. It takes blame for what it receives, for it would be humbling to the mind's vanity to admit that the only thing it is doing is experiencing, and, in fact, only experiencing experiencing. The mind does not even experience the world, but only sensory reports of it. Even brilliant thoughts and deepest feelings are only experience; ultimately we have but one function: to experience experience.

Identification solely with the content of consciousness accounts for the experience of self as limited. In contrast, to identify with consciousness itself is to know that one's actual self is unlimited. When such circumscribed selfidentifications have been surmounted, so that the sense of self is identified as consciousness itself, we become 'enlightened.'

One characteristic of the experience of pure consciousness is a perception of timelessness. Consciousness is experienced as beyond all form and time and seen as everywhere equally present. It is described as 'Is-ness' or 'Being-ness' and in the spiritual literature as I-am experience-ness.' Consciousness

---

[42] Ibid, pp.104-105.

does not recognize separation which is a limitation of perception. The enlightened state is a 'Oneness' in which there is no division into parts.

Another attribute of pure consciousness is cessation of the ordinary flow of thoughts or feelings, a condition of infinite power, infinite compassion, infinite gentleness, and infinite love. In this state self becomes Self with a capital 'S.' This awareness of self as Self is the culmination of the process of eliminating limited identification of self.

The steps one should take in order to facilitate the awareness of one's Self as pure consciousness have been well detailed historically. Many techniques and behaviors have been prescribed to facilitate removal of obstacles to expanded awareness; these can be found in the practice of various spiritual disciplines. The one process common to all such teachings is the progressive elimination of the identification of self as finite. [43]

The Power of Now

Richard Alpert changed his name to Ram Dass in the 1970s due to the life-changing experiences he had while in India Ram Dass was inspired to write the contemporary spiritual classic, *Remember Be Here Now*, in which he teaches that everyone is a manifestation of God and that every moment is of infinite significance. The 'Love Serve Remember Foundation' was organized to preserve and continue the teachings of Neem Karoli Baba and Ram Dass, and to work with Ram Dass on his writings and other future plans.

Ram Das has been spreading ancient spiritual teachings since the 70's, focusing on Meditation to still the mind and stay in the Moment by use of chanting a mantra, repeating a phrase over and over, until all other thoughts drift out of the mind and a person is in a heightened state of awareness, calmness and peace in his body. Being at peace and in the Moment with yourself helps you to let go of worries and stresses in your life, bringing you joy, healing, health and happiness.

In his book, *The Divine Feminine,* Rabbi Rami Shapiro points

---

[43] David Hawkins. *Power Versus Force: An Anatomy of Consciousness.* New York: pp. 209-211.

out the importance of applying our inner wisdom to the experiences of each moment as expressed below:

"This is what Wisdom teaches: Life is this moment, and this moment, and this moment. Each moment is both means and end; fulfilling the conditions of the precious moment and setting the conditions for the next moment There is nothing you need to add to the moment. No why, just what.

Wisdom frees you from the obsession with why. Wisdom frees you for the wonder of what. What is the moment at hand; healing, mourning, dancing, tearing mending, and so on. Wisdom simply says that when the moment is for crying - cry! But do not cry when crying time has passed.

Each moment has its own integrity. Living with wisdom means you live in that integrity. It doesn't mean you don't suffer, it means that you don't suffer a moment longer than necessary. It means you don't laugh a moment longer than appropriate. Wisdom reveals the truth of the moment. It is up to you to engage it." [44]

Eckhart Tolle, in his book, *The Power of Now*, points to the importance of accepting the reality that we are not just a physical mind which is primarily concerned with material things but that we also possess a higher consciousness that enables us to experience peace of mind and a happier and healthier existence. By focusing our attention on each moment, 'the now,' we can learn to shift our attention away from the debilitating effects of the ordinary analytical, conscious mind with its attachment to our ego and achieve a higher state of being. The following excerpts from his book provide some of the powerful insights which can lead in the direction of freeing ourselves from the limitations of the ego dominated mind:

End the delusion of time - To be identified with your mind is to be trapped in time: the compulsion to live almost exclusively through memory and anticipation. This creates and endless preoccupation with past and future and an unwillingness to honor and acknowledge the present moment and *allow it to be*. The compulsion arises because the past gives you an identity and the future holds the promise of salvation.

---

[44] Rabbi Shapiro. *The Divine Feminine in Biblical Wisdom Literature.* Vermont: Skylight Paths Publishing, p. 80.

Both are illusions…The more you are focused on time - the past and the future - the more you miss the NOW, the most precious thing there is.

Why is it the most precious thing? Firstly, because it is the only thing. It's all there is. The eternal present is the space within which your whole life unfolds. The one factor that remains constant. Life is now. There was never a time when your life was *not now,* nor will there ever be. Secondly, the now is the only point that can take you beyond the limited confines of the mind. It is your only point of access into the timeless and formless realm of Being.

The reason why some people love to engage in dangerous activities, such as mountain climbing, car racing, and so on, although they may not be aware of it, is that it forces them to into the Now - that intensely alive state that is free of time, free of problems, free of thinking, free of the burden of the personality. Slipping away from the present moment, even for a second, may mean death. But you don't have to engage in those activities in order to be in the state of Now.

What is needed and what we are concerned with is a permanent shift in consciousness. Make it your practice to withdraw your attention from past and future whenever they are not needed. Step out of the time dimension as much as is possible in everyday life. …

The enlightened person's main focus of attention is always the Now, but they are still peripherally aware of time. In other words they continue to use clock time but are free of psychological time. …

You will not have any doubt that psychological time is a mental disease if you look at its manifestations. They occur, for example, in the form of ideologies such as communism, national socialism, or any nationalism, or rigid religious belief systems, which operate under the implicit assumption that the highest good lies in the future and that therefore the end justifies the mean.

In the normal, mind-identified state of consciousness, the power and infinite creative potential that lie concealed in the

Now are completely obscured by psychological time. Your life then loses its vibrancy, its freshness, its sense of wonder. The old patterns of thought, emotion, behavior reaction, and desire are acted out in end-less repeat performances, a script in your mind that gives you an identity of sorts but distorts or covers up the reality of the Now. The mind then creates an obsession with the future to escape from the unsatisfactory present.

All negativity is caused by an accumulation of psychological time and denial of the present. Unease, anxiety, tension, stress, worry - all forms of fear - are caused by too much future and not enough presence. Guilt, regret, resentment, grievances, sadness, bitterness, and all forms of non-forgiveness are caused by too much past, and not enough presence.

As soon as you honor the present moment, all unhappiness and struggle dissolve and life begins to flow with joy and ease. When you act out of present moment awareness, whatever you do becomes imbued with a sense of quality, care, and love—even the most simple action.

So do not be concerned with the fruit of your action—just give attention to the action itself. The fruit will come of its own accord. When the compulsive striving away from the Now ceases, the joy of being flows into everything you do. The moment your attention turns to the Now, you feel a presence, a stillness, peace. You no longer depend on the future for fulfillment and satisfaction. Therefore you are not attached to the results. Neither failure nor success has the power to change your inner state of being.

As far as your life situation is concerned, there may be things to be attained or acquired. That's the world of form, of gain and loss. Yet, on a deeper level you are already complete, and when you realize that, there is a playful, joyous energy behind what you do. Forms are born and die, yet you are aware of the eternal underneath the forms. You know that 'nothing real can be threatened.' When this is your state of Being, how can you not succeed? You have succeeded already. [45]

---

[45] Eckhart Tolle. *The Power of Now.* Novato, CA: New World Library, 48-70.

Awareness of the fact that we do possess a consciousness which is not just physical but also spiritual has a powerful influence on achieving peace of mind as described in the URANTIA BOOK:

"The fact of self-conscious existence, associated with the reality of spiritual experience constitutes man a potential son of the universe. A human mind, built up solely out of the consciousness of physical sensations, could never attain spiritual levels; this kind of material mind would be utterly lacking in a sense of moral values and would be without a guiding sense of spiritual dominance which is so essential to achieving harmonious personality unity. The supremely happy and unified mind is the one wholly dedicated to the doing of the will of the Father in heaven. Unresolved conflicts destroy unity and may result in mind disruption. Peace of mind can be achieved in the overcoming of evil with the potent force of good." [46]

There are a number of excellent methods to achieve peace of mind, strength, and freedom from illness by changing our thought patterns. From the Bhavagad Gita and from many other sources we learn that the mind is conditioned to harbor negative thoughts about ourselves due to our early childhood experiences. Parents, usually with the best of intentions, say or do things which plant negative thoughts in our mind. Other children frequently poke fun at one another calling attention to each other's apparent weaknesses, adding to the feelings of fear or guilt about ourselves. These unpleasant thoughts, which persist as a constant reminder that something is wrong with ourselves, because of the way we look or act can cause us to feel inferior and can manifest in physical pains and serious illnesses.

We come to believe that this is an unchangeable condition which we just have to accept as an unpleasant part of our life. We think that this poor image of ourselves is what we really are; not realizing that it is merely an illusion based on a false perception of who we really are. In most cases of very painful past memories, the original incident causing the painful memory is filed in a part of the mind called the subconscious or reactive

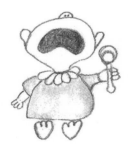

---

[46] URANTIA, channeled. Chicago: Urantia Foundation, 1955, p. 1298.

mind. Some people turn to psychologists or psychiatrists for help which is usually given in the form of medication. This situation will continue on and on as a source of mental disturbance and physical weakness until we become aware that this condition needs to be faced and corrected by our own efforts.

If you want to try doing what you can on your own, you can make use of the following steps which have been found to be very helpful. First identify which thought really bothers you the most; the one that intrudes on your feelings and makes you feel bad. Then take the following actions: First, order the disturbing thought to go away. Do it with authority. After all, it is your mind and you have the right to make choices as to what you want to think about. Repeat this as often as you feel the need. Keep in mind that you are perfect in the eyes of the Creator. You have a higher mind which is linked to the Divine and can bring about anything you focus on with faith that it can be done.

Next, 'replace' the negative thought with positive thoughts. Think of something or someplace where you have had very pleasant memories. **Change the channel!** This powerful statement was made by my 10 year old granddaughter, Lysandra, during a conversation about her experience the night before at a movie theater. The movie had a scene in it which showed a person dying. At breakfast, the following morning, I asked Lysandra how she liked the movie. She replied that she had a nightmare which kept her awake thinking about the dying person in the movie. She felt sad and unhappy and couldn't fall back to sleep until she decided to think about something pleasant in order to get her mind off of the unpleasant thoughts. She then said, "I changed the channel to a happy memory and shortly after that, I fell soundly asleep."

Affirmations

You can also think or say out loud a phrase, affirmation or mantra which is uplifting and makes you feel good. By doing this, as often as you feel the need, you will gradually get rid of the thoughts which disturb you. Use affirmations from any source available to you. Affirmations which I use on a regular basis follow below:

- There is nothing to fear but fear itself.
- I am not my body, I am free. I'm still just as God created me.
- Every day in every way I'm getting better and better.

Gary Null, one of the founders of the health food movement in the 1970's, recognizes the importance of using affirmations in order to maintain a peaceful state of mind thus reducing stress. He provides an excellent list of affirmations in his most recent book, Power *Aging*. A few of his recommended affirmations are quoted below:

- I easily release negativity from my life.
- I expect the best from life.
- I live with integrity.
- I am a person who always chooses to see the good in others, as I know we are all individuals on our own spiritual journey.
- Every night I give thanks for everything I now have and for all the blessings I am receiving.
- I visualize success! If I can see it, I can achieve It.
- I am willing to release all my resistance to change.
- I vow to eliminate all toxic circumstances from my life.
- I value my body and commit to only nourishing it with healthy nourishing foods.
- I look at each crisis in my life as an opportunity for growth and learning.

Gary Null has the following suggestions on how to resolve pain and resentment: "Don't make excuses for the person who hurt you. Don't use shame, guilt or revenge. Just forgive them. Forgive—and gain. Once again, when you for-give, an equal and opposite energy will come your way. This is just a rule in life that must be accepted and observed. So when you give, you will receive. You have no control over when and what you will receive but rest assured there is the ecology of Karma. [47]

Sandra Agazzi devotes most of her book, *The Real Me,* to the use of 'Positive Affirmations for Empowering your Life.' She offers excellent suggestions on how to handle stressful situations in your life as described below:

Our most challenging moments in life usually create our best lessons for our spiritual growth. Truly experiencing your present emotions without judging yourself or others allows you to flow with life and whatever is here. After feeling your emotions and allowing them to pass through you, it becomes easier to affirm new loving beliefs about yourself and others. By creating some new beliefs and repeating them as positive affirmations (aloud in front of a mirror or silently), you may become empowered with their real meaning.

Believing loving messages about your real self helps you consciously choose to stop the negative self-talk and 'stories.' This allows you to embrace your true potential, experiencing real freedom and openness to life. Through kinder beliefs and positive self-talk about your true self, you may create a more accepting and loving life for yourself that extends to others, uniting everyone.

I encourage you to awaken to the infinite love that is already present in each of us and in each moment to create a more peaceful, fulfilled, and happy life - the kind of life you truly deserve to give yourself. May your positive thoughts create inner peace and renewed health as you say to yourself:

*'I now choose to awaken to God's always present Divine love that is in me and in all of God's creations. I now choose to always honor the **real** me.'*

Do something positive for yourself. Enjoy life and have fun. As you are kind to yourself, you are able to be kind to others. Share your thoughts and concerns from a place of love –not fear. Realize that you are responsible for your life. You have the power within you to create happiness and joy. The more you surround yourself with moments that uplift you, the

---

[47] Gary Null, PhD. *Power Aging.* New York: New American Library, 2003, pp. 326-328.

more energy and peace you may feel. When you feel happy and peaceful, you are better able to fulfill your life purpose. By re-leasing painful thoughts and returning to your loving presence, you are able to release strife and enjoy life.

Everything is made up of energy, including your thoughts and beliefs. Your life matches how you are thinking. Whatever you believe inside will show up in your world in some way. So as you change your thoughts, you change what you see in your life.

Since your thoughts form your views about life, it is important to know your current beliefs. Writing your beliefs about life helps you to see how you are thinking. By looking at your self-talk, you can decide which beliefs are healthy and which ones are not.

Wherever you are, you are abundantly blessed. Whatever you focus on, you receive as a blessing. When you share your gifts and talents to help others, you create more blessings for everyone, including yourself. May you manifest and enjoy happiness, health, freedom, and wealth in its many wonderful forms. The following affirmations help welcome wealth to you:

- I am WEALTHY and I am a kind and caring person.
- I am WEALTHY and I give to others and myself.
- I am WEALTHY and I am a loving person.

{ Sandra offers the following affirmations for your health: }

- I enjoy life by doing less and being more.
- I am happy, healthy, and at peace.
- It is healthy to laugh and to cry.
- I am surrounded by positive thoughts, and people. [48]

A Course in Miracles

A revealed source of wisdom that contains deep insights into how to achieve a life of peace and happiness is a collection of three books known as *A COURSE IN MIRACLES*. They consist of a

---

[48] Sandra A, Chimenti. *The Real Me: Awakening Your True Self.* Rochester Hills, MI: Creative Books, 2007.

Workbook, a Textbook and an Instruction Book for Teachers of the Course.

The Workbook contains 365 lessons, one for each day of the year. Each lesson is based on one thought for the day which is to be repeated in your mind a number of times each day. The thoughts are simple statements or **affirmations** which, when used as instructed, have a profound effect on your state of mind. The results are phenomenal bringing about such things as: complete release of tensions; freedom from fears; awareness of what is real and what is an illusion, a deep understanding that we are all children of one God who loves us all equally regardless of our race color or beliefs.

The purpose of the workbook is to train your/the mind in a systematic way to have a different perception of everyone and everything in the world...The overall aim of the exercises is to increase your ability to extend the ideas you will be practicing to include everything. This will require no effort on your part. The exercises themselves meet the conditions necessary for this kind of transfer. The following excerpts from the Workbook give you some insights into what the Course can do for you:

LESSON 5: 'I am never upset for the reason I think'

This idea can be used with any person, situation or event that you can think is causing you pain....Search your mind to identify a number of different forms of upset that are disturbing you. Apply the idea for today to each of them. Examples are:

'I am not worried about.....................for the reason I think.'
'I am not depressed about.................for the reason I think'

Three or four times during the day are enough.

LESSON 8: 'My mind is preoccupied with past thoughts'

This idea is the reason why you only see the past. No one really sees anything. He sees only his thoughts projected outward. The mind's preoccupation with the past is the cause of the misperception about time from which your seeing suffers. Your mind cannot grasp the present, which is the only time there is.

The only wholly true thought one can hold about the past is that it is not here. To think about it at all is therefore to think about illusions.

The purpose of the exercises for today is to begin to train your mind to recognize when it is not really thinking at all.

The exercises for today should be done with eyes closed. This is because you actually cannot see anything, and it is easier to recognize that you are actually not seeing anything. Introduce the practice period by saying:

'I seem to be thinking about------------------.'

Name each of your thoughts specifically, concluding with:

'But my mind is preoccupied with past thoughts'

LESSON 76: 'I am under no laws but God's.'

Think of the freedom in the recognition that you are not bound by all the strange and twisted laws that you have set up to save you. You really think you would starve unless you have stacks of green paper strips and piles of metal disks. You really think a small round pellet or some liquid pushed into your veins through a sharpened needle will ward off disease and death. You really think you are alone unless another body is with you.

It is insanity that thinks these things. You call them laws, and put them under different names in a long catalogue of rituals that have no use and no purpose. You think you must obey the 'laws' of medicine, of economics and of health. Protect the body, and you will be saved.

These are not laws, but madness. The body is endangered by the mind that hurts itself. The body suffers just in order that the mind will fail to see it is the victim of itself. The body's suffering is a mask the mind holds up to hide what really suffers.

It would not understand it is its own enemy; that it attacks itself and wants to die.

It is from this your 'laws' would save the body. It is for this you think you are a body.

There are no laws but the laws of God. This needs repeating over and over, until you realize it applies to everything that you have made in opposition to God's will.

Your magic has no meaning. What it is meant to save does not exist. Only what it is meant to hide will save you.

The laws of God will never be replaced....There are no laws but God's. Dismiss all foolish magical beliefs today, and hold your mind in silent readiness to hear the Voice that speaks the truth to you. You will be listening to One Who says there is no loss under the laws of God. Payment is neither given nor received. Exchange cannot be made; there are no substitutes; and nothing is replaced by something else. God's laws forever give and never take. ...We will repeat today's idea until we have listened and understood there are no laws but God's. Then we will tell ourselves, as a dedication with which the practice period concludes:

'I am under no laws but God's'

We will repeat this dedication as often as possible today; at least four or five times an hour. It is our statement of freedom from all danger and tyranny. It is our acknowledgement that God is our Father, and that His Son is saved.

LESSON 77: 'I am entitled to miracles'

You are entitled to miracles because of what you are. You will receive miracles because of what God is. And you will offer miracles because you are one with God. Again, how simple is salvation! It is merely a statement of your true identity.

Your claim to miracles does not lie in your illusions about yourself. It does not rely on any magical powers you have ascribed to yourself, nor any of the rituals you have devised. It is inherent in the truth of what you are. It is implicit in what God your Father is. It was ensured in your creation, and guaranteed by the laws of God.

...Begin the practice periods by telling yourself quite confidently that you are entitled to miracles. Closing your eyes, remind yourself that you are asking only for what is rightfully yours.

After this brief introductory phase, wait quietly with the assurance that your request is granted. ..You will receive the assurance that you seek. Tell yourself often today:

'I am entitled to miracles'

Ask for them whenever a situation arises in which they are called for. You will recognize these situations. And since you are not relying on yourself to find the miracle, you are fully entitled to receive whenever you ask.

LESSON 107: 'Truth will correct all errors in my mind'

What can correct illusions but the truth? And what are errors but illusions that remain unrecognized for what they are? Where truth has entered errors disappear. They are gone because, without belief, they have no life.

Can you imagine what a state of mind without illusions is? How it would feel?

Try to remember when there was a time –perhaps a minute, maybe even less - when nothing came to interrupt your peace; when you were certain you were loved and safe. Then picture what it would be like to have that moment be extended to the end of time and to eternity. Then let the sense of quiet that you felt be multiplied a hundred times, and then be multiplied another hundred times more.

And now you have a hint, not just more than the faintest intimation of the state your mind will rest in when the truth has come. Without illusions there can be no fear, no doubt and no attack.

"Truth will correct all errors in my mind" [49]

---

[49] *A Course in Miracles, channeled.* New York: Foundation for Inner Peace, 1975.

'I' AM Discourses

Another channeled source of revealed wisdom is a series of books titled *The 'I' AM Discourses.* By applying the insights gained from reading the 'Discourses,' it is possible to achieve an inner calm and peace of mind that sustains us during the ups and downs of life marked by a state of well-being and joy of life. Certain statements can be used as affirmations to be used over and over again to guide our minds to accept the benefits of accepting the reality of the statements. The following excerpts from the book can open the mind to an understanding of the immense benefits that can be obtained by those who are receptive to receive the divine blessings that are there for the sincere seeker:

> The condition of the outer world at the present time is such that those who sincerely seek the Light and want the constructive way of Life *must have more **than** human help* if they are to survive over the present period of chaos—which is the accumulated discord generated by humanity en masse through the centuries, and which is pressing heavily upon the outer experience of individuals today.

> The need of protection and help for the children of earth is so great at the present hour that the Great Ascended Masters and Legion of Light have 'Let the bars down,' so to speak, and have released this Inner Understanding of the 'Mighty I AM Presence' into the outer life of mankind, that all who want the Light and will make conscious effort to attain their own Freedom and Mastery may have the Assistance which will give them the help they need. In this day, no sincere, reasoning mind, once turned its attention and keeping it firmly fixed on the 'I AM Presence,' can argue, doubt, or question the Omnipotence of that 'I AM Presence.'

> The constant use of your 'I AM Presence' does impel you forward in spite of any activity of the outer self. So long as this single Idea is held firmly, storms, distress and disturbance may rage about you, but in the Consciousness of the 'I AM Presence,' you can and are able to stand serene, unmoved by the seething vortex of human creation which may or may not be about you.....It is only when the outer becomes sufficiently obedient, giving all power to the Great Inner Presence, that one

finds peace and rest in this Mighty Acknowledgement.

In that peace and rest flows a Mighty River of Energy, like a mountain stream flowing through a fertile valley, lined with flowers and perfect vegetation.

So in the Peace that passeth understanding do you move more and more, finding that Eternal River of Energy flowing into and through your Being, spreading its blessing and opulence into your Life and experience everywhere you go.

When you say and feel 'I AM" you release the spring of Eternal, Everlasting Life to flow on Its way unmolested. In other words, you open wide the door to Its natural flow. When you say 'I AM not,' you shut the door in the face of this Mighty Energy. 'I AM' is the Full Authority of God.

The student, endeavoring to understand and apply these mighty, yet simple Laws, must stand guard more strictly over his thought and expression—in word or otherwise; for every time you say 'I AM not,' 'I have not,' 'I cannot,' you are, whether knowingly or unknowingly, throttling that 'Great Presence within you.

Everyone who manifests in the physical form today has made plenty of mistakes, so let no one take the attitude, 'I AM more holy than thou,' but each one's first attitude should be to call on the Law of Forgiveness; and if he be feeling or sending criticism, condemnation, or hate to another of God's children, he can never have enlightenment or success until he calls on the Law of Forgiveness.. Further than this, he must say to that person to whom he was feeling disturbed in any way—silently: I send to You the fullness of the Divine Love of my Being to bless and prosper you.' This attitude is the only release and Freedom from the seeming failures of the outer activity.

For individuals to continually revolve in their minds and discussion critical thoughts will surely in the end destroy themselves—if they do not face about, and through calling on the Law of Forgiveness find complete conscious release from the entire situation.

When critical or disturbing thoughts try to find entrance into your consciousness, slam the door quickly and command them to be gone forever. Do not give them a chance, nor time to gain a foothold, remembering always that you have the Strength and the sustaining

Power of the 'Mighty I AM Presence' to do this. Should you have difficulty in holding the door shut, talk to your 'I AM Presence' and say here! I need help! See that the door is closed, and kept closed forever.'

I want you to get fixed in your consciousness that you can talk to your 'I AM Presence' the same as you could talk to Me, believing that I had limitless Power, because I tell you, it is no idle comment when I say *you can cause this Mighty Presence to handle every condition in your entire experience and raise you into its Freedom and Dominion of all things.*[50]

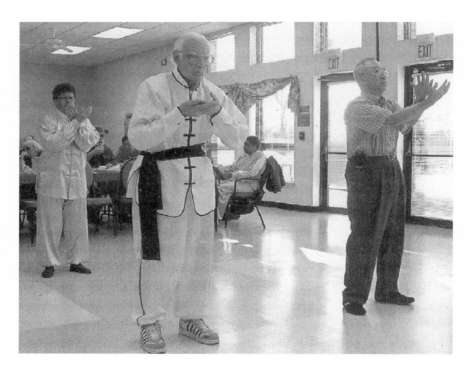

Dr. Singer teaching Tai Chi at the Piscataway Senior Center

---

[50] *The "I AM" Discourses.*

Water Crystals and Thoughts

In his book, *The Hidden Messages in Water,* Masaru Emoto tells us how he discovered that crystals formed in frozen water reveal changes when specific, concentrated thoughts are directed towards them. He found that water from unpolluted sources such as pure spring water formed beautiful and complex snowflake patterns. He also found that pure water exposed to loving words, either spoken or written, would form brilliant, complex and colorful patterns. In contrast, polluted water, or water exposed to negative thoughts would form incomplete, asymmetrical patterns with dull colors.

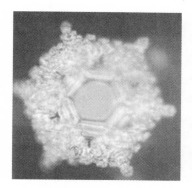 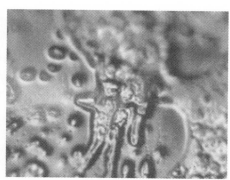

Love / Appreciation   *"You make me sick, I hate you"*

The influence of thoughts is demonstrated by photographs of water crystals (see images above and below) taken by Dr. Emoto showing the beautiful colors and designs that each water crystal formed depending on the source of the water and the thoughts that surrounded the water at the time the photographs were taken.

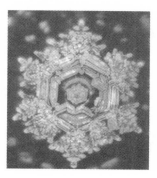 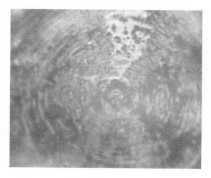

Prayer   *Heavy Metal Music.*

The implications of this knowledge point to the importance of how our thoughts and words affect not only water but everyone and everything around us. We should be aware of just how important it is to maintain a pure water supply and how our thoughts impact the earth and our personal health.

Dr. Emoto conducted studies of water crystals in different parts of the world. In order to produce samples of frozen water in different locations he needed a battery-operated freezer with a very low range of temperatures which he then proceeded to invent and manufacture. He found that there were universal laws at work that produced the same results regardless of different climates, cultures or languages. The following quotations from his book illustrate the deep insights that were produced by his studies:

Water is the mirror of the soul. It has many faces, formed by aligning itself with the consciousness of human beings that gives water its ability to reflect what is in people's souls? In order to answer that question, I would like to make sure that you understand this fact: Existence is vibration. The entire universe is in a state of vibration, and each thing generates its own frequency, which is unique. All that I have to say in this book is based on this one fact. My years of research into water have taught me that this is the one fundamental principle of the universe.... The science of quantum mechanics generally acknowledges that substance is nothing more than vibration. When we separate something into its smallest parts, we always enter a strange world where all that exists is particles and waves.

Human beings are also vibrating, and each individual vibrates at a unique frequency. Each one of us has the sensory skills to feel the vibrations of others.

All things vibrate, and they vibrate at their own frequencies. When you understand this, you will significantly broaden your understanding of the universe.

But how can we interpret the phenomena of crystal formation being affected by words written on paper and shown to water? The written words themselves actually emit a unique vibration that the water is capable of sensing. Water faithfully mirrors all the vibrations created in the world, and changes these vibrations into a form that can be seen with the human eye.

Water exposed to the words 'Thank you' formed beautiful geometric crystals, no matter what the language. But water exposed to 'You fool' and other degrading words resulted in obviously broken and deformed crystals.

We can surmise that when a complete geometric crystal is formed, water is in alignment with nature and the phenomenon we call life. The crystals do not form in water that has been polluted by the results of our failure to remember the laws of nature. When we tried taking photographs of crystals from Tokyo's tap water, the results were pitiful. This is because the water is sanitized with chlorine, thus damaging the innate ability of water to form crystals.

The words *gratitude* and *love* form the fundamental principles of the laws of nature and the phenomenon of life. Therefore, water in its natural form is required to create the hexagonal form. By contrast words such as 'You fool' do not exist in nature and are instead unnatural elements created by people. Words that revile harm, and ridicule are the result of the culture created by humans.

Humans are the only creatures that have the capacity to resonate with all other creatures and objects in nature. We can speak with all that exists in the universe. We can give out energy and also receive energy in return. However, this ability is a two-edged sword. When people act out only on their own greed, they emit an energy that serves to destroy the harmony within nature.

The defiling of our earth is the result of an unrelenting hunger for convenience and the fulfillment of greed, initiated by the industrial revolution. This has led to lifestyles of mass consumption that seriously threaten the global environment.

We have embarked on a new century, a time in history when we must make serious changes in the way that we think. Only the human can resonate with the rest of the world, and this is why it is so essential that we change our thinking, so we can live in harmony with nature and not go on destroying the earth. What vibration we give to the earth and what kind of planet we create depends on each one of us as individuals.

If you fill your heart with love and gratitude, you will find yourself surrounded by so much that you can love and that you can feel grateful for, and you can even get closer to enjoying the life of health and happiness that you seek…The life you can live and the world you live in are up to you.

There is an increase in interest in holistic medicine—not only treating the symptoms of the illness, but overseeing the patient's lifestyle and psychological wellbeing …The days of believing only that which can be seen with the naked eye have passed, and we are now starting to open our eyes to the importance of the soul.

The human body is essentially water, and consciousness is the soul. Methods that help water to flow smoothly are superior to all other medical methods available to us. Can you imagine what it would be like to have water capable of forming beautiful crystals flowing throughout your entire body? It can happen if you let it.

Among all medicines, there are none with the healing powers of love. Since I came to this realization, I have continued to tell people that *immunity* is love. What could be more effective at overcoming negative powers and returning vitality to the body? Emoto goes on to add another dimension to the power of love. He points out the importance of including gratitude along with love.

I have mentioned that water shown the words *love* and *gratitude* forms the most beautiful crystals. Of course the word *love* alone has the ability to create wonderful crystals, but *love* and *gratitude* combine to give the crystals a unique depth and refinement, a diamond-like brilliance.

I suggest that having twice the amount of gratitude as love is the balance we should strive for. At a seminar, after I had mentioned this in my presentation, two young women came up to me and said 'We were very impressed. Weren't you saying that people have one mouth for speaking and two ears for listening?' Of course the grandeur of love cannot be denied, and most people do have a general understanding of the power of love. However, we have been raised in a culture where all of our focus is placed on the energy of love, while the other side of the formula receives little attention. The focus of the human race has been drawn away from that which cannot be seen, and towards the obvious physical world. And in order to make so much of the physical world our own as soon as possible, we have cut down forests and fought back deserts in an effort to insure the supreme domination of our culture.

Such advancements by human society may indeed be the result of love - for our families and our countries - but as long as we continue to live our lives based on this strategy, there will be no end of conflict. The history of the twentieth century was the history of fighting and warfare.

Perhaps we are finally beginning to see that the direction we are moving in leads nowhere. We have sacrificed too much in order to secure the riches of life. Forests have been destroyed and clean water lost, and we have cut up and sold the earth itself.

What the world needs now is gratitude. We must begin by learning what it means to have enough. We need to feel gratitude for having been born on a planet so rich in nature, and gratitude for the water that makes our life possible. Do we really know how wonderful it is to be able to breathe a big breath of clean air?

If you open your eyes, you will see that the world is full of so much that deserves your gratitude. When you have become the embodiment of gratitude, think about how pure the water that fills your body will be. When that happens, you yourself will be a beautiful shining crystal of light.

It's often said that if something happens twice it will happen again. According to this theory, when the same thing repeats itself, a *morphic field* is formed and resonance with this morphic field increases the likelihood that the event will happen. When I first attempted to take photographs of crystals, I had no success at all for the first two months, but once I was able to capture the first photograph, other researchers also started to succeed. Perhaps this is also a result of morphic resonance. Everything in the world is linked. Whatever you are doing right now is being done by someone else at the same time. So what type of morphic field should we be interested in creating? Are we creating fields of pain and viciousness, or are we creating a world filled with love and gratitude?

Whenever you sit in front of water and send out messages of love and gratitude, somewhere in the world, someone is being filled with love and gratitude. You don't need to go anywhere. The water right in front of you is linked to all the water in the world. The water you're looking at will resonate with water everywhere, and your message of love will reach the souls of all the people in the world. [51]

The Power of Attraction

As mentioned in the Introduction of this book, the concept that we can create our own reality is clearly presented in the book *The Secret* The basic premise of this concept is that we can bring about anything that we desire by making use of the three essential things that must be done in order for the law to work. The three essentials are: Desire, Belief and Acceptance. These essentials appear simple enough and are, in fact, simple when you know how to apply them properly. Desire is the first step in the process. We all have many desires for things that we wish would happen or come to us such as a new car or house or freedom from cares or better health, etc., etc. It is very important to focus on just one thing at a time. This requires that

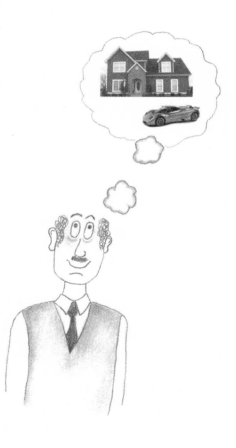

[51] Masaru Emoto. *Hidden Messages in Water.* Pp. 39-80.

we put aside all other needs or desires while we focus on the one thing that we want to happen. Picture this thing as clearly as possible. Look at pictures or go where you can actually see the thing that you wish for. Close your eyes and visualize exactly how the desire looks in great detail. Keep this up until you get what you desire. Be careful to avoid focusing on anything negative such as illness or anger at someone or something. The Law works to bring about what we focus our attention on so if we are constantly thinking about an illness it will prolong the illness and make it worse. It would be better to focus on how you would look and feel when you are free of an illness. Dwell on the desired result not on any perceived weakness or inability to overcome obstacles to your desire. There are many examples of miraculous healings taking place which leads us to the second step in the Law of Attraction, the need to believe that your desire can and will be achieved.

Belief involves complete trust or faith that what you desire can take place and will happen. It may happen quickly or after some time has passed. Do not allow any doubts to take place in your mind. If you think that your desire is too difficult or impossible to happen then it will certainly not happen. The most powerful thing you can do is to let go of any thoughts about how your desire can be achieved. It may occur in a way that you could not possibly think of or expect to take place. The best way I can think of to express this idea is to *LET GO AND LET GOD*. If you don't believe in God then express the idea in your own words. The main thing is to let go in complete confidence that your desire will happen because you know that the source of all Life has the power to bring about whatever you desire. This idea is expressed as a fact in *The Course in Miracles*. "There is no order of difficulty in miracles." In other words, you can be cured of cancer just as easily as a common cold when you ask for help in complete faith that it will happen.

The third essential in the Law of Attraction is the acceptance or receptivity on your part in order to receive your desire. It may seem impossible that anyone would refuse to accept their desire or place any blocks on their desire when it is about to take place. This can and does happen when doubts are allowed to enter your mind or when you are so preoccupied with negative thoughts such as guilt that you think you are not worthy of receiving the desire you wished for. Because of beliefs in being sinful or unworthy due to early conditioning as a child this can block your desire from taking place. It is also possible that you may become so immersed in your daily activities that your mind cannot accept anything that appears to be unusual or of a spiritual nature. You might simply take the attitude that this thing that is happening cannot possibly be true. Rhonda Byrne, author of *The Secret,* lists the following concepts and tips on how to make use of the Law of Attraction:

The Great Secret of Life is the law of attraction.

The law of attraction says like attracts like, so when you think a thought you are also attracting Like thoughts to you.

You are like a human transmission tower, transmitting a frequency with your thoughts. If you want to change anything in your life, change the frequency by changing your thoughts.

Your current thoughts are creating your future life.

What you think about the most or focus on the most will appear as your life. Your thoughts become things. [52]

You get to fill the blackboard of your life with whatever you want.

The more you use the power within you, the more power you will draw through you.

Do what you love. If you don't know what brings you joy, ask, "What is my joy?" As you commit to your joy, you will attract an avalanche of joyful things because you are radiating joy.

Now that you have learned the knowledge of the Secret, what you do with it is up to you. Whatever you choose is right. The power is all yours. [53]

The Universe offers *all* things to all people through the law of attraction. You have the ability to choose what you want to experience. Do you want there to be enough for you and for everyone? Then choose that and know, 'There is abundance of all things. There is an unlimited supply. There is so much magnificence.' Each of us has the ability to tap into that unlimited invisible supply through our thoughts and feelings, and bring it into our experience. So choose for You, because you're the only one who can.

Everything that you want - all the joy, love, bliss, abundance, prosperity, - it's there, ready for you to grab a hold of it. And

---

[52] Rhonda Byrne. *The Secret.* New York: Atria Books, 2006, p. 25.
[53] Ibid, p. 184.

you've got to get hungry for it. You've got to be intentional. And when you become intentional and on fire for what you want, the Universe will deliver every single thing that you've been wanting. Recognize the beautiful and wonderful things around you and bless and praise them. And on the other side, the things that aren't working the way you want them to work, don't spend your energy faulting or complaining. Embrace everything that you want so that you can get more of it. [54]

As you become aware of the power of *The Secret*, and begin to use it, all of your questions will be answered. As you begin to have a deeper understanding of the law of attraction, you can start to make asking questions a habit, and as you do, you will receive the answer to each one. If you are seeking an answer or guidance on something in your life, ask the question, believe you will receive, and then accept the answer when it comes.

The truth is that the Universe has been answering you all of your life, but you cannot receive the answers unless you are aware. Be aware of everything around you, because you are receiving the answers to your questions in every moment of the day. The channels these answers can come through are **unlimited.** A lot of people feel like they're victims in life and they'll often point to past events, perhaps growing up with an abusive parent or in a dysfunctional family. Most psychologists believe that about 85 percent of families are dysfunctional, so all of a sudden you're not so unique.

If you go over your past life and focus on the difficulties, you are just bringing more difficult circumstances to you now. Let it go no matter what it is. Do it for you. If you hold a grudge or blame someone for something in the past, you are only harming yourself. You are the only one who can create the life you deserve. As you deliberately focus on what you want, as you begin to radiate good feelings, the law of attraction will respond. All that you have to do is make a start, and as you do, you will unleash the magic.[55]

Think thoughts of perfection. Illness cannot exist in a body

---

[54] Ibid, pp. 150-151.
[55] Ibid, pp. 165-166.

that has harmonious thoughts.

You can see that beliefs about aging are all in our minds. Science explains that we have a brand new body in a very short time. Your body is casting off millions of cells every second and it's also creating millions of new cells at the same time.

Aging is limited thinking, so release those thoughts from your consciousness and know that your body is only months old no matter how many birthdays you have chalked up in your mind.

Unfortunately, Western society has become fixated on age, and in reality there is no such thing.

You can 'think' your way to the perfect state of health, the perfect body, the perfect weight, and eternal youth. You can bring it into being by your consistent thinking of perfection. [56]

The Power of Intention

Dr. Wayne Dyer wrote a book titled *The Power of Intention* in which he presents substantial evidence to support his theory that the chief obstacle to achieving our goals in life is being unaware of our inner intentions which frequently conflicts with what we think we want. He makes a number of powerful statements about the reality of the spiritual aspects of life and how we can access this universal power. He states: "The power of intention is to have in mind a purpose or plan, to direct the mind to aim. With intention we draw upon all the forces of the universe to manifest even the most impossible as possible. You have innate power to attract to yourself anything you want to manifest in your life." Dr. Dyer offers practical steps to help bring into reality our goals as follows:

Get clear about something and write it down.

Share your intention with someone in a way that will support and hold you accountable to taking action.

Do something today to demonstrate your commitment to your intention.

Acknowledge that you did what you said you would and then take the next step.

Dr. Dyer also describes Seven Laws of the Power of Intention,

---

[56] Ibid, pp. 130-131.

as follows:

1. Law of Creativity-recognize the face of creativity. You can create something from nothing using the power of your mind.

2. Law of reciprocity-any great purpose that can bring energy and thought into physical form must come out of kindness, with an intention to do good.

3. Law of Love-think of this power of intention as the face of kindness filled with the emotion of love.

4. Law of Beauty-is the truth, honesty and a knowing that what 'is' is exactly as it should be. Reframe any negative attitude you may have towards others and replace them with an 'I' appreciate you (a thankfulness) attitude towards them.

5. Law of Expansion-this is the power of spirit to help you expand your awareness of what is possible. Whatever you think about expands. Listen to your inner spirit guidance.

6. Law of Abundance-the face of unlimited abundance. Believe in unlimited abundance and you can have it.

7. Law of Receptivity-the flow of abundance is open to everyone without any judgment. Believe in yourself and be receptive to unlimited possibilities. Focus on your positive intentions towards others and yourself to tap into this energy. [57]

In the book, *Secret of the Millionaire Mind,* Eker has this to say about the power of intentions:

One of the principles we teach in our course is the power of intention. If you are saving money for a *rainy* day, what are you going to get? Rainy days! Stop doing that. Instead of saving for a rainy day, focus on saving for a *joyous* day or for the day you win your financial freedom. Then by virtue of the law of intention, that's exactly what you will get.

Many people who come from poor families become angry and rebellious about it. Often they go out get rich about it or at least have the motivation to do so. But there's some little hiccup, which is actually a big burp. Whether such people get rich or work their buns off trying to become successful, they are not usually happy. Why? Because the root of their wealth or motivation for money is anger and resentment. Consequently, money

---

[57] Dr. Wayne Dyer. *The Power of Intention.* New York:

and anger become linked in their minds, and the more money such individuals have or strive for the angrier they get.

Eventually, the higher self says, 'I'm tired of being angered and stressed out. I just want to be peaceful and happy.' So they ask the same mind that created the link what to do about this situation. To which their mind answers, 'If you want to get rid of your anger you're going to have to get rid of your money' So they do. They subconsciously get rid of their money.

They overspend or make a poor investment decision or get a financially disastrous divorce, or they sabotage heir success in some other way. But no matter, because these folks are now happy. Right? Wrong! Things are even worse because now they're not just angry, they're broke and angry. They got rid of the wrong thing!

They got rid of the money instead of the anger, the fruit instead of the root. Meanwhile, the real issue is, and always was the anger between them and their parents. And until that anger is resolved, they will never be truly happy or peaceful regardless of how much money they have or don't have.

The reason or motivation you have for making money or creating success is vital. If your motivation for acquiring money or success comes from a non-supportive root such as fear, anger, or the need to 'prove' yourself, your money will never bring you happiness.

Why? Because you can't solve any of these issues with money. Take fear, for instance. Most people believe security is their chief concern. But, get this - security and fear are both motivated by the *same* thing. Seeking security comes from insecurity, which is based on fear.

So will more money dissolve the fear? You wish! But the answer is absolutely not. Why? Because money is not the root of the problem, fear is. What's even worse is that fear is not just a problem, it's a habit. Therefore making more money will only change the kind of fear we have. Once we make it, however, our fear usually changes to 'What if I lose what I've made? Or 'Everyone's going to want what I have' or 'I'm going to get creamed in taxes.' In short, until we get to the root of this issue and dissolve the fear, no amount of money will help.

As with those of us driven by fear, many people are motivated to achieve financial success to prove they are 'good enough.' Money can't make you something you already are. Again, as with fear, the 'always having to prove yourself' issue becomes your habitual way of living. You don't even realize it's running you. You call yourself a high achiever, a hard driver, determined, and all these traits are fine. The only question is why? What is the root engine that drives all this?

For people who are driven to prove they are good enough, no amount of money can ease the pain of that inner wound that makes everyone and everything in their life 'not enough.' No amount of money or anything else, for that matter, will ever be enough for people who feel that are not good enough themselves.

Again, it's all about you. Remember, your inner world reflects your outer world. If you believe you are not enough, you will validate that belief and create the reality that you don't have enough. On the other hand, if you believe you are plenty, you will validate that belief and create plenty of abundance. Why? Because 'plenty will be you root,' which will then become your natural way of being.

By unlinking your money motivation from anger, fear, and the need to prove yourself, you can install new links for earning your money through *purpose, contribution, and joy*. That way, you never will have to get rid of your money to be happy. [58]

A very important aspect of attitude is being lighthearted. Most centenarians (people who live to 100 or beyond) exhibit a joy of life and a sense of humor. Dr. Brownstein's study of centenarians revealed the following:

"Most centenarians I have met, although they are unique individuals, share a common bond in how they lived their lives. Most have eaten moderately, kept active, enjoyed good sleep, rested when necessary, stayed involved with family and friends, and generally enjoyed life. Although many of them had to endure extreme hardships over the course of their long lives, including the loss of their closest loved ones and fami-

---

[58] T. Harry Eker. *Secrets of the Millionaire Mind.* New York, Harper-Collins, 2005, pp.29-33.

ly members; still. Most of these people have exhibited what I would call a "lighthearted attitude. It's rare to meet a centenarian without a great sense of humor and a smile on his or he face. An example of this was the world's oldest living Western woman, a French woman who lived to 122 years of age. Although she had lost her eyesight and recently had come to rely on a wheelchair, she still kept her sense of humor. When interviewed about the secrets of her longevity, she replied that the only thing she knew was that. 'I only have one wrinkle on my entire body and I'm sitting on it.' This kind of lighthearted attitude typifies those who have reached the age of 100 or beyond.

The well known comedian, George Burns lived to be more than 100 years old, and he continued to perform and act in movies until his passing. He never stopped smiling and telling jokes! His positive attitude helped to strengthen his immune system and enable his body to restore its' natural state of health after illness.

Many people come into my office and tell me that they are 'getting old and falling apart!' I have had people in their thirties and forties tell me this. Conversely, I have seen many other patients who are learning to surf and water ski at the age of seventy; others who are taking yoga in their eighties and are more supple and graceful than people less than half their age, and still others who are dancing and gardening daily well into their nineties. (That describes me, by the way, at my present age of 93.) Youth and health appear to be more connected to our states of mind, and reflect our attitudes more than pure chronology. A positive attitude and a zest for life are critical for enhancing and fortifying your healing system." [59]

---

[59] Ibid, pp. 19-20.

CHAPTER FOUR

POWER OF BELIEFS

Spirituality and belief in a Universal Creator

There is no doubt in my mind, based on my own experiences and research, that our health and wellbeing require a solid belief in God. Add one "o" to God and it spells good. When we take time to think about it all of our many blessings, our 'good things', are provided for us. Things exist. Life is real. It cannot be created by humans. Our DNA can be analyzed but it cannot be created. The infinite wisdom that created all of the essentials for survival can be seen in the following examples:

-   There is the gift of life through the miracle of conception and birth.
-   The air we breathe contains vital elements such as oxygen and prana which sustain our life.
-   Our minds are capable of miraculous inventions and creative thoughts which provide us with all of our basic needs plus luxuries fit for a king.
-   There is the miracle of chlorophyll which is created in plants through the reaction of sunlight on plant leaves. Our entire food chain depends on green plants.
-   All of the elements which are essential for our survival were placed in the air and the earth before humans were created.
-   All of the natural herbs and foods that sustain us, and also provide cures for every ailment, were created without any human intervention.

Science cannot explain creation. The theory of the 'big bang' simply states that there was a point in time in the very distant past when a tremendous burst of energy occurred setting off in motion waves of energy that led to the creation of the universe. The theory does not reveal where the elements essential to creation of the material universe came from nor does it offer any plausible explanation for the tremendous wisdom and power behind the creation of galaxies and solar systems in the organized fashion which exists. Of course, the fact that living intelligent organisms from the single cell to the myriads of living beings including humans, that exist cannot be duplicated by science. Life itself had to be created by something or someone with infinite creative power.

If we look about us, we see many things such as houses, cars, airplanes, appliances, etc. We know that all of these things were created by someone with the intelligence to conceive of these things and also with the ability to produce them. Nothing exists that wasn't created. The basic materials that provide the means to make all of these things were placed in and on the earth so that we humans could make use of them. The only logical explanation is that there is an all-wise, all-powerful being who created the wonderful universe we live in.

When we accept the fact that there is an infinite wisdom involved with creation and in sustaining life throughout the universe, then we can either attribute that awareness to a divine source, God, an all-wise, all-powerful, infinite being or whatever other explanation we choose to believe in. All of the great religions are based on a belief in God. All of the great prophets were inspired to teach that there is one God and that all humans are children of God. A simple code of laws, such as the 'ten commandments' was taught by each prophet to be followed as a means to maintain peace and harmony among people. The fact that chaotic conditions exist on planet Earth does not necessarily reflect on God's wisdom. Humans were created with a superior intelligence and with free will with no restraints on their thoughts and actions. In order to use our free will, we have to be free to make choices and learn from our mistakes. Prophets and angelic beings were created to help guide us in the ways of peace, love and harmony. Man's inhumanity to other humans results in wars and pestilence. We have no one to blame but ourselves when things go wrong. We should learn from our mistakes and make the changes necessary to improve the situations that require change.

This book does not get into a thorough discussion about the many reasons why the world we live in is chaotic as it would take another book to treat this topic fully. The author has conducted seminars on this important issue, and is presently writing another book that will present the powerful influences on human behavior exerted by customs, myths and religions. As stated before, this chapter deals with the value and benefits of a belief in a loving, compassionate God. This belief opens our minds to the unity of all things; to the realization that we are all children of the One Universal Creator.

Oneness and Consciousness

In Western societies, the emphasis is on a belief in 'dualism.' This belief gives rise to conflicts of all kinds. There is the concept that 'I am me' as separate from everything else. Concern for the welfare of the body predominates in one's thinking. The ego judges everything from the standpoint of its own perception of reality which is largely based on its perceived need for things, such as acceptance by others; possessions; etc.

In Eastern societies the emphasis is on a belief in non-dualism. This is the belief in the concept that 'I am one.' This belief frees the mind of the perceived needs of the ego and instead accepts the unity of everything plus the awareness that 'I am consciousness.' From this point of view, our reality is not our body but is actually our consciousness. Our consciousness enables us to make use of all of our senses to appreciate all of our experiences without being encumbered by the limited perception of the dualistic mind. We just accept what is without the ego's need to judge each experience on the basis of the perceived needs of the ego. The following excerpt from the book, *That Which You Are Seeking Is Causing You to Be Sick,* describes the limitations of the ego:

What is ego?

It's the illusion that I am separate from everything else; the part of me who's always comparing, the part who feels superior, or inadequate, or deprived. It is the one who clings and resists, who sees me as subject and everything else as object. It is the source of my suffering.

Why is it an illusion?

You are separate aren't you? How can you be more than you are? You're a person—and a very specific one at that. You're not your Uncle Bob. You're not a cat, a tree, a rock, and everything else that is. You are you.

Yes, I am me, but what animates Uncle Bob, the cat, the tree, the rock, and all that is. We are packaged differently, but we share the same essence. There are many of us and we are not the same, but we are all one."

Letting go does not mean 'not having' although egocentricity thinks it does....If I let go I'll never get what I want. We let go of our 'attachment to getting' what we want. We aren't required to let go of the what,' the object of our desire. And if we let go of that attachment, the odds of getting what we want will be just as good as ever. The only real difference will be that we won't suffer if we don't get it."

Joy is not the product of what you want. Joy is compassion turned inward—the end of struggle, the end of competition. Get current, make sure you're not still carrying around old ideas about yourself that aren't really applicable to your present life....and perhaps never were![60]

How can we change something by being one with it? What about social injustice and cruelty—how can we bring about change if we aren't making choices, if we just go around accepting everything? How can we change something by being one with it?"

How can we change something in any other way? By being one with the present moment, we experience full acceptance. Nothing escapes us; nothing is denied. We see it all and we move with it. And in moving with it we are able to respond appropriately to what is happening 'right now.' We have food to share with someone who is hungry. Saddened by cruelty to animals? We stop eating meat. Interested in helping out in the ghettos? We volunteer. We offer ourselves in love and oneness, out of a sense of us all being in this together.

Change that arises from duality is change in content only - the whats change but the hows remain the same. The oppressed become the oppressors. We only change roles. Profound change - in 'how' we do, not what we do—happens only with complete acceptance. Acceptance which goes beyond the dualities of right and wrong, them and us, good and bad. Complete acceptance and profound change are inseparable.

Letting go is releasing our grip on delusion, allowing us to see what is. When we stop resisting what is, when we stop clinging to our beliefs and assumptions about how things should be, we are letting go, we are opening ourselves to the present moment. Letting go goes hand in hand

[60] Cheri Huber *That Which You Are Seeking is Causing You To Seek.* Mountainview, CA: Zen Center, 1990, pp. 21-33.

with acceptance. One does not occur without the other. Letting go is opening the hand. Acceptance is what the open hand receives.

We hide things from ourselves when we are afraid to see what's there. When we're willing to accept ourselves just as we are, we have nothing to fear. We stop identifying with the process that maintains our suffering when we stop judging ourselves, when we stop holding a club over our heads to make sure we do things right. The moment we drop all of that, we have dropped the only thing that can cause us to suffer. [61]

When we're living in the present moment, life is very easy. It's not that living in the present means only good and pleasant things happen to us. It is an attitude of mind as well as an actual experience of seeing that whatever happens is perfect.

In the present we see that life is happening exactly as 'it should'— exactly as it 'is.' When we realize that we are part of that perfection and realize it's not possible to be separate from it, except through our own delusion of separation (ego), then we experience our lives as easy.

When we separate ourselves out, when we identify with a small, egocentric separate self, then life becomes hard. Because that's when we're trying to 'make' life happen.

I get an idea about how life should be, and then I set out to make that happen. A great deal of the time my idea about what should be is just not what's going on in the universe. And so I'm constantly in conflict. People are not behaving the way I want them to; my car breaks down; I'm late for an appointment. I'm comparing the way I think life should be to the way life is.

As soon as we get rid of the notion that there is the possibility of a life other than the one that is, we move from suffering and into a deeper level of peace and acceptance. [62]

Another excellent book, *The Teachers of One,* presents the underlying principles behind the power of non-duality. Excerpts from the book follow:

And now, in the 21st century, the emphasis is on self-investigation— not blind adherence to a religious or philosophical party line. And inasmuch as the essence of Eastern teaching is still the transience of 'I'—an

---

[61] Ibid, pp.44-62.
[62] Ibid, pp. 83-84.

inconsequential bundle of rising and falling thoughts and perceptions—the invitation is to transcend the veil of 'I' and go beyond it. What lies beyond is not a meaningless emptiness but the very consciousness of the universe itself. Self-realization, the ultimate goal and end of ignorance, is the understanding that 'I' is not a separate identity but merely a filter of mind; that God or consciousness is the animating life force in which the 'I' arises. Consciousness therefore comes before 'I'. And if I am not intrinsically this 'I', I must be the consciousness in which the 'I' manifests. Thus essence precedes existence; I am conscious. I am God.

To know that 'I am consciousness' is the basic tenet of Advanta, non-dualism—I am One, existing without a second. Indeed it is the fundamental principle of all Eastern teachings, its source being found in the ancient texts of the Indian Vedas, the oldest scripture known to mankind. And it is this teaching that has become available once more in the 20th and 21st centuries, initiated through the life and teachings of Bhagavan Sri Ramana Maharshi, and now through teachers in the West. Using the method of Self-Inquiry, it is possible to see through the veil of illusion and find an answer to the most elusive question of all - Who am I?" [63]

Another source of deep insight into the question of Who am I, is revealed in the teachings of Lao Tsu, in his book *Tao Te Ching*. An excerpt from the Introduction to the book follows below:

"A mind that is full of content knows a universe that is full of things. To go behind the apparent universe requires that we go behind the apparent mind. This may be called 'opening to non-being.' At the same time, what Lao Tsu called *non-being* is a force of irresistible, ultimate power. It is most certainly not 'nothing' in the usual sense of the word. Nor is it 'existence' in the usual sense of the word. Similarly, for ourselves: What lies behind the glittering surface of our mind or ordinary sense of self are not simply other fabulous 'things', such as the psychological 'black holes' that modern psychology has revealed to us under the designation of the 'unconscious.'

What lies behind the appearances in ourselves and in the universe—is not another world, another 'thing' or collection of 'things.' Not new stars, planets, or black holes; not new desires, sensations, or insights. What lies behind the ten thousand things is the awareness of the ten thousand things. What lies behind the ego is the awareness of the ego.

---

[63] Paula Marvelly. *The Teachers of ONE*. London: Watkins, 1988, pp. XI-XII.

The 'other world,' the 'real world out there and in here is *simply* this world illumined with the inconceivably powerful and subtle energy of consciousness—which we perhaps are beginning to recognize as love itself.

All phenomena everywhere depend upon the harmonious relationship of these forces called *yin* and *yang,* female and male, return and expression. To be fully human is to develop a power of attention that allows this relationship to take place within one's own psychophysical organism. A man in whom this attention is highly developed is called a sage, an enlightened human being—although here too there are levels and degrees of inner attainment.

As has been suggested, the study that leads to the emergence of this consciousness within us is known as the path. *Tao*, understood as the Way of inner spiritual practice….At every stage of the practice, the truth one needs to experience is hidden and dark, and bears the marks of death. This is the death of all that has been built up by the automatism of the mind and ego. It is the death of forms and the momentary release or appearance of a formless energy. The seeker must allow himself or herself to be the female in relation to that which is waiting to pour itself into the seeker from above—whether it be called truth or the ultimate energy.

To see the Tao's message as a permissive, self-calming 'going with the flow' in the way some modern writers have is to make a mere fantasy out of a profound, subtle doctrine that blends into one vision the truth of Mercy and the truth of Rigor, to use the language of the Kabbalah. To make non-doing into non-struggling is to be an advocate of what has come to be one of the world's great half truths….we find in the *Tao Te Ching* and the countless other esoteric spiritual teachings of the world: the need to struggle for an attention or consciousness that can embrace two opposite forces without being swallowed by either." [64]

Additional insights into how to apply the awareness of *consciousness* into our daily lives are found in the writings of Joel Goldsmith. Excerpts from his writings follow below:

Since God is Spirit, Spirit is real; spirit is vital, alive. But although this is true, there must be a conscious awareness of the reality of Spirit. In that conscious awareness, we have the power that produces the harmonies of our daily experience. Today most of us are limited by our

---

[64] Lao Tzu. TAO TE CHING. New York: Vantage Books, 1989, pp. xxiv-xxix.

sense of body; we believe wherever we are at this moment is the extent of our being. Actually that limitation has as little foundation as the limitation imposed on those who thought the earth was flat. A few have had the actual realization that they are not confined to a body.

If we do not have a conscious awareness of the presence and power of Spirit, it does no healing work for us. That is the reason one person is able to do successful healing work, while another fails....

Our great purpose in life should be the development and enfoldment of our spiritual consciousness or spiritual awareness. It is absolutely necessary first, to understand that we exist as consciousness; and secondly, to become conscious of this reality of existence.

Physical or mental healing is based on the belief that we are somewhere between our feet and our head, and it attempts to do something about a physical existence. Spiritual healing has an entirely different basis. Spiritual healing is dependent on the individual's becoming consciously aware of the truth that we do not exist in the body or as the body, but that we exist as infinite, divine consciousness. [65]

Another source of knowledge that helps us achieve inner peace and enlightenment can be found in the book, *The Spiritual Teaching of Ramana Maharshi*. Excerpts from this book follow below:

"Beyond that which you think is that which you are. Realizing this does not involve specific practices or attitudes other than Understanding. No withdrawal is necessary—no change of present time, place or condition—only a change of viewpoint, which you bring about yourself, for your Self.

Sri Ramana declares unmistakably that the real purpose of spiritual practice is the dissolution of the 'I'. Ramakrishna however shows a hesitating attitude in this respect. Though he says, 'As long as the 'I' sense lasts, so long are true knowledge and Liberation (Mukti) impossible,' yet he must acknowledge the fatal nature of *ahamkara*. He says. 'How very few can obtain this Union (*samadhi*) and free themselves from this 'I'? It is very rarely possible. Talk as much as you want; isolate yourself continuously, still this 'I' will return to you." [66]

In the book, *Power Versus Force: An Anatomy of Consciousness,*

---

[65] Joel Jacobson. *The Infinite Way*. New York, pp.244-249.
[66] Ramanu Maharishi. *The Spiritual Teaching of Ramana Maharishi*. Boston: Shambala publications, 1988, p.x.

Dr. David Hawkins presents an in-depth presentation of the power of being aware of the fact that our consciousness should not be identified with our ego since that limits our ability to be receptive to the unlimited power of the universe. The following excerpt from his book provides an insight into how we can achieve unlimited blessings by becoming aware of whom and what we are:

The mind identifies with its content. It takes blame for what it receives, for it would be humbling to the mind's vanity to admit that the only thing it is doing is experiencing, and, in fact, only experiencing *experiencing*. The mind does not even experience the world, but only sensory reports of it. Even brilliant thoughts and deepest feelings are only experience; ultimately we have but one function: to experience experience.

Identification solely with the content of consciousness accounts for the experience of self as limited. In contrast, to identify with consciousness itself is to know that one's actual self is unlimited. When such circumscribed self-identifications have been surmounted, so that the sense of self is identified as consciousness itself, we become 'enlightened.'

One characteristic of the experience of pure consciousness is a perception of timelessness. Consciousness is experienced as beyond all form and time and seen as everywhere equally present. It is described as 'Is-ness' or 'Being-ness' and in the spiritual literature as I-am-ness.' Consciousness does not recognize separation which is a limitation of perception. The enlightened state is a 'Oneness' in which there is no division into parts.

Another attribute of pure consciousness is cessation of the ordinary flow of thoughts or feelings, a condition of infinite power, infinite compassion, infinite gentleness, and infinite love. In this state self becomes Self with a capital 'S.' This awareness of self as Self is the culmination of the process of eliminating limited identification of self.

The steps one should take in order to facilitate the awareness of one's Self as pure consciousness have been well detailed historically. Many techniques and behaviors have been prescribed to facilitate removal of obstacles to expanded awareness; these can be found in the practice of various spiritual disciplines. The one process common to all such teachings is the progressive elimination of the identification of self as finite. [67]

Another technique for releasing disturbing thoughts which are hidden in your subconscious mind is regressive hypnotism. One of the foremost practitioners of this method is Dr. Brian Weiss. He found that bringing suppressed memories to the awareness of the conscious mind resulted in the reduction or elimination of tensions that were the cause of many illnesses. His findings were based on his personal experiences with thousands of his own patients. Patients were cured of serious ailments that had not responded to conventional psychiatric or medical methods.

In about 70 percent of the cases, patients had memories of what appeared to be past lives. Weiss came to the following conclusion: "There is no doubt in my mind that past-life regression therapy offers a rapid and effective way of treating physical and emotional symptoms, in addition to offering many other benefits.

… Regressing to significant childhood events, to infancy, or even to past lives may provide significant relief and benefit in the present time." [68]

Dr. Shakuntala Modi is another psychiatrist who learned of the harmful effects of past-life memories through the use of regressive hypnotism. He gives an excellent presentation of the subject, based on his own clinical experiences and research, in his book, *Remarkable Healings,* as follows:

Through time, practitioners have tried everything in an attempt to heal their patients. Psychiatrists have gone through a range of vain attempts, from ancient times to modern, to find answers in psychiatric treatment. They have drilled holes in skulls, performed surgery to literally destroy frontal brain tissue, used shock therapy, insulin therapy, nutrition therapy, and chemical therapy. In all these attempts, psychiatrists have met with little true success. At best they have masked symptoms, giving patients a false sense of well-being that goes away with the therapy.

The human psyche is not a physical entity; it is a spiritual manifestation of our soul's connection to 'the source.' Whether we refer to that source as God, Allah, Buddha, Shiva, Mohammed, Jesus

---

[67] Hawkins, op.cit., pp.209-211
[68] Dr. Brian Weiss. *Mirrors of Time. New York:p.13.*

Christ, Messiah, or Jehovah is not the issue. The issue is simple. We are all souls (spirits), pieces of our creator, on a journey through eternity.

And what is the goal? Consistently my patients affirm one thing; our destiny is with Our Creator and our longing is to return to Him. Understanding this, we can understand how treating mental illness—feelings of isolation, loneliness, despair—must be a spiritual, soul restoring process. The early shamans and medicine men understood this. Humans are spiritual beings; we can operate on them, and remove their stomachs, their hearts, and their kidneys. We cannot, however, remove their spirit. Organs can cease to function; bodies die; but the spirit, the soul, lives on. It is eternal, and it is linked to its creator.

In recent years, some psychiatrists, and other mental health professionals have 'happened upon' evidence that tells them it is time to return to the age-old practice of dealing with the spiritual essence of patients, and they are finding through regression of patients, that our psychological problems are based on the 'history of our souls,' both in this life and in past lives. In dealing with this spiritual side of patients, mental health professionals are finding not only lasting cures for mental illness, but so much more.

Consistent experiences with my hypnotized patients have fostered my understanding that mental illness can be attributed to several sources that include:

- Current Life traumas including prenatal and birth traumas.
- Past life traumas.
- Possession or attachment by earthbound spirits.
- Possession or attachment by earthbound spirits or demon spirits.
- Soul fragmentation and soul loss.

During the sessions with my hypnotized patients, I have found that a major source of mental illness finds its roots in prenatal and birth traumas. The experiences of the fetus are far more dynamic and penetrating than we have ever suspected. The scars the fetus sustains in the prenatal months and during birth carry over later in life. The fetus in the womb tunes in to its mother's emotional, mental, and physical feelings and accepts them as its own. The baby, upon its birth feels rejected and cast out into a cold world from the warmth and security of the womb. I find problems and feelings of separation, anxiety, rejection, inferiority, inadequacy, anger, remorse, depression, fear, paranoia, claustrophobia, headaches, asthma, and sinus problems can stem from prenatal and birth traumas. To heal the patients of these problems, we need to help them in recalling, releasing, understanding and resolving these prenatal and birth traumas.

It would seem that one must believe in reincarnation to accept past life traumas as a cause for mental illness. Interestingly, it does not require that the patient or the therapist believe in reincarnation or past live for this therapy to be effective.

Several of my patients have reported finding inside them another spirit, a human soul separate and distinct from their own soul. This soul is reported by the patients to be a visitor or, as we say, an attached or possessing earthbound spirit who did not make its transition to the light (heaven) after the death of its physical body and has remained on the earth plane. The hypnotized patients report that the visiting or possessing spirits are influencing them and causing them problems, either intentionally or unintentionally. Before there can be any resolution of the patient's symptoms and problems, all possessing earth bound spirits must be treated and released from the patients.

This approach is not in keeping with the psychiatric tradition and definitely is not part of my training. This information also is not based on my beliefs and personal experiences, but solely on the experiences reported by my patients while under hypnosis.

Frequently, the spirits' experiences are seen by the patients as part of their own current or past experiences. The experiences of the possessing spirits frequently cause physical and emotional problems for the patients. Usually, it is a possessing spirit's death experience and its cause that contributes to the patient's problem. Possessing spirits' thoughts, experiences, and voices can be very distressing to patients, who may think they are insane because they hear and react to these thoughts and voices.

By recognizing all these possibilities, we can clearly understand that any emotional, mental, or physical disease is in fact a disease of the soul. To heal the mind and body, we need to heal the soul by removing all the possessing earthbound and demon spirits from the soul of the living being. Then we need to heal the traumas from the current and past lives by recalling, releasing, and resolving them. By healing the soul we can heal the body from its emotional, mental, physical problems.

None of this theory is based on any religion or spirituality. It is based on the information given by patients, under hypnosis. If the patient has a basis in religion, and spirituality, that basis may of course influence what the patient's subconscious is telling us. No claims are made for the accuracy of the religious or spiritual information provided by the patients. [69]

Life after Death

Confirmation of the fact that life goes on after death is supported by extensive research which I conducted into such subjects as near-death experiences; out-of-body experiences; and contacts with the deceased as presented in my earlier book, *Life Beyond Earth; The Evidence and its Implications.* The following excerpts from my book demonstrate the reality of life after death:

Robert Monroe

Robert Monroe is an inventor, author and successful businessman. He is known for his extensive knowledge and first-hand experiences with out-of-body experiences (OBEs). In my book, *Life Beyond Earth* (see the Bibliography), as described in his own words his unusual abilities which led to his discovery, among other things of proof of 'life after death' and out of body experiences:

He learned that he had what he called a 'Second Body' which was able to function in what he called the 'Second State.' These descriptive terms were used by him instead of the 'astral body' and astral realm". He learned that certain techniques were very effective in achieving the state of deep relaxation which enabled him to have conscious control of his spontaneous OBEs.

He also made himself available to scientists who were inter-

---

[69] Shakuntala Modi, M.D. *Remarkable Healings.* Charlottesville, VA: Hampton Roads Publishing Co., 1996, pp. 43-49.

ested in investigating his unusual abilities. The tests showed that Monroe could have OBEs without going into a deep trance as is the case with most psychics such as Edgar Cayce.

As Monroe gained more control of his journeys, which he used as a descriptive term instead of astral projection, he found that he could journey into three different realms of existence while in his Second Body and eventually could journey to visit persons or places within these realms at will. He described the different realms as follows: Locale I is the physical world of our planet. Locale II is the space just above the Earth where the human personality survives the transition of death and continues to exist. Locale III includes distant realms beyond the Earth including other planets and other beings. Most of Monroe's journeys were within Locale II.

He found that the Second Body contained a very high level of awareness which functioned at its best in Locale II. He was able to identify several levels or areas within Locale II. The one closest to Earth contained discarnate humans who refused to accept the fact that they had died and remained in the locations which they were most attached to. A level just above this one contained discarnate humans who held strong beliefs and attachments to a particular sect, creed or interest. They congregated with those of like mind and were reluctant to accept the fact that they could leave that level and go to higher realms if they chose to. Another area he was able to identify was an extremely beautiful place which he called the Park. After a number of journeys to the Park, he became aware that this was a place where newly deceased persons were received by already departed friends and relatives and helped to adjust to their new life in the spirit world. There were other beings present of a higher order who were able to simulate the environment for the benefit of those who had just experienced 'death' so that they would find themselves in familiar surroundings, at least temporarily. After a period of adjustment, each new-comer was taken to a place where he or she 'belonged.' Monroe found that thought is the driving force in Locale II, which he described as follows:

Superseding all appears to be one prime law. Locale II is a state of being where what we label thought is the well-spring of existence. It is the vital driving force that produces energy, assembles matter into form, and provides channels of perception and communication. As you think, so you are.

In this environment, no mechanical supplements are found. No cars, boats, airplanes or rockets are needed for transportation. You *think* movement and it is fact. No telephones, radio, television, and other communication aids have value. Communication is instantaneous. No farms, gardens, cattle ranches, processing plants, or retail outlets are in evidence. In all experimental visits, no food energy needs were indicated. How energy is replaced— if it is truly spent—is not known.

Mere thought is the force that supplies any need or desire, and what you think is the matrix of your action, situation, and position in this greater reality....A facet learned in this medium of thought explains much. It is: Like attracts Like. I didn't realize there was such a rule that acted so specifically.

Project this outward, and you begin to appreciate the infinite variations found in Locale II. Your destination seems to be grounded completely within the confines of your most *constant* motivations, emotions and desires. You may not consciously want to go there, but you have no choice. Your Supermind (soul?) is stronger and usually makes the decision for you. Like attracts Like.

When Monroe's wife, Nancy, died, he made several attempts to find her in the astral realm. He finally found her in the Park. They were able to see each other and communicate their love for each other. It was very difficult for Monroe to leave his wife and return to his physical body but he was made to understand that he had work to complete on Earth while his wife had to continue her destiny in the other realm.

Monroe continued to intensify his efforts to learn more about his OBEs. In 1968 he found that certain patterns of sound could induce altered states of consciousness. In 1971 he created a separate Research and Development division of his radio business called the Monroe Institute. In his book, *Ultimate Journey,* Monroe describes what took place at the Institute as follows:

Among the techniques developed at the Institute was the Hemi-Sync, a trade name for an audio wave system which helps synchronize the brain waves between the two hemispheres of the brain. Specific sound patterns help the listener achieve various states of consciousness, enhancing the ability to achieve an OBE whenever desired. It was discovered that certain rates of frequency produced different results.

For example, listening to the sounds on a tape called Focus 21 through headphones produced the subjective experience of being mentally carried to a location other than where the physical body was, with the conscious awareness shifted almost entirely to the non-physical realm. On the other hand, the Focus 12 tape is useful for facilitating telepathic communication while still remaining in close contact with the physical realm.

Another series of audio-tapes were developed to induce complete relaxation by use of countdown techniques. These audio-tapes, together with other techniques developed by Monroe, were used the U.S. Dept. of Defense in the training of army personnel to conduct espionage using a form of projection now known as 'remote viewing'. At the present time, the Monroe Institute offers a one week course of training which prepares the participants to conduct their own controlled OBEs. The courses are given at the Monroe Institute, Route 1, Box 175, Faber, Virginia.[70]

Further confirmation that life goes on after so-called death are the following accounts of first-hand personal experiences that occurred after my wife, Ruth passed on in March, 2005. She reappeared to me and also to many other people, making her presence known in ways that were unmistakably her. The following quotations are from the people who were visited by Ruth and described what actually took place:

After Death Visitations of Ruth Singer

Bernie, Ruth's husband

"Shortly after Ruth's death she appeared to me in a most unusual manner. I was fast asleep when I was awakened by a strong feeling that someone was standing next to the bed. I struggled to open my eyes and I saw what appeared to be a figure of a person right next to my bed. Then I heard Ruth's distinctive voice say to me in a loud assertive tone, 'Bernie open your eyes and look at me.' As I opened my eyes I could then see

---

[70] Bernard Singer. *Life Beyond Earth: The Evidence and its Implications.* Piscataway, NJ: Eloist Press, 2001, pp. 36-38.

Ruth's face staring at me. She appeared to be in the prime of life and was vibrantly alive. Then her face moved closer and closer to my face and I felt her press her lips to mine in a fervent kiss. The pressure on my lips was so strong that I was surprised by its intensity. Then I suddenly felt the weight of her body as she laid herself right on top of me. I embraced her in my arms and I basked in the glow of joy and happiness at having her close to me again. Then she said, "I love you" and suddenly disappeared. I fell back into a deep sleep.

Several months later, I was awakened from my sleep one morning by hearing Ruth's voice say "Bernie, get up." It was so real and typical of the way Ruth often awakened me after a night's sleep that I turned to the side of the bed where Ruth usually slept and I said, "Yes Dear." Not seeing her there I realized that this was just another way of Ruth letting me know that she was still around.

Lana, cleaning woman

On June 1st, 2004, Lana called me and stated that Ruth had come to her in her sleep (the night before). Ruth appeared to her vividly staring at her with her dark brown eyes She said very sternly; "How come you didn't come to my house to clean for a long time? You better do it now!"

She appeared to be very angry. Lana said "I'm sorry, I'm sorry" and then she woke up. She was so startled that she couldn't fall back to sleep. Lana called me early the next morning to tell me what had happened. She told me that she had never had a dream in her entire life and that if she did she never remembered it. This incident was very typical of the way my wife would act. She took great pride in her home. She would never leave the house until all the beds were made and all the dishes washed and put away.

Arnie, son of Roz

While talking to Barry during Roz's 90th Birthday Party, he saw Ruth's face instead of Barry's. His deceased aunt appeared young, vibrant and happy. The thought came to Arnie that Ruth was happy to be able to see the family at Roz's party even though she wasn't there in her physical body.

Arnie, Just before Roz's death

Arnie called me to tell me that my sister had just died (April 14, 2008.) He went on to tell me that he had a wonderful experience while sitting at Roz's bedside the day before. She had awakened from the coma she was in and was able to speak to him for several minutes before lapsing back into the coma.

Roz said to him, "It's true. There is life after death. I see angels and departed loved ones." After a little while she said excitedly, "I see Mary Lou. She tells me that she will help me." There was a peaceful smile on Roz's face as she dozed off.

Arnie was delighted to be present when his mother spoke about her awakening to the reality of life after death. Prior to that moment, Roz had never believed that life could go on.

Kimberly, Ruth's Granddaughter

Sunday, the day after her trauma (aneurism), my grandmother came to me in spirit stating that I was going to be okay. She seemed to ask me whether or not she could go. I told her that she didn't have to stay for me. It evoked such emotion from me. I don't ever recall crying like that. It was so hard to be completely selfless. I knew she was going at that time.

By Wednesday, I no longer felt the pain of detachment. Although she was still in a coma, I knew she was gone. She didn't actually pass until the following Monday night, but she left her body on that Wednesday. That was confirmed to me when our friend Diane said to me that she 'was told' that Ruth left her body on Wednesday. I don't recall how she knew that; if Grandma had told her she was going or some other spiritual force told her. But, she didn't know that I knew that, so it wasn't something she was 'trying' to back up for me.

On another occasion, I was in Cozumel, Mexico. I had a dream that I saw her and she was standing with my grandfather, Bernie, who is still alive. She was so tall and young looking. He looked the same as he does now. All I could manage to say to her in the dream was "Grandma, you are so tall." Her response was, "We don't take our bodies with us". And that was the end of the visit!

David Singer, Ruth's son.

David, who is a physician, had been trying desperately for over a week to bring her out of the coma that she was in. He expressed the thought to her that he gave her permission to leave her body and pass over. After her death, she appeared to him in a dream and said to him, "David, I did not need your permission. I had already decided to leave my body several days ago."

Other Peoples Experiences

Brian, Roz's grandson

Brian woke up early one morning to find himself crying with co-pious tears flowing. He didn't know why! His grandfather had died recently after being incapacitated by a series of strokes but Brian had not grieved his passing. He then noticed a strong fragrance. It was the aroma of cologne that his grandfather had used. The cologne was a special blend of flowers that was prepared at a specialty store and his grandfather was the only one in the family that used it. As Brian walked around his bedroom, he noticed that the fragrance was very strong no matter which part of the room he was in. It then dawned on Brian that this was his grandfather's way of letting him know that he was present and was still very much alive in the spirit realm.

Ellen, Viola's niece

Ellen communicates with her deceased father. Her aunt, Viola, told me that Ellen was in a severe depression over the loss of her father. Ellen was given a copy of my book, *Life Beyond Earth: The Evidence and Its Implications.* After Ellen read my book, she realized that her father could still be alive in the spirit world. She gradually overcame her depression and started to get on with her life. She has been able to communicate with her deceased father on a regular basis in recent months and is now happy and well-adjusted again.

Mary, Arnie's wife

Mary frequently communicates with her deceased mother. Mary also told me that my book, *Life Beyond Earth* trans-formed her life. Before reading my book, she had a deadly fear of being abducted by aliens (ET's). When she learned what their purpose was in abductions (observation, communication & impregnation) she was able to get rid of her fears. And knowledge of the facts about life after death eased her fears of death and of being judged in regards to what she thought were sinful deeds.

Consider these facts: When we enter the spirit world after death we are no longer subject to the limitations of a physical body. We no longer experience physical pain since we no longer have a physical body. We do have a spirit body which is capable of doing things in the spirit realm and we do retain our memories.

Death and Angels

There are also angels who are assigned to assist us. The following excerpts from my book, *Life beyond Earth: The Evidence and Its Implications* provide some insights into the realities of the universe:

Spirit guides were created to aid in opening our minds to the reality of the spirit worlds. They are commonly known as angels. The word "angel" is used to designate the offspring of the Universe Mother Spirit who are chiefly involved with the plans of mortal survival. There are a number of classifications of angels based on their different levels of experience and their particular assignments. Some are assigned to be in contact with human beings as guardian angels. Some act as escorts of the soul as it leaves the body at death bringing it to a reception center in the lower heavens. Some of the angels are involved with the educational programs established for the benefit of the ascending mortals who have entered the spirit world. There are three primary groups of angels: the seraphim and the aids of the seraphim, the cherubim and the sanobim, all of whom comprise the angelic corps of a local universe.

The angels have certain aspects that have not been accurately portrayed in the myths and legends of the past. For example angels do not have wings. They don't have physical bodies. They do not respond to prayers. They do not invade the human mind nor manipulate the will of humans. It is a rule throughout all levels of the universe that the free will of every being is respected and is not to be infringed upon. The role the angels play with humans is that of guardians. They protect us and try to guide us within the limits of our own free choices. Angels do have feelings. They experience spiritual emotions that are somewhat similar to human emotions. They take great interest in our spiritual progress and when humans make choices that lead to spiritual growth they are joyful.

Every effort is made to ease the transition from life on a planet to life in the spirit world. For example, a subjective heavenly plateau was prepared for the early American Indians many years ago with beautiful mountains and plains together with the kinds of animals they were fond of hunting. This heavenly plateau came to be known among the Indians as the "Happy Hunting

Grounds." This, of course, was only a temporary dwelling place. It was used by the guardian angels as a means of inducing the Indians to accept the fact that life continues on in the spirit world.

Immediately after death the newly deceased, as mentioned earlier, are brought to a reception center where they are usually greeted by family members, friends and others who may wish to be present. Every effort is made to ease the adjustment from the earthly experiences of each person to that of the new life in the next realm. Angels, with the help of mortals who have already adjusted to the spirit environment, offer support and guidance to the mortal survivors. Conditions are controlled to the extent that the new spirit body appears to be very similar to the deceased earth body except that all previous ailments are gone and the new spirit body appears just as when they were in the prime of life. The spirit body is not subject to any illnesses. For example, vision is extended to include greater distances and wider scopes. A broader range of colors and sounds is also included in the heightened senses.

In spite of all of the efforts made to ease the adjustment of the newly dead to their new surroundings and new conditions, there are still large numbers of new arrivals who refuse to relinquish their ties to earth. They continue to remain on earth in their spirit bodies frequenting the places where they had strong ties while alive on earth. They become known as sleeping survivors and they can remain earthbound for many years until such time as they respond to their guardian angels and make the decision to leave their attachment to earth.

Earthbound souls are not permitted to remain on earth forever. At the end of a dispensation (about every millennium) there is a general resurrection of souls when most of the earthbound souls are gathered up and removed from earth. They are helped to become aware that they are no longer alive on earth. Any earthly survivor who makes the irrevocable decision to stop living will have the request granted and will cease to exist. The records of such a person will still be available in the universal memory records. [71]

---

[71] Ibid. pp. 158-164.

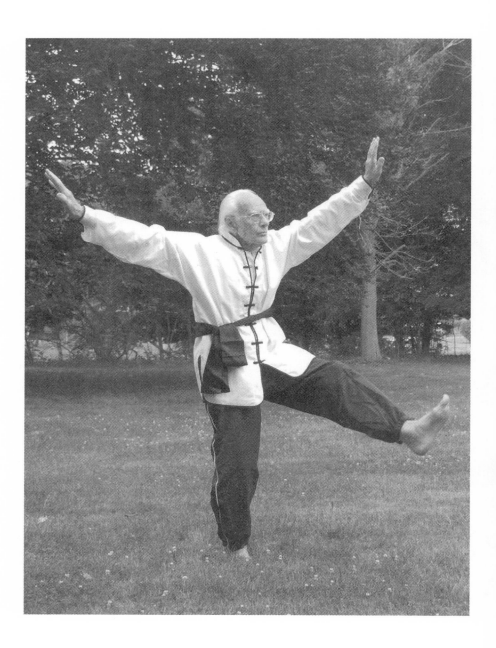

PART TWO

ALTERNATIVE HEALTH CARE

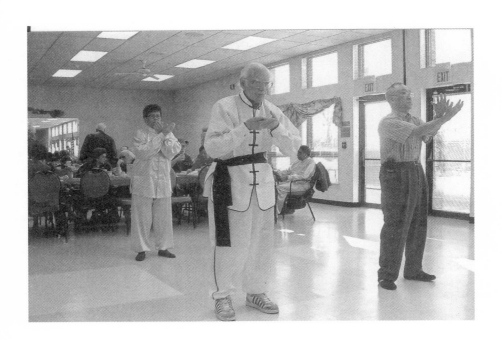

CHAPTER FIVE

NEED FOR ALTERNATIVE HEALTH CARE

Failure of Western Medicine

There has been a very large increase in the numbers of people in the United States who have turned to alternative health care providers in recent years. This, no doubt, is the result of the failure of organized medicine to find cures for the deadly illnesses such as cancer and heart disease and because of the many dangerous side effects of prescription drugs. On top of this, as pointed out in other parts of this book, the chemical and pharmaceutical industries have been pushing toxic poisons in medicines, flu shots, vaccinations and even in the foods and water we consume. In the book, *Poisoned Nation: Pollution, Greed and the rise of Deadly Epidemics,* the author, Loretta Schwartz-Nobel had this to say about the situation in 2007:

"Whether it is contamination from air, water, food, or the everyday things we buy and use, the patterns are the same. We are surrounded by life-threatening contaminants and carcinogens that we cannot avoid or control. Most of us have relatively little knowledge of the threat and, of course, we had nothing to do with making the decisions that have set these chemical events in motion. We were not protected by those in authority, and we were not consulted. In fact, we were deliberately misinformed. What science conceives, industry makes possible. Government and big business give lip service to protecting us, but often they do just the opposite, and do it knowingly. According to *USA Today,* the U.S. Department of defense is the largest polluter in the world, producing more hazardous waste than the five largest U.S. chemical companies combined." [72]

Loretta goes on to review some of the more deadly poisons that have been and still are polluting our planet. Some of the deadly poisons, such as thimerosal, perchlorate, mercury and many others are also discussed in the following pages.

Dr. John Baillor II, a professor of epidemiology and biostatics at McGill University pointed out in 1993, "More than 20 years and $25 Billion after President Nixon declared war on the disease, and the cancer mortality rate continues to rise." He goes on to say at a later date, "Although information released by the media give the impression that serious diseases such as cancer are decreasing, the facts remain that the most serious illnesses such as cancer and heart disease are actually increasing. It is generally acknowledged that obesity is increasing year by year among the general population...Again I conclude, as I did seven years ago, that our decades of war against cancer have been a qualified failure.

"Dr. Bailor and the Cancer Institute agree: Most of these deaths are preventable. What this means to you and me is that despite a worldwide crusade against it, our chances of surviving cancer today are not much better than they would have been thirty years ago – unless we take matters into our own hands. There are documented, effective preventive measures that can work to keep a body free for a lifetime.

The NCI estimates that about a third of all cancers could be brought on by the patient's diet. Other scientists say that figure could go as high as 60 percent." [73]

In the book, *Ascorbate: The Science of Vitamin C,* Dr. Steve Hickey points out the fact that the medical establishment, for the

---

[72] Loretta Schwartz-Nobel. Poisoned Nation: *Pollution, Greed, and the Rise of Deadly Diseases.* New York: 2007, p. 23.

[73] William Fischer. *How to Fight Cancer and Win.* Baltimore: Agora Health Books, 2001, pp.23-27.

most part, has ignored the enormous amount of evidence that supports the value of properly administered amounts of vitamin C as the cure for practically every major disease. Not only have they ignored the evidence but efforts have been made to prevent the use of effective cures and treatments. Here is what he has to say:

"At the time of writing, there is an international plan, called the Codex Alimentarius, to restrict the availability of vitamins and other nutrients, based on assumptions of safety and trade. The successful implementation of laws based on the Codex will mean that people who believe in prevention of disease with vitamins and associated nutrients will be unable to supplement themselves.

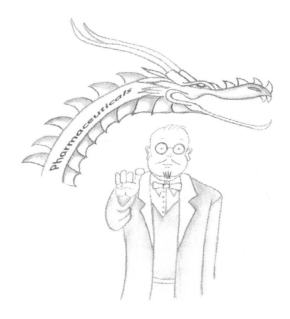

The Pharmaceutical industry wants you...and your money!

Restriction of supplements will clearly mean that any disease resulting from vitamin deficiencies will continue, by law. The result will be regular profits for the pharmaceutical and related medical industries, which are involved in the treatment and management of unnecessary illness and death. Some doctors and alternative health experts have described this as genocide." [74]

---

[74] Dr. Steve Hickey. *Ascorbate: The Science of Vitamin C.* New York: p.215.

Since medical doctors rely heavily on the use of drugs and surgery as the preferred methods of treatment and have practically no background in the field of nutrition, it is no wonder that people, who are aware of the problem, are taking steps to protect their health by turning to alternative health care.

There are basically two types of health care available. We have the conventional (current) medical approach to disease which is based on treating the symptoms of each illness. The most common treatments are prescription drugs, chemo-therapy, radiation and surgery. The treatments are based for the most part on the theory that germs are the cause of most diseases. The need to fight germs became the main focus of modern medicine beginning with the discovery of germs by Louis Pasteur

Pasteur's Germ Theory

Western medicine concentrates on symptoms, while Eastern medicine treats the patient as a whole. Doctors in America focus on the diagnosis and elimination of symptoms. They have placed an emphasis on destroying harmful bacteria based on the discovery of germs by Louis Pasteur. They became too narrow in their diagnoses and treatments in the belief that most diseases are caused by harmful bacteria. It is now known that both good and harmful bacteria are present in the body all of the time. The only time that harmful bacteria can harm us is when our immune system has been weakened to the point that the bacteria can inflict harm. The body will spring into action to destroy harmful bacteria by activating scavenger cells (white blood corpuscles). The body will also increase its temperature (fever) in order to destroy the harmful bacteria.

Outside intervention by physicians is helpful when the body can no longer restore itself to health on its own. The common practice of destroying harmful bacteria with the use of antibiotics such as penicillin has the side effect of destroying beneficial bacteria in our digestive systems at the same time. Unless the beneficial bacteria are restored by ingesting probiotics such as acidophilus our digestive systems cannot function properly leading to many illnesses. In spite of this knowledge, Western doctors still rely heavily on killing germs. The reason for this strong reliance on the use of antibiotics lies in the early success with the use of penicillin. The problem now is the fact that antibiotics no longer work effectively because over the years bacteria have developed into highly resistant types which cannot be destroyed by the original antibiotics. Many people became highly sensitive to the antibiotics because of their widespread use. We now have different types of antibiotics in use to counteract the resistant bacteria. These kinds of antibiotics are of a synthetic nature which causes serious side effects in the human body. Because of the concern of the meat industry to prevent diseases in animals raised for slaughter, the feed of hogs, chickens, and beef have been laced with antibiotics which eventually wind up in the people who consume these products.

The new, more powerful antibiotics result in the destruction of larger numbers of the beneficial bacteria that are vital for the proper functioning of the digestive and elimination systems in our bodies. Pasteur was aware of the importance of the beneficial bacteria but the emphasis in our current medical system is to destroy harmful bacteria no matter how many dangerous side-effects there are.

Another aspect of the problem is the fact that most of the serious illnesses in recent times are caused by viruses which cannot be eliminated by antibiotics. In spite of this, many doctors continue to use antibiotics as a treatment for illnesses caused by viruses.

Eastern medicine, on the other hand, concentrates on the whole person, practically ignores symptoms, treating them as a side effect of a basic imbalance in the patients' way of life. The principle of Yin and Yang is applied to correcting any imbalances in the physical, mental or spiritual condition of each person. There are no harmful side effects to their treatments

Alternative health care is known as the holistic or traditional method which relies on treatments other than those of the medical approach. It includes herbs, nutrition, breathing techniques, exercise, yoga, chiropractic, acupuncture, Reiki and other natural methods of healing. Alternative health treatments are based on the theory that the body heals itself when it is in balance. This is known as a state of homeostasis. It can be accomplished by making use of such things as: diet, reduction of stress, meditation, increasing the strength of the immune system and prayer. There is an urgent need for as many people as possible to become aware of the need for change in the present medically-oriented health care system and to make use of the proven alternative methods that are available.

Failures of the Modern Medical System

The medical approach to health care has turned out to be a disaster due to a number of factors that everyone should be aware of. The major problem is the domination of conventional medicine by the drug industry which has not been controlled by government agencies which were supposed to protect the public such as the Food and Drug Administration (FDA).

Two authors, Kallet and Schlink, who did research for Consumers' Research, wrote a book which was published in 1933 in which they called attention to the widespread use of dangerous chemicals that were commonly used by an unsuspecting public. The book, *100,000,000 Guinea Pigs*, became a best seller. The title of the book refers to the fact that known chemical poisons were being placed in foods, drugs, pesticides, toothpaste and even the water we drink without any protection from the government agencies such as the FDA which were supposed to protect the consumer. The problem exists because the Food and Drug Act allows producers and manufacturers of foods and drugs freedom to use any chemical as additives or preservatives that they want to without any restrictions when they introduce a new product. The only time that the manufacturers are asked to do something about the safety of their products is after a large number of complaints have been filed with the agency in regard to illnesses and deaths that were caused by a particular product. When a decision is finally reached about the danger posed by a poisonous chemical in a particular product, the manufacturer is usually asked to place a warning on the label which most consumers don't read or, if they do, have no idea of how dangerous it is. When a substance has been identified as very dangerous, the FDA may place a fine on the company which is insignificant when compared to the huge profits that were made by the sale of their products. When enough people are clamoring for more drastic action a product may be banned. What happens in many cases is that the same ingredients are brought back under a new name and continue to be sold with the same dangerous consequences. The book contains solid evidence of how dangerous substances continue to be sold with little or no warning to the public. False and misleading advertising produces public acceptance of dangerous products and huge profits to the companies even after the danger has been exposed. A few examples follow below:

Acetphenetedin and *acetanilide* are two common constituents of drug store headache cures which have been responsible for thousands of cases of poisoning and many deaths. The Food and Drugs Act requires that the presence of these drugs be shown on labels. It is evident, however, that naming a drug on the label is not sufficient protection when the dangerous properties of the drug are not recognized by the average person. The label should obviously include also the words 'a dangerous drug' or a similar statement. *Bromo-Seltzer,* a headache remedy which is not only sold at the drug counter but is also frequently dispensed at the soda fountain, is one of the many preparations containing acetanilide. The drug which probably causes an abnormal reaction more frequently than any other drug is acetylsalicylic acid—ordinary aspirin. This drug is one of the most popular drugs and has become a household word with little awareness of its dangerous effects. [75]

The artificial sweetener, *saccharine,* was used in many different products for many years causing many illnesses and many deaths before it was finally banned. It has since been replaced by a more deadly sweetener, *aspartame.* Dr. Wiley, who tried to help protect the public by bringing about the enactment of the Food and Drug Act in 1906, was present in President Roosevelt's office at a hearing regarding the use of saccharine. The president relied on his personal physician's advice, Dr. Rixey, who believed saccharine was safe. When Dr Wiley stated that saccharine was injurious to health, "President Roosevelt said, 'Anybody who says saccharine is injurious to health is an idiot.' There are many who will rate as idiots by the standard of President Roosevelt's ill-advised assertion. [76]

A tremendous burden of disease and suffering, the loss of thousands upon thousands of lives each year, and economic losses running to billions of dollars—this is the toll being paid today by 125,000,000 Americans for the ignorance, the

---

[75] Arthur Kallet and F. Schlink. *100,000,000 Guinea Pigs.* New York: Vanguard Press, 1933, pp. 71-73.
[76] Ibid, p. 201.

indifference, and the avarice of the manufacturers of food and drugs, and for the laxity of governmental officials. In the year 1932, a quarter century after the passage of the national Food and Drug Act, dangerous foods and drugs are being produced by the most reputable of our manufacturers; a hundred different poisons are being fed and dosed to millions of men, women and children daily, worthless medicines and drugs are being sold everywhere, through drugstores, department stores, and the mails, for the treatment of serious diseases; hundreds of thousands of persons are being persuaded to risk their health and, in many cases, their lives by trusting antiseptics that make pretty streaks of color but won't kill germs; poisonous hair dyes, depilatories, and other cosmetic preparations; the most respectable of American Drug manufacturers are selling dangerous drugs...so runs the list.

Judging from the frantic scramble for vitamins to preserve health and for medicines to restore it, we confess our doubts that the public likes to be *poisoned;* or that 125,000,000 Americans want to act as laboratory guinea pigs for a small group of manufacturers each of whom insists that his particular poison, be it arsenic or carbolic acid, is safe and not *really* a poison, and who will try it out on the public—with full sanction of laws, courts, and regulatory agencies, city, state, and national.[77]

The Failure of Protection

The control of foods and drugs in America has been characterized by inexcusable official indifference and negligence; that such control has been hamstrung by a weak and nearly useless body of laws; that there has been a progressive weakening of official activity and concern for the public health through the pressure of concealed commercial forces in close touch with food and drug administrators; that control has been further weakened by unfavorable court decisions. Dr. Harvey Wiley spent four hundred pages in his "History of a Crime Against the Food Law,' in a rapid and incomplete survey covering the period from 1906 up to 1929. Decline in public control of food and drug poisoning, adulte-

---

[77] Ibid, pp. 251-252.

ration, and misbranding has gone far worse since that time. [78]

Other, more recent, authors such as Kevin Trudeau and Byron Richards have provided the public with the startling evidence that known cures for major diseases have been suppressed and alternative health care doctors have been threatened and in some cases have been stripped of their licenses.

An example of a cancer cure that was suppressed is that of a treatment that made use of a beam of light which cured cancer, as reported by Primrose Cooper, noted color-therapist and author: "Royal Rife developed a microscope which illuminated specimens with polarized light that showed each organism has its own resonant frequency. He developed a device, known as the Rife Beam Ray, which produced an electromagnetic field tuned to the frequency of each organism. By using the principle of vibratory resonance, Rife was then able to destroy bacteria or viruses and cure infectious diseases. Rife believed that cancer was caused by a virus or micro-organism, and by isolating this organism from cancer tissue, he was able to discover its resonant frequency. In 1934, he took part in trials at the University of Southern California, which resulted in a success rate in curing all types of cancer of over 90 percent.

Unfortunately, Rife's research was suppressed by the medical authorities; after they failed to buy into his company, and doctors who were successfully using the Rife Beam Ray had to stop for fear of being blacklisted. A laboratory built to study the Ray mysteriously burned to the ground, while Rife, himself faced trumped up charges in the California courts.

These incidents are just the tip of the iceberg as pointed out by Randall Fitzgerald in his book, *The Hundred-Year Lie*. He provides evidence that the major problem is the widespread contamination of our food, water and air by synthetic toxic chemicals, such as those manufactured by huge chemical companies like Monsanto and Dow Chemical.

---

[78] Ibid, pp. 195-196.

Randall Fitzgerald presents important facts for each year from 1900 to 2000 showing how the increased use of synthetic chemicals paralleled the increase of many diseases during that time period. The following excerpts are from his book *The Hundred Year Lie*:

1900-Cancer is responsible for only three percent of all **Deaths.** By the end of the twentieth century, cancer will be the cause of twenty percent of all deaths in the United States.

Breast cancer in women is very rare; by 2005, one in three women will develop breast cancer.

Refined sugar replaces molasses in the average American diet... Diets high in refined sugar will lead to diabetes, heart disease, gastric and duodenal ulcers, chronic infections and tooth decay.

1901-The Monsanto Company is formed by a chemist to manufacture **saccharin,** the first artificial sweetener.

1908--A Japanese chemist identifies a chemical called MSG that enhances the flavor of food.

1909--German chemist Fritz Haber invents chemical fertilizer.

1910-Margarine, a chemical synthesization of vegetable oil, is introduced as a substitute for butter. This was the beginning of **highly saturated trans fats** entering the U.S. diet through processed foods, bringing with them higher cholesterol levels.

1911-The first partially hydrogenated vegetable shortening, **Crisco**, is introduced to the public.

A new **grain-milling** process is discovered in which the germ and outer layers of wheat are removed and refined flour is created, allowing the manufacture of white bread, thus eliminating a source of Vitamins **E and B.**

1920 From this date forward to 2000, U.S. production of **Synthetic chemicals** will increase from less than one million pounds a year to more than 140 billion pounds a year.

1923 Despite concerns about health hazards, tetraethyl **lead is added to gasoline** sold in the U.S. Over the next few decades air-borne lead will **toxify soil, water and food.** The lead will lodge in human bones and cause prenatal damage to children's brains.

1929 PCBS are first manufactured. By 1977, studies will find that PCBs bioaccumulate as a toxin in body tissues; 94 percent of fish nationwide will contain PCB residues; most women tested will show PCB residues in their breast milk.

An additive used as a preservative in vaccines, Thimerosal, is found to cause death in laboratory test subjects. Despite this finding, the additive will continue to be used in most children's vaccines.

1931 In this year a girl named Virginia is born. She will become the oldest child diagnosed with the **new disease called autism;** her birth year is also the first year that **thimerosal** is used in vaccines.

1933 A muckraking book, *100 Million Guinea Pigs: Dangers in Everyday Foods,* Drugs, and Cosmetics, is published and becomes a bestseller. It reveals many cases of **harm and death** from such products as eyelash liners, that blind women, hair removal creams made from rat poison, and a weight-loss program that causes cataracts.

An *American Journal of Medicine* paper identifies a **new type of diabetes resistant to insulin,** called Type 2 diabetes, which is becoming an epidemic in the U.S.

1937 A Danish scientist publishes a book, *Fluorine,* describing hundreds of scientific studies indicating **fluoride poisons** human and animal life, and especially affects the central nervous system.

1938 A new Federal law, the Food, Drug and Cosmetics Act takes effect. The FDA chooses to focus enforcement on the accuracy of information on product labels.

A powerful new pesticide called **DDT** is discovered and also a **synthetic estrogen** called **DES.**

1939 The first proposal to add **fluoride to** public water is made by a scientist under a grant from the Aluminum Company of America.

1941 The FDA approves **DES** for use as a treatment for menopausal women.

Nerve Gas Research conducted during the war results in the development of **chemicals toxic to insects,** producing an explosion of the production of pesticides.

1947 Sex hormones are introduced into **livestock** production adds more fat and **weight** on the animals. Several decades later one of those hormones **DES will be found to cause cancer.**

1948 Use of MSG in Processed foods will double every decade, including **baby food.** By the end of the century, MSG is found to trigger dozens of toxic reactions in the human body.

1953 Fluoride in water can cause acute and **painful allergies** according to Dr. Waldbott. Whenever his own patients stop drinking fluoridated water, they no longer headaches, muscle weakness, and stomach upsets.

1956 Medical researcher Ancel Keys finds that the consumption of trans fats in partially hydrogenated vegetable oil is connected to heart disease. Perfluorochemicals used in Teflon and other non-stick products are first introduced; by 2004, blood tests will reveal that **96 percent of U.S. children** have one of these nonbiodegradable chemicals in their blood streams.

1961 The FDA approves a medication called Ritalin for use by **children with behavior problems.** By 1975 about six million U.S. children will be using Ritalin.

1965 A chemist working for G.D. Searle & Company discovers aspartame, an artificial sweetener.

1968 A scientist at Washington University gives doses of MSG to laboratory mice and discovers widespread brain damage especially in immature and newborn animals.

1974 The FDA approves the artificial sweetener aspartame.

A year later an FDA task force will find that some of the data submitted by the G.D. Searle C Company had been falsified to hide results showing animals fed aspartame had developed seizures and **brain tumors** but no recall or ban will be enacted.

1979 The EPA **bans the manufacture and use of PCBs,** citing them as hazardous to human health PCBs are detected in **30 percent of human breast milk.** This is more than the level that triggers an FDA recall of cow's milk contaminated with PCBs.

1980 Testing by the FDA finds 38 percent of all **grocery foods sampled contain pesticide residues;** by 1998 the FDA will discover that 55 percent of all foods sampled contain pesticides.

1983 A neuroscientist reports that the **artificial sweetener aspartame** may actually increase body weight because it stimulates a craving for calorie-laden carbohydrates.

1985 The medical journal *The Lancet* reports a study in which **79 percent of hyperactive children** improve when **artificial colorings and flavorings** are eliminated from their diet.

1986 The results of a four year study in 803 New York City public schools found students raised their mean academic scores by 15.7 percent when a diet that **reduced the amounts of artificial food colors, flavors and preservatives** they consumed in school cafeterias.

1987 A study by the EPA estimates that everyone alive carries within his or her body at least **seven hundred chemical contaminants,** most of which have not been well studied.

1989 A laboratory study in Boston finds that rats given moderate amounts of **fluoride** in their drinking water give birth to **hyperactive babies**, while baby rats exhibit retardation and other **cognitive defects.** Many Americans are routinely exposed to higher levels of fluoride than the levels administered to the rats.

1992 A University of Utah study finds that water **fluorida-**

tion weakens bones and increases the risk of hip fractures.

The FDA announces a finding that 65 percent of women's **cosmetics** sampled contain **carcinogenic** contaminants.

Application of pesticides on vegetation reaches 750 million pounds a year or three pounds for every man, woman and child in the nation.

Two studies in the *Journal of the Medical Association* report having examined seventy-four thousand men with vasectomies and finding their **prostate cancer risk** has been increased by up to 66 percent as a result of the procedure. Testing conducted by the U.S. Department of Agriculture finds 72 percent of fruits and vegetables contain detectible levels of pesticides. One sample of peaches contained the residues of 14 separate pesticides. DDT was detected in 25 of *food* samples even though it had been banned decades earlier.

1997--A study published in the *Journal of the American Medical Association* reveals that 106,000 people die each year in American Hospitals from the **side effects of prescription medications.**

Adverse drug reactions have become the fourth leading cause of death in the United States.

1998 As of this year, more than 25,000 cosmetics chemicals are in use. Less than 4 percent of these cosmetic have been tested for side effects. The United States Public Health Service issues a warning that **vaccinations are exposing many infants to quantities of mercury** well above safe levels.

2000-*The American Journal of Epidemiology* reports that after five decades of usage, the anti-**depressants** imipramine and amitriptyline are associated with increased rates of breast cancer.

Three drugs previously approved by the FDA - Lotronex for irritable bowel, Propolsid for heartburn, and Rezulin for diabetes—are **withdrawn** after patients experience intestinal damage, heart arrhythmia, and liver toxicity.

Physicians for Social Responsibility releases a report describing an **epidemic of developmental, learning, and behavioral disabilities** affecting an estimated twelve million children in the United States. Evidence suggests the epidemic may be the result of **toxic chemicals affecting the central nervous system of** these children.

2002 -The U.S. pharmaceutical industry now employs 675 lobbyists, including 26 former members of Congress, and spends $91 million a year on influencing decisions made by Congress.

The combined **profits of the ten largest U.S. Drug companies** reach 35.9 billion, a sum higher than the combined profits for all of the 490 corporations on the Fortune 500 list of largest corporations.

For the first time since 1958, the **infant mortality rate increases.** It is now twice that of Japan and most other industrialized nations.

2003-As of this date, 80 percent of the soy and 38 percent of the corn planted in the United States are **genetically engineered** and show up in 70 percent of all **processed foods.**

The Centers for Disease Control and Prevention reports that of all the babies born in the United States in 2000, at least **one-third will become diabetic.**

2005--Two science studies in the journal, *Circulation,* turn up evidence that the **entire class of painkillers known as COX-2 inhibitors puts users at risk of heart attacks and strokes.** The drugs studied were Bextra and Celebrex, both of which remain on the market.

Breast milk sampled from women in 18 states is found to contain traces of perchlorate, a toxic component of rocket fuel.

The journal, *Health Affairs,* reports that about One-half of all personal bankruptcies that occur each year are due to medical bills.

Yale School of Medicine researchers report that low doses

of the contaminant Bisphenol A (BPA), used to make many plastics found in **food storage containers, can lead to learning disabilities in children and neuro-degenerative diseases in adults.**

The FDA reports that two thousand women who used the **acne drug Accutane** while pregnant either had **miscarriages or abortions** because the drug caused severe birth defects in the fetuses.

In the largest study of chemical exposure ever conducted on humans, the Centers for Disease Control finds more than **one hundred toxic substances in the bodies of the 2400 people tested.** Children are found to carry higher levels of these synthetic chemicals in their bodies than adults.

The United States spends more than **twice as much on health care than any other industrialized nation** in the world--$6100 per year for every man, woman, and child.

Fifteen percent of the economy is now devoted to medical care, up from 10 percent in 1987. Yet, the United States ranks forty-sixth in life expectancy and forty-second in infant mortality among the nations of the world. [79]

Other authors such as Kevin Trudeau made great contributions to our knowledge of the dangers of the chemicals that pervade our society as described below:

Virtually everything you put in your mouth has pesticides, herbicides, antibiotics, chemical additives, growth hormone, or genetically altered foods. All of our fruits, vegetables, grains, nuts and seeds are grown with highly poisonous chemical fertilizers, pesticides and herbicides. Many have been genetically modified, turning them into poisonous material.

The same conditions apply in the meat industry. Like farmers and other food producers, the meat industry needs to create a lot of product cheaply and quickly, and sell it as high a profit as possible. To that end, the meat industry uses

---

[79] Randall Fitzgerald. *The Hundred-Year Lie.* New York: Dutton, 2006.

growth hormones to speed up the animals' growth (contributing to the record levels of obesity and early puberty in children); antibiotics to keep the animals healthy in unsanitary and inhumane conditions, feeds the animals unnatural feed diets that not only pump more chemicals into the meat, but also so upset the animals systems that they become out of balance and diseased, and pass the imbalances and diseases along to those who consume the meat. Remember, if it's not organic, if man made it, don't eat it.

The same holds true with dairy products. Because of the use of drugs, growth hormones, pasteurization and homogenization, dairy products today are a major health concern. The problem is homogenized and pasteurized milk, and all dairy products, are unnatural. The clusters of molecules in the treated milk are so small that when you ingest them they virtually scar your arteries. They clog up your digestive system, making it very hard to digest food, which is one of the major causes of acid reflux disease obesity, allergies, and constipation. And the scarring of the arteries causes the LDL cholesterol to attach itself to the artery, which is one of the major causes of arteriosclerosis, which is one of the major causes of heart disease. The bottom line is pasteurized and homogenized dairy products are unnatural.

When you eat fish you are only slightly better off. Many kinds of fish are 'farmed,' meaning that highly toxic feed and chemicals are used to make the fish grow unnaturally fast to unnaturally large sizes. Other poisonous chemicals are used in the processing of the fish before sale to consumers. When you consume this 'man-made fish you are also taking in all the poisons and toxins that have been use in their production. Fish in the wild are much better. However, because of the massive dumping of poisonous chemicals into our lakes, rivers and oceans, many wild fish have been found to have abnormally high levels of toxic chemicals in them as well.

What else do we put in our body through our mouth? If it's in a box, if it's in a jar, if it's in a can, it's been processed by the food industry. The food industry, keep in mind, consist of publicly traded corporations that have one objective; to make more money and increase shareholder value. And the way they do that is sell more food, and produce that food at a lower cost. Always remember, it's all about the money. [80]

A chemical barrage has been hurled against the people on earth by the unrestrained use of chemicals and by the pollution of industrial waste. Our government leaders have failed in their responsibility to protect the earth and the people all over the world are suffering as the result. The illnesses and destruction of many life forms, as evidenced by the increasing number of endangered species, must be brought under control before all life forms will be destroyed. There are those who say the issues are too complex or that we need to do more research before we take any action. As you can see from the evidence presented above there is an urgent need to take action now. Fortunately, there are groups of concerned people who are taking action by forming organizations to protect the environment such as the National Religious Partnership for the Environment founded in1992. The need for action NOW is eloquently expressed by Loretta Schwarts-Nobel as follows:

We stand at a dangerous crossroad. But we still have the capacity to think, to see, to understand, to express outrage, and to act on it collectively. The choice, after all, is still ours.

This is the time for action and outrage. The efforts of every parent, every person of faith, and every person of goodwill must continue and increase. We must all become pivotal in shaping new doctrine. Religious groups and leaders must increase the strength of their power, their numbers, and their voices, because the earth has become a battlefield that is chaotic, unmanageable, and impossible to control without their wisdom and collective leadership.

It is time for the politicians, businessmen, scientists, and watchdog agencies at the highest levels, which are 'playing God' or yielding to bribes and pressure to be restrained. It is time for the military to stop telling us its job is to protect us while it poisons our water, food, and air and sickens and kills our children.

It is time for the drug companies to stop injecting the innocent children of the world with vaccines containing thimerosal, a known neurotoxin, and lying about it simply because it allows them to pro-

---

[80] Kevin Trudeau. *Natural Cures 'They Don't Want You to Know About.'* Elk Grove Village, IL: Alliance Pub., 2004, pp. 78-81.

duce vaccines in bulk and increase their profit.

It is time for the cancer industry to stop misleading women with deadly conflicts of interest, ionizing radiation, and false representations of the effectiveness and safety of mammograms. It is time the cancer industry began the real search for the environmental causes of cancer.

It is time for every single one of us to fight as if our lives depend upon it - because they do!

I still believe that there is hope, even a bright side, and an opportunity that awaits us if we collectively and passionately choose to take it....We must not throw up our hands, and we cannot remain indifferent. Why should we accept, as if there were no alternative, the casual and careless and ever –increasing contamination of the world we have been given simply for profit? Why should we allow our lives and the lives and health of our children, born and yet unborn, to be compromised and stolen by a ruthless few? Surely we have the strength and wisdom not to be mesmerized and controlled and fed like animals to our own slaughter. [81]

It is apparent from the documented evidence presented above that many of the diseases and irrational behaviors occurring in our society are due to the contamination of our food, medicines and water by the widespread use of synthetic chemicals.

Children are more vulnerable than adults to these chemical poisons and it is reflected in the large increase of children being diagnosed as having ADHD. The following section deals with this problem and offers suggestions as to what can be done to help these children.

---

[81] Op. cit., Loretta Schwarts-Nobel, pp. 177-178.

CHAPTER SIX

ADD & ADHD

Causes and Cures

Attention deficit hyperactivity disorder, ADHD, is a label being placed on an alarmingly large number of school children. There are several problems associated with this labeling of children. First of all it is not a disease. It is a behavior problem that includes such annoying behavior (mostly to teachers and some parents) such as poor school or work performance, hyperactivity, lack of attention, and misbehavior. Much of this problem is caused by the synthetic chemicals that children are exposed to such as the artificial colors, sweeteners, and flavorings which are used in cookies, candies and many other foods that children consume. A study reported in the medical journal, The Lancet, in 1985 found that 79 percent of hyperactive children improved when artificial colorings and flavorings were eliminated from their diet. Other studies indicate that toxic chemicals such as mercury and thimerosal used in vaccinations are linked to ADHD. Other important factors to consider are diet, exercise and environmental things such as TV, electronic games and lack of sunshine.

As a teacher of children with learning disabilities, I can tell you from my first-hand experiences that there have been an ever larger number of children being labeled each year as having learning problems and/or behavior problems. My own experience with these children is that they usually respond very well to a supportive teacher who makes use of positive reinforcement and methods that provide for successful experiences for the child. An improved diet for these children also helped them considerably.

There are alternative ways of successfully helping children over-come their disabilities which will be gone into after the following presentation of the serious drug problems associated with ADHD. Instead of looking into the causes of the problem, the usual procedure is to refer the child to a school's learning disability specialist and/or Child Study Team for evaluation and then to a psychiatrist who in most cases will prescribe a drug such as Ritalin to control the prob-lem. The harmful side-effects of these drugs have been well-documented. There are so many dangers involved with the giving of drugs to children that it is of the utmost importance that everyone be made fully aware of the full extent of the problem. The results of recent studies illustrate the extent of the problem and point the way to overcome the problem. You cannot depend on school authorities or doctors in this situation. They have failed miserably as the records show, but armed with the information that is provided below positive steps can be taken by anyone who is willing to be responsible for the welfare of children and for society at large.

The following information about drugs and ADHD was pre-sented in the May, 2008 issue of the Douglas Report:

Candy from a doctor: cocaine, lollipops and morphine, bub-ble gum....

Surprised? You shouldn't be - not when you consider their well-documented side effects. This list should scare the you-know-what out of any parents with children on such drugs. I won't take six pages to describe the deadly side effects, but I'll hit a few of the more serious ones. Take a look: heart attacks, growth problems, blood disorders, and psychosis. (That's right— we're talking a severe mental disorder that brings about delusions and hallucinations.)

Travis Thompson, Ph.D., from the University of Minnesota and Klaus R. Unna, M.D., from the University of Illinois re-ported that 'perhaps the best-known effect of chronic stimulant administration is psychosis. Psychosis has been associated with chronic use of several stimulants, such as, amphetamines, me-thylphenidate, phenmetrazine, and cocaine.'

It gets worse. Children who are or have been on ADHD drugs

have an increased risk of committing suicide.

Remember Tom Cruise's shameless attack of Brook Shields for taking the post-natal anti-depressant drug Paxil? I don't necessarily agree with his approach, but I do agree with the message—any drug that alters your brain chemistry should be avoided like the plague. There's no end to the potential damage it could do. And when it comes to kids taking ADHD drugs, the effects can be especially devastating.

Even the American Psychiatric Association admits that suicide is the major adverse reaction of withdrawal from these drugs. Clarke reports that "symptoms usually peak within two to four days after withdrawal of the drugs although depression and irritability may persist for months. Suicide risk can persist for years. Studies have shown that approximately 15 percent of the children on ADHD drugs will threaten, attempt, or actually commit suicide by the age of 18." He goes on to explain that most psychiatrists blame the withdrawal effects on "underlying mental illness coming to the surface." What quackery!! These ghouls are killing our children! How dare they blame it on the parents' or the child's genes!

But even the kids who are lucky enough to escape such "side effects" are still faced with increased risks of drug abuse and a criminal lifestyle.

Want specifics? Here's the nightmarish truth about what I like to call the King of Speed (from a National Institute for Mental Health study mentioned in Clarke's essay):

46 percent of the children raised on these drugs are charged with at least one major felony by the time they reach 18.

30 percent are charged with two or more such crimes by the age of 18.

25 percent of these children are locked up in mental institutions or prisons by age 18 (remember that psychosis is a known side effect)

15 percent will threaten, attempt, or actually commit suicide by age of 18.

Susan Schenk, a psycho-pharmacologist from Texas A&M

University, conducted a study of 5,000 children with ADHD from adolescence to adulthood and concluded that children treated with ADHD drugs are three times more likely to use cocaine.

When you put it that way, it becomes painfully obvious why children experience such drastic withdrawal effects when coming off such drugs. Imagine force-feeding a child cocaine multiple times a day for years, trying to "wean" him off the drug, and then blaming the inevitable withdrawal effects on an underlying brain disease! Yes, I know. It's absurd. That's my whole point.

This is your brain on drugs...

The drug makers say that no studies have been done showing that ADHD drugs are safe or unsafe to use long-term. I have two things to say about that. First, if they really have no idea whether they're safe to take the drugs for long periods of time, WHY on earth are they giving them to children for years on end?

But besides that, long-term studies HAVE been done on the drugs. They're not telling you about them because not one of them came out the way they would like.

Doctor Joan Baizer, a professor of physiology and biophysics at the University of Buffalo, led a study on brain changes due to methylphenidate, the generic name for a number of ADHD drugs. "Clinicians consider [methyphenidate] to be short-acting," she said. "When the active dose has worked its way through the system, they consider it 'all gone.' Our research with gene expression in an animal model suggests that it has the potential for causing long-lasting changes in brain cell structure and function." Just like long-term use of any Schedule II stimulant drug.

Most parents and teachers think the drugs are necessary in order for the children to learn and to be successful in school. In reality, studies have shown that they lead to brain shrinkage. Brain shrinkage!! One of the studies, published as far back as 1986 in Psychiatry Research, showed that young male adults who had taken methylphenidate drugs for a period of time actually had mild cerebral atrophy (a.k.a., brain shrinkage).

Ten years later, another study, this one published in the Archives of General Psychiatry, found that "subjects with ADHD had a 4.7 percent smaller total cerebral volume." Ninety-three percent of the subjects (53 of 57) had been treated with psycho-stimulants.

At the American Society of Adolescent Psychology in 1998, a psychologist named James Swanson reported on research that showed brain atrophy in children with ADHD. Interestingly, the brain atrophy did not show up in controls. I can only assume that by "controls," he means children not "diagnosed" with ADHD—and not taking any methylphenidate drugs.

Sure, there was shrinkage all right. But it had nothing to do with ADHD and everything to do with the drug. When neurologist Fred Baughman, M.D., questioned Swanson on this point, Swanson reluctantly admitted that 93 percent of the subjects in the study had been on chronic stimulant therapy.

With this research, Swanson and his colleagues had proven the case that methylphenidate is the disease producer and is a cure for nothing. Dr. Baughman said, "Instead of confirmation of brain atrophy due to ADHD ...we had strong, replicated, evidence that it was the stimulant therapy (methylphenidate, amphetamine) that was the cause of the brain atrophy."

Of course, this acknowledgment was conveniently left out of Swanson's lecture and was also missing from his review of this research in a February 1998 Lancet article. To admit this would be shooting himself in the foot, and shooting a serious—if not fatal—blow to the Big Pharma methylphenidate money machine.

Here's a novel idea: State medical associations should introduce to their legislatures a bill that will require all patients being put on ADHD drugs to have a brain scan before treatment is initiated. The tragic result—brain shrinkage—would prove, once and for all, that psychiatrists have been assaulting and killing our children for decades. It would be hard to cheat on a test like this. Radiologists are generally neutral on these medical issues. Besides, they're obsessed with accuracy in their reports. As they should be.

Put a stop to psychiatric witch hunts...

How did it get this bad? What parent would allow his child to put such a mind-altering, life-shattering substance into his body?

And not just allow his child to do so—but actually force him to?

The lies told to parents about ADHD drugs are outrageous and criminal. They are panicked into believing their children are mentally ill and need early treatment to avoid a life of crime, drug addiction, and early death. Despite all the evidence, this drug has survived (even though many of its young victims have not) only because the criteria for making the diagnosis of attention deficit disorder are vague and unscientific labels created by medicine's step-children, the sorcerers of psychiatry.

If parents knew the actual "criteria" that comprise the so-called mental disorder, and if they knew the facts about the drug, there would be an outright rebellion and millions of lawsuits. The result would be death to ADHD drugs and, hopefully, the professional death to all of the psychiatrists involved in this mass felony committed against our children.

Everything about this disorder is contradictory. They say it's a neurological brain disorder, which is what justifies the use of the stimulant drugs to treat it. Therefore, the only people qualified to diagnose children suspected of having ADHD are neurologists. Instead, school teachers suggest the diagnosis and send the unfortunate children to psychiatrists—the people responsible for emotional and behavioral pr problems—to confirm the diagnosis and write the prescription.

If ADHD is REALLY the neurological disease the medical world wants you to think it is the people diagnosing your children are the ones LEAST qualified to do so. And it shows in their drastic over-diagnosis and misdiagnosis of the disease.

Baughman said, "Throughout the eighties and nineties, I witnessed the exploding ADHD epidemic. Just as it was my duty to every patient to diagnose actual disease when it was present, it was equally my duty to make clear to them that they had no disease when that was the case—when no abnormality could be found. That was the case with every child and adult referred with a diagnosis of ADHD...

Neither could I find validation of ADHD in the medical scientific literature...In 40 years of pseudo-scientific research, 'biological psychiatry' has yet to validate a single psychiatric condition or diagnosis as an abnormality/disease, or as anything neuro-logical, biological, chemically imbalanced or genetic.

Drug companies should be held criminally libel for running ads with the false message of a chemical imbalance among our children. What chemical imbalance have they proven to exist? None. Unless Dexedrine, Alderall, or Ritalin deficiency is a newly discovered disease.

The whole scam is incredibly medieval, if you ask me. It reminds me of the 17th century witch-hunts. To determine if a woman was a witch, the accusers would tie a large rock to her ankles and throw her in a lake. If she survived the test, she was declared guilty. And if she didn't survive, well...

Today's psychiatric witch hunters believe that if the child becomes adequately brain numb and malleable, the medicine is working. But if he kills his parents, well, the medicine just brought out an "underlying psychopathology," and it would have happened eventually anyway. It's a win-win situation for the drug makers. Mighty convenient, if you ask me.

Think outside the box: alternatives to the King of Speed...

If you have children or grandchildren in first grade or higher, they are in great danger from health authorities in the school system. These people—nurses, social workers, teachers, psychologists, psychiatrists, etc.—are, in general, fanatical about getting your child doped up. No surprise there: It makes everyone's job easier to subdue the hyperactivity of a child through drugs.

I'm not denying that many, if not most, of today's children are hyperactive with a short attention span—and that it's enough to drive any levelheaded teacher to the brink of insanity. But can you really blame the children? When their diets consist mainly of sugary stimulants (soda, candy, fast food, you name it), it's no wonder they're bouncing off the walls and are unable to concentrate! And when you add that to the startling lack of discipline doled out by insecure parents who just want to be "friends" with their children, teachers don't look quite so bad for wanting to take the easy route. I'm still not letting them off the hook, though.

Most of the problems of these boisterous and aggressive

children (usually boys) can be solved by dietary modifications. If you're a regular reader of The Douglass Report, this needs no elucidation. If you're not a regular reader, I'll summarize it in one sentence: Eliminate all sugar and starch, sodas like Coke and Pepsi, and diet drinks, and feed your children and grandchildren a diet of fat (Omega fish oil and flaxseed oil) and protein. If that's not specific enough for you, read Nourishing Traditions by Sally Fallen of the Weston A. Price Foundation. (You can order it by going online at (westonprice.org)

Put a stop to widespread OTC drug abuse...By now, it should be obvious to you that it's plenty dangerous for children to take even the prescribed dose of an ADHD drug. But it doesn't end there. An increasing number of children are abusing their pre-scriptions—or are peddling them to those who are more than willing to trade their lunch money to get a fix. These days, teens and preteens across the country are snorting crushed methyphe-nidate and popping Adderol like Altoids just to stay up late and cram for a test or to stop eating long enough to fit into their prom dresses.

I can just imagine their thought process: My mom gave it to me. It can't be that bad.

From there, it's just a small step to intentionally abusing other prescription and over-the-counter medications to get high. In fact, the Partnership for a Drug-Free America (PDFA) reports that this is now "an entrenched behavior" among today's teen population. They say that nearly one in five teens (19 percent, which totals about 4.5 million) report abusing prescription medi-cations (whether it's the speedy ADHD drugs in question or painkillers like Vicodin and Oxycontin) to get high, and one in 10 (that's about 2.4 million) report abusing cough medicine to get high. These statistics are even higher than those for the abuse of ecstasy, cocaine, crack, and methamphetamine combined.

This study removes any doubt that intentional abuse of medi-cations among teens is a real issue threatening the health and well-being of American families," said Steve Pasierb, president and CEO of the partnership. (This report has no attribution and is believed to be a press release from the Partnership for a Drug-Free America.)

There is a shocking indifference of government, schools, the Environmental Protect Protection Agency, the Surgeon General (who is nothing but a mouthpiece for the president), and the Centers for Disease Control and Prevention (CDCP). It's alarming, to say the least. These statistics provided by the PDFA say it all:

1. Two in five teens (40 percent or 9.4 million) agree that Rx medicines, even if they are not prescribed by a doctor, are much 'safer' to use than illegal drugs;

2. Nearly one-third of teens (31 percent or 7.3 million) believe there's "nothing wrong" with using Rx medicines without a prescription "once in a while;"

3. Nearly three out of 10 teens (29 percent or 6.8 million) believe prescription pain relievers——even if not prescribed by a doctor—are not addictive; and

4. More than half of teens (55 percent or 13 million) don't agree strongly that using cough medicines to get high is risky."

It's obvious that today's teens have a false sense of security about abusing prescription and OTC drugs. The good news is that because of the vigorous efforts of the PDFA, there's a downward trend in the abuse of these dangerous compounds. They have taken the wise course of informing parents so that they can enlighten their children. This is freedom of action at its best (a nice change of pace, since we both know that government action is usually counterproductive).

Support the Partnership for a Drug-Free America with your time and your money. I do. And I believe that you could never make a better investment. [82]

The above information provides dramatic proof of the relationship between inadequate diet and the saturation of our foods and medicines with synthetic chemicals as the chief causes of the high incidence of ADD and ADHD. Instead of relying on medications to control these ailments we should put to use our knowledge of healthy nutrition and keep synthetic chemicals from entering the bodies of our children. Pregnant women should make use of the knowledge contained in this book to help create normal, healthy children. Also,

---

[82] William Douglas II, MD. *The Douglas Report.* May, 2007, pp.1-8.

avoid shots and vaccinations, both for yourself and for your children. (see section in this book on Immunization)

The Feingold Diet

A pediatrician, Dr. Ben Feingold, became interested in the relationship between diet and hyperactive, learning disabled children back in the 1970s. He wrote two books, the first one was titled *Why Your Child is Hyperactive.* The second book, *The Feingold Cookbook for Hyperactive Children,* includes many recipes based on his recommended diet which came to be known as the "Feingold Diet.' Parents who followed his advice were delighted with the results. His books became very popular. He received numerous letters from all over the world from parents who wanted to thank him for the improvement in their children's lives, as described below:

No longer are all the letters plaintive cries expressing desperation (For God's sake, please help!) or guilt (What have we done wrong?). There are now growing numbers of success stories, often dramatic, in response to dietary management. Instead of distraught parents and a disrupted home, the family life is now serene and happy; instead of conflict with peers, the children enjoy the companionship of playmates; instead of failure and frustration at school, the children's scholastic performance is not only satisfactory but frequently reported as excellent. All this is achieved without the crutch of medication, which masks the underlying condition and cures nothing. The experiences of the many thousands of children, their parents, and their teachers have led to a sharpening of our understanding of this complex clinical pattern. We have learned from the many questions and problems that at times confront parents when they undertake dietary management for their children. Those questions are the basis for many of the answers that follow. How do you know your child is hyperactive? If a child's behavior is extremely disturbed, no professional advice may be required to make a diagnosis. Symptoms of sleeplessness, hyperactivity, aggressiveness, destructiveness, abusiveness, short attention span, and inability to concentrate for more than a few moments are obvious. Occasionally, the child may not be particularly hyperactive but may have an assortment of other deficits, for example short attention span, inability to concentrate, aggression, etc. Such children may fail to do well at school.

An estimated 10 to 15 percent of pupils in the United States were diagnosed with some form of attention deficit disorder, ADD or attention deficit hyperactivity disorder, ADHD. Though scientists disagree on the exact causes of ADD and similar disabilities, an increasing body of research supports the theory that the highly organized music of Mozart can greatly benefit children and adults who suffer from them. This is welcome news to parents of the more than one million American children who take Ritalin, an amphetamine, for ADD every day.

Dr. Feingold identified two major groups of foods and additives which his research indicated were the chief causes of hyperactivity and learning problems. He offers very detailed explanations of why each item must be removed from the diet in order to achieve the benefits of his diet. He describes the two groups as follows:

Group One is made up of all foods that contain synthetic colors and synthetic flavors plus two preservatives: the anti-oxidants: butylated hydroxytoluene (BHT) and *butylated* hydroxyanisole (BHA).

Synthetic (Artificial) colors may be listed as <u>U.S. certified, certified, FD&C approved, or USDA approved). Each of these terms indicates synthetic or artificial color.</u> *Synthetic (artificial) flavors* may be listed as 'flavoring' or 'artificial flavoring.' Both types should be eliminated. Note: Vanillin is usually a synthetic product. Caramel is usually chemically treated and should be eliminated. Most pediatric medications contain artificial coloring or flavoring or both. Malt flavoring should be eliminated.

BHT and BHA are antioxidant preservatives used to prevent oils and fats from going rancid. They are very commonly incorporated into cooking fats, and cooking oils. Be sure to read labels carefully. *If in doubt do not use the product.*

In addition the following sundry items should be eliminated: Practically all pediatric medications. Most of the over-the-counter medications. All toothpastes and tooth powders. All mouth-washes, cough drops, and lozenges. Perfumes and most aromatic sprays, for example, deodorizers, disinfectants, and insecticides. All chewing gums contain BHT, and sugar-less gum also contains synthetic sugars, synthetic flavors and, at times, colors. Finger paints and play dough used by children at home or at school contain artificial coloring.

Group Two of the diet eliminates a number of fruits, vegetables, beverages, and medications with a salicylate radical which many children are highly sensitive to. There are many foods that cause adverse reactions in individuals who are predisposed or allergic to, but they are not necessarily salicylate-containing foods. The question is frequently raised, 'Does cane sugar cause hyperactivity?' The answer is, sugar does cause hyperactivity in some individuals. We are unquestionably in a 'sweet tooth' culture. Cane sugar consumption over the last one hundred years has increased over twenty-five fold, from four pounds to over one hundred pounds per person per year. Short term and long-term ill effects have been indicated.

In addition to the immediate problems of behavioral disturbance, one must be mindful of the long-term detrimental effects of sugar, for example, predisposition to obesity, diabetes, dental caries, and perhaps even heart disease with hypertension. [83]

It has also been observed that getting outside to play outdoors for at least 20 minutes each day works as well as drugs in kids with attention problems. This is no doubt due to the importance of being exposed to sunlight which provides the best source of vitamin D3 which is essential to health and well-being. Everyone needs an adequate amount of vitamin D3, especially growing children. The need to accept children with learning problems as they are, without placing them under undue stress, is a very important aspect of the problem. Parents should make every effort to prevent their children from being labeled.

---

[83] Ben Feingold, MD and H. Feingold. *The Feingold Cookbook for Hyperactive Children*. New York: Random House, 1979, pp.3-16.

Dr. Jacob Liberman does an excellent job of summarizing the true nature of the learning disabilities problem in his book, *LIGHT: Medicine of the Future,* as follows:

Any treatment should be considered from the perspective of whether it is aimed at the *cause* of the problem or the *effect* of the problem. Having been a non-reading, hyperactive child with all the symptoms of a learning disability, I can fully appreciate how miraculous it would have felt to me as a child if I had been, all of a sudden, able to read easily. The real question, however, is what caused me to shut down that part of my learning ability as a child. Why was it that most of the children with whom I went to school with didn't like school? Could our teaching methods, or the high demands placed on children to learn to read early, have something to do with their learning problems? Having worked with thousands of children and adults with learning difficulties, it has become increasingly evident to me that they *all show signs of fear.* Is it the learning difficulty that causes the fear or the fear that causes the learning difficulty? And, if the latter, what causes the fear?

For years we have been labeling and relabeling children who appear to have difficulties we do not understand. We test and tutor them continually, only to find out that they are usually bright but, that for some reason outside of our understanding, they do not achieve in the expected manner within the traditional learning environment. Although the labels for these children have changed from dumb, stupid, and lazy to dyslexic, minimally brain dysfunctional and learning disabled to ADD and ADHD, the labels nonetheless scar them for life. Einstein, Beethoven and Edison were thought to be hopeless, stupid, or mentally slow. How many of these so-called learning-disabled individuals will it take to show us that what we think describes a learning problem may be characteristic of a different creative expression of intelligence? Many truly brilliant individuals consistently achieve below their potential level because they get frightened and freeze up in an academic environment. [84]

---

[84] Jacob Liberman, OD, PhD. *LIGHT: Medicine of the Future.* New York: Bear & Co., 2001.

Dr. Lieberman also provides the results of research showing that natural light plus various color therapies can improve the behavior and learning abilities of children with learning disabilities. (See Chapter 12 pp. 315-322)

The author of the best-seller, *Heal the Body,* Louise Hay, came to the conclusion that practically all illness and disabilities are due to negative patterns of thinking about ourselves. Much of this negative thinking is instilled in early childhood by poor parenting, poor schooling and social conditioning which inculcates fear and guilt in the mind. She spent many years studying techniques for undoing the damage of negative thinking and came up with specific instructions on how to replace negative thoughts with positive thoughts. She found specific cures for each of the illnesses. Here is what she had to say:

How often have we said, 'that's the way I am' or that's the way it is.' What we are saying is that is what we 'believe to be true for us.' Usually what we believe is only someone else's opinion we have accepted and incorporated into our own belief system. It fits in with other things we believe. If we were taught as a child that the world is a frightening place, then everything we hear that fits in with that belief, we will accept as true for us. 'Don't trust 'strangers,' 'People cheat you,' 'Don't go out at night,' etc. On the other hand if we were taught early in life that the world is a safe and joyous place, then we would believe other things. 'Love is everywhere,' People are so friendly,' 'Money comes to me easily,' and so on. Life experiences mirror our beliefs. For instance, I could ask myself, 'Why do I believe it is difficult for me to learn? Is that really true? Is it true for me now? Where did that belief come from? Do I still believe it because a first-grade teacher told me over and over? Would I be better off if I dropped that belief?

Stop for a moment and catch your thought. What are you thinking right now? If thoughts shape your life and experiences, would you want this thought to become true for you? If we want a joyous life, we must think joyous thoughts. Whatever we send out mentally or verbally will come back in like form. Be willing to change your words and thoughts and watch your life change. The way to control your life is to control your choice of words and thoughts. No one thinks in your mind but you.

We have learned that for every effect in our lives, there is a thought pattern that precedes and maintains it. Our consistent thinking patterns create our experiences. Therefore, by changing our thinking patterns, we can change our experience.

Take full responsibility for your own health without either reproaching yourself or feeling guilty. Begin to learn how to avoid creating thought patterns of disease in the future. In order to permanently eliminate a condition, we must first work to dissolve the mental cause. This can be done by making use of positive affirmations that have been identified as curative for specific ailments. This book provides a helpful guide for building new thought patterns that can heal disease.

The mental thought patterns that cause the most disease in the body are CRITICSM, ANGER, RESENTMENT, and GUILT. For instance, criticism indulged in long enough will often lead to diseases such as arthritis. Anger turns into things that boil and burn and infect the body. Resentment long held festers and eats away at the self and ultimately can lead to tumors and cancer. Guilt always seeks punishment and leads to pain. It is so much easier to release these negative thing patterns from our minds when we are healthy than to try to dig them out when we are in a state of panic and under the threat of the surgeon's knife. A few examples of specific ailments with their probable cause and positive thought patterns that are known to help cure the condition are shown below:

High Blood Pressure (Hypertension)

Probable Cause: Long standing emotional problem, not solved.

New Thought Pattern: *I joyously release the past. I am at peace.*

Boils

Probable Cause: Anger. Boiling over Seething.

New Thought Pattern: I express love and joy and I am at peace.

Bladder Problems

Probable Cause: Anxiety. Holding on to old ideas. Fear of letting go. Being *pissed off.*

New Thought Pattern: *I comfortably and easily release the old and welcome the New in my life. I am safe.*

Cataracts

Probable Cause: Inability to see ahead with joy. Dark future.

New Thought Pattern: *Life is eternal and filled with joy. I look forward to every moment.*

Candida (Yeast Infections)

Probable Cause: Feeling very scattered. Lots of frustration and anger. Demanding and untrusting in relationships. Great takers.

New Pattern: *I give myself permission to be all that I can be and deserve the very best in life. I love and appreciate myself and others.*

Cancer

Probable Cause: Deep hurt. Longstanding resentment. Deep secret or grief eating away at the self. Carrying hatreds. 'What's the use'?

New Pattern: *I lovingly forgive and release all of the past. I choose to fill my world with joy. I love and approve of myself.*

Eye Problems

Probable Cause: Not liking what you see in your own life.

New Pattern: *I now create a life I love to look at.* [85]

---

[85] Louise Hay. *Heal Your Body.* Carlsbad, CA: Hay House, 1982, pp. 4-23.

CHAPTER SEVEN

DANGEROUS THINGS TO AVOID

Antibiotics

There are a number of reasons why antibiotics should be avoided. The first problem is that antibiotics can only kill bacteria. They do not have any effect on viruses although they are used for that purpose. In the process of killing bacteria, important strains of beneficial bacteria in the body are killed off together with harmful bacteria. The second problem is that harmful bacteria that survive become drug resistant and over time cannot be killed by antibiotics. As a result of the weakening of the good bacteria and the strengthening of the bad bacteria, our immune systems go haywire leaving us more vulnerable to infectious diseases.

A lack of good bacteria in the body has been linked to many illnesses such as: diarrhea, ulcers, allergies, asthma, celiac, cancer, food poisoning, and obesity. The message is clear, stay clear of antibiotics. The best thing to do is to boost your immune system and increase the number of good bacteria by taking probiotic supplements daily. The best kinds of probiotics are the ones that have many strains and have at least 30 billion active cells. They can be found in health food stores and in health mail order company catalogs.

Fluoride in water and toothpaste

The discovery of fluoride's ability to fight cavities and tooth decay began with experiments by Dr. Basil Bibby, MD, in the early 1940's. Bibby found that if a little bit of fluoride was put on a cotton swab and applied to a decayed tooth, the tooth could be saved. Although the benefits of fluoride are topical, its risks are primarily systemic. Medical literature reveals many study results which indicate that there are negative health effects of fluoride. Most of us have had fluoride in our drinking water for many years. Why? The following excerpt from the book *Ultimate Healing* presents the historical background of how fluoride came into use:

"As early as the 1930s, the manufacturers of aluminum needed something to do with the sodium fluoride that was a by-product of the aluminum smelting process. When they became aware of Dr. Bibby's research, a campaign was mounted to convince the American Dental Association to accept fluoride as a topical anti-cavity treatment so that it could be advocated for general use in toothpaste. In 1950, the Public Health Service authorized the use of fluoride in water systems as a way to get fluoride to the general public as a tooth-decay preventative agent.

During the 1960s and 1970s, heavy phosphate mining for fertilizers produced another type of fluoride as a by-product - fluorosilic acid. This time, the industry got rid of the new type of fluoride by marketing it to municipalities as a less expensive alternative to sodium fluoride and most municipalities in the US bought it. *Scary:* 89 percent of communities now fluoridate with the less expensive fluorosilic acid instead of the traditional sodium fluoride. A water specialist, Dr. conducted water tests and learned that the combination of fluorosilic acid with low level chlorine added to water resulted in a high level of lead." [86]

In 1955, Dr. Benjamin Nesin, director of laboratories for the New York City Water Dept. summed up his views by saying:

"Never in the history of water supply has a substance so toxic in nature, with such a high degree of physiological potency and associated with so much adverse evidence affecting the health of the public, been seriously considered for introduction into public water

---

[86] Editors of Bottom Line. "*More Ultimate Healing.*" Boardman, 2007, p. 242

supplies." [87]

Fluoridation has now been linked to Alzheimer's disease according to Dr. Douglas in his article in the Summer 2009 issue of the Douglas report. For further information see the section in this book on Alzheimer's disease. Additional dangers of fluoridation are described by Dr. Bruce West as follows:

Is the alarming rise in cases of hypothyroid and diabetes related in any way to **fluoride?** Lots of experts think so. Fluoride is the most active of the halogens, which also include iodine and chlorine. In fact fluoride displaces iodine in the thyroid hormone, making it unusable in your body - the definition of hypothyroidism. Fluoride also disrupts certain proteins in your body that are critical in getting hormones into your cells - a definition of type 2 diabetes. So how did we get duped into mandating fluoride in the form of *hydrofluosilicic acid* for medicinal use? How did we get duped into having this toxic acid, defined by the Environmental Protection Agency as an 'extremely hazardous waste,' added to two-thirds of our public water systems by gullible cities? How did we get duped into having this fluoride chemical, which is so toxic and radioactive that it can't be legally dumped into any body of water, used in our mouths by dentists? How did we get this extremely toxic waste sold as a remedy to stop tooth decay?

The answer is simple, as always - follows the money. The sale of this poison has turned some corporations' financial red ink into profits. Their industrial waste is sold **unrefined** to be diluted and dumped into municipal water supplies with **no scientific support of its safety or effectiveness in preventing tooth decay.**

What does all this mean for you? It means that if you have any kind of thyroid disease, such as hypothyroidism, or if you have type 2 diabetes, osteoporosis, or kids or infants in the house, **you need to get rid of the fluoride** in your water. And if you have thyroid disease, you also **need to get the chlorine out of your water.** Fluoride and chlorine displace iodine in your thyroid hormone, making it useless in your body. This means that the thyroid hormone that should contain iodine, contains toxic fluoride instead causing or making thyroid disease, osteoporosis, and/or diabetes worse. And

---

[87] Leonard Wickenden. "*Our Daily Poison*". Devin-Adair, 1956, pp. 96-97.

give your kids a chance. Their developing glands and bones need real food and water, not a mash of toxic waste. Never ingest dental fluoride products. And ensure a good supply of pure water without fluoride or chlorine. Unfortunately, this is difficult to do. About the only safe approach is to use a **reverse osmosis water purifier.** [88]

Health Screening

There are periodic free health screenings offered at Senior Citizen Centers and at other locations. Many of the people who are screened are told to have follow-up tests done by their own doctor because some abnormality shows up during the screening. Mammograms are given and many women wind up having more tests done leading in many cases to medication and/or surgery.

An article appeared in the *Washington Post* on November 17, 2009, which was widely quoted in other newspapers around the country with bold front page headlines saying: **"Cut back on mammograms, fed panel urges."** The article went on to say:

"In its first reevaluation of breast cancer screening since 2002, the panel that sets government policy on prevention recommended the radical change, citing evidence that the potential harm to women having annual exams beginning at age 40 outweighs the benefits. We are recommending against routine screening There are important and serious negatives or harms that need to be considered carefully."

Dr. West called attention to the potential dangers of a recent medical practice of offering free screenings for many of the common illnesses. On the surface it would seem that this is a worthy endeavor designed to help people, but the facts are just the opposite as Dr West points out in an article in the *Health Alert Newsletter,* as follows:

Health Screenings can be a good tool when they catch something that can be treated early to avoid a catastrophe. Unfortunately, these are the rare instances. For the most part, screenings are moneymaking promotional efforts. They benefit doctors, nurses, medical equipment makers, hospitals, surgeons and most of all, the pharmaceutical companies.

Health screenings in themselves are not too hazardous to your health. But when the findings are false, or when a non-

---

[88] Dr. West. *Health Alert.* Monteray, CA: June, 2009, p.6.

disease is diagnosed as arterial disease, dangers abound. If this happens, you will be referred to your doctor or some other professional for more aggressive testing, followed too frequently by surgery, and or a lifetime of toxic drugs. Therein lies the danger.

One of our patients wrote me a note saying, "Dear Dr. West, my 80 year old mother wants to go to a free health screening sponsored by our church. Is there any danger to her? My answer: there are no **free** health screenings. Rather these are promotional endeavors paid for by the drug companies, medical equipment makers, doctors' unions, and others - who then pass on the cost to you based on the increase in business they garner through these screenings.

"As for your mom, I answered, 'it is probably safe as long as she isn't shuffled into some unnecessary and dangerous follow-up testing and treatment.' A few months later, I heard again from my patient. The following is what happened:

Mrs. Mom was an active, healthy, jovial loving grandmother who had a close relationship with her family and friends. She was not taking any prescription drugs—a miracle for an 80 year old. The health screening would end that miracle quickly.

During the screening she was told that she had high cholesterol at 265 (total), and high blood pressure at 140/90. She was referred to her family physician for further testing. Despite the fact that after age 80, the **higher** your cholesterol the longer you live she was placed on the cholesterol-lowering drug Lipitor. And despite the fact that 140/90 is **normal** at her age, she was put on the blood pressure drug Toprol.

Within days she became completely weak, somnolent (having trance-like sleepiness, depressed, and dizzy. She began to suffer from dyspnea (labored breathing) and lost all interest in life. Alarmed our patient brought his mother to see another doctor. This doctor did not even ask what drugs she was taking. When our patient informed the doctor of her prescriptions, he made no change. Rather, he added a prescription for Zoloft to help with her 'depression.'

The following day Mrs. Mom was so very weak and dizzy that she fainted, fell and broke her hip. Off to the hospital. She was admitted and x-rays revealed that she also had osteoporosis. She was further prescribed the osteoporosis drug Fosamax. This drug was prescribed despite the fact biophosphonate drugs do not help older women maintain and build strong bones—that they are, in fact, implicated in causing irreversible horrifying cases of **necrosis of the mandible** (rotting of the jawbone).

Now Mom was in a life-threatening situation. She struggled along in the hospital through hip replacement surgery and ended up in excruciating pain. Pain medications were started, and she was in the final stages of a downward medical spiral.

Barely able to breathe, she was put on oxygen, later ventilated, and finally incubated (had a tube inserted for breathing). That night, less than 14 days after this still spry, healthy grandma with a twinkle in her eye, had the medical screening, she died. Her blood pressure just before death was 80/40.

It almost seems like this was made up. Unfortunately, over 30 years, I have been witness to hundreds of such cases. Across the country the numbers are absolutely mindnumbing. And very, very few of these cases are ever statistically recorded as medical errors.[89]

Heart Surgery

Julian Whitaker, M.D. calls attention to the failure of heart surgery to benefit heart patients as follows:

Way back in 1983—long before angioplasty became the revenue generating darling of cardiology—the Coronary Artery Study (CASS) was published. This definitive clinical trial was expected to confirm the benefits of bypass surgery in patients with significant heart disease.

Instead, CASS showed that bypass was a bust. Rates of heart attack and death from heart disease were no lower in pa-

---

[89] Dr. West. *Health Alert.* Monteray, CA, Dec., 2006, pp. 2-3.

tients who had surgery than they were in a similar group without surgery. The death rate in the patients who did not have bypass surgery was a surprisingly low 1.6 per cent per year. The chance that any surgery will improve on a death rate this low is virtually nil. It boils down to one indisputable fact. You cannot save the life of someone who is not going to die.

When you weigh the certain pain and cost of surgery against the slim chance of benefit, it's an easy call. Yet today, bypass, angioplasty, and other 'lifesaving' heart procedures continue to be foisted upon more and more folks who don't need them. If hard science and patient benefit were central factors here, these procedures would be a rarity. But invasive surgery has nothing to do with science. It has nothing to do with saving lives or improving quality of life. It has to do with money. Period! [90]

Immunization Shots, Vaccinations

An extensive investigation of the effects of vaccinations on children was made by Dr. John Riker. In a report titled *POLIO VACCINE: MIRACLE OR MYTH,* he summarizes the results of his findings as follows:

"My studies have led me to the following conclusions: (1) vaccinations are dangerous; (2) vaccinations do not work as well as the medical profession and the media have made us believe; and (3) some of the great epidemics of the past have been iatrogenically produced... Iatrogenesis is a term that many medical people do not like to hear. When broken down, we have the term 'iatric,' which is defined as referring to medicine, the medical profession or physicians ; and 'genesis,' meaning the origin of something. Hence, the term, 'iatrogenetic disorder' is defined as any adverse mental or physical condition induced in a patient by effects of treatment by a physician or surgeon. When speaking of this term in conjunction with the polio epidemics of the past, there are two common medical procedures that should come to mind-tonsillectomy and vaccination itself.

"Statistics are one of the pillars of modern science The medical profession very often uses statistics to back up the 'success' of their

---

[90] Dr. Julian Whittaker, MD. *Health and Healing. Vol 17:2,* pp.2-3.

vaccination programs. When properly done, statistics are an invaluable way of assessing a particular program or situation. However statistics are easily manipulated, and when they are, they become an honest person's way of telling a lie.

Professor Bernard Greenberg, former head of biostatistics at the University of North Carolina School of Public Health and chairman of the Committee on Evaluation and standards of the American Public Health Association makes the following statements on the statistical analysis of the efficacy of the Salk vaccine: "...my primary concern, my only concern is the very **MISLEADING** way that most of this data has been handled from a *statistical* point of view... a scientific examination of the data, and the manner in which the data were **MANIPULATED**, will reveal the true effectiveness of the Salk vaccine is UNKNOWN and GREATLY OVERRATED."

One of the scare tactics the American Medical Association used on people via television, radio, and newspapers was to tell them that the attack rate among unvaccinated children was much higher than for those who were vaccinated. This concept was based on statistics that the United States Public Health Service had accumulated.

The following statement by Dr. Greenberg shows the inadequacies of these statistics: "First of all, the unvaccinated population figure for 5 to 9 year old children used in the Public Health Service report was the number given in the 1950 census minus the numbers of children vaccinated. The number of children aged 5 to 9 in 1955 was estimated, however, to be 101,000 more than it was in 1950. The Public Health Service did not take this into account. This omission of 101,000 children from the unvaccinated population would have increased the latter roughly from 236,000 to 337,000 children. Hence, the attack rate for unvaccinated children was **over estimated by 40 percent.**

Dr. Richard Moskowitz, M.D. reached the following conclusions about the polio vaccine: "...it is evident that natural immunity to poliovirus was already as close to being universal as ever it can be. "It is dangerously misleading and, indeed, the exact opposite of the truth to claim that a vaccine makes us 'immune' or protects us against an acute disease If, in fact it only drives the disease deeper into the interior and causes us to have it chronically, with the result that our responses to it become progressively weaker and show less tendency to heal or resolve themselves spontaneously.

"Immunization programs against flu, measles, mumps, polio, and so forth, may actually be seeding humans with RNA to form latent proviruses in cells throughout the body. These latent proviruses could be molecules in search of diseases. When activated, under proper conditions, they could cause a variety of diseases including rheumatoid arthritis, multiple sclerosis, systemic lupus, Parkinson's disease, and perhaps more." [91]

Parents have a right to be angry with the medical profession. Tonsillectomies make a child more susceptible to the most severe forms of the disease, and it was known as far back as 1928 that this procedure increased the risk of getting it – yet, the medical authorities continued to allow this procedure to be recklessly performed on millions of helpless children.

Another iatrogenic link to the polio epidemics of the past was vaccination, not only the polio vaccine itself, but also vaccinations against other diseases….A study published in the *British Medical Journal* in 1950 shows that an immunization drive against diphtheria and pertussis contributed to an outbreak of polio in Great Britain in 1949. During this outbreak, the children who had been vaccinated had a greater incidence of paralysis than those who were not vaccinated.

The article comes to the following conclusion: 'Whichever way we choose to set out the statistics, they clearly reveal an association between recent inoculation and paralysis….We must conclude, therefore, that in the 1949 epidemic of poliomyelitis vaccinated children were at greater risk than the unvaccinated children.

Tonsils are defined as a mass of lymphatic tissue located in the depression of the fauces and the pharynx. Their function is to act as a filter to protect the body from invasion of bacteria, and to aid in the formation of white blood cells. A common childhood ritual, which is still being performed today, is a procedure known as tonsillectomy or removal of one's tonsils.

The late Dr. Mendelson made the following statement about this procedure: 'For decades tonsillectomies were the bread-and-butter surgery for surgeons and pediatricians. During the 1930's, doctors

---

[91] Ibid, pp. 1-10

were doing between 1.5 and 2 million tonsillectomies a year. Few children reached their teens with their tonsils intact, despite the fact their removal could rarely be justified on legitimate medical grounds. For millions of children, the consequences of this purposeless surgery were emotional trauma, loss of natural defense against disease, and in some cases, death. ..I doubt that more than one child in 10,000 requires this surgery, yet hundreds of thousands of tonsillectomies are still performed each year. They result in 100 to 300 deaths, with a complication rate of 16 per 1,000 procedures... This information is enough to discourage one from having this procedure performed on them or their children, but it must also be known that the removal of tonsils makes a child more susceptible to becoming a victim of paralytic poliomyelitis.

An article in the *American Journal of Diseases of Children* (July 1944) comes to the same conclusion: 'tonsils are absent in a significantly high percentage of patients who have bulbar or bulbospinal poliomyelitis. The absence of tonsillar tissue apparently increases the likelihood that the bulbar centers will be involved when a susceptible person becomes infected with the virus of poliomyelitis....It is recommended that the tonsils be no longer removed unless their removal is specifically indicated.' [92]

Vaccine for Chickenpox linked to Shingles

If you have had shingles or know someone who has, you know that it can be a serious, painful, sometimes life-changing, and occasionally deadly event. What you may not know is that a great deal of this suffering, and even death, is a direct result of the never-needed, rejected-by-all-medical-boards, but politically-mandated-for-all-kids-anyway *chickenpox vaccine.*

Both chickenpox and shingles are caused by the same virus—the varicella-zoster virus (VZV). Getting chickenpox provides natural immunity to its close cousin, shingles. And as you get older, this immunity is naturally boosted by contact with children who have chickenpox. But since 1995, when the chickenpox vaccine was mandated, there are fewer and fewer children getting chickenpox, therefore older people are not provided this natural immunity booster. The result of opening this Pandora's vaccine box is fewer children

---

[92] Ibid. p. 8.

with chickenpox, and an epidemic of adult cases of shingles, which have resulted in three times as many deaths and five times the number of hospitalizations as for chickenpox.

I said in 1995 that "chickenpox in kids was not a problem, but that the chickenpox vaccination {which is now the law} debacle could backfire and produce chickenpox in adults (shingles)." And I added, "but unlike the typical impact of the disease in childhood (remember chickenpox parties?), chickenpox poses *serious risks to adults,* such as pneumonia, inflammation of the brain, and some truly nasty cases of shingles and post-shingles neuralgia."

According to public health experts, there would be 42% fewer shingles cases in older adults if the chickenpox vaccine was never instituted. And what are "experts" thinking about all this mess? They are hoping that any shingles epidemic associated with the chickenpox vaccine can be offset by treating adults with a *shingles vaccine."*

Sounds OK, right? And Merck, the maker of the new shingles vaccine, is counting on you to think it is OK. But what do the real experts have to say about all this? "Using a shingles vaccine to control shingle epidemics in adults would likely fail because adult vaccination programs, have rarely proved successful."

This debacle ushers in a whole new era of treating the side effects of vaccines with a new vaccine! Enter *Zostavax*, the shingles vaccine, now approved by the Food and Drug Administration (FDA). Great business for the vaccine makers—Merck estimates that there are 50 million potential American customers over age 50.

This is a fiasco already happening. And it will become standard in the future, even as other vaccines backfire. This cash cow for pharmaceutical companies will result in a *continuous treatment cycle* as a Pandora's Box is opened farther and farther. As natural immunity declines—all thanks to vaccines—a 30% to 50% increase in serious problems like shingles will become routine. But not to worry—as each one develops, another vaccine will be developed to treat its side effects. And who knows there may even be a third and fourth vaccine created to treat problems caused by the second and third. The real way to handle the epidemic of shingles will never come to be. For starters, it would require that we end the ridiculous chickenpox vaccine.

But just what can you do? There is no cure for shingles. But you can prevent and even treat this condition naturally. Maintaining the level of useable (ionized) calcium in your skin and lower skin layers is the key. This is done by using the best calcium supplement in addition to the best calcium delivery supplement *Calcium Lactate* is the best, most easily digested, and most usable form of calcium. *Cataplex F* is the best nutritional delivery system for calcium. These products can be obtained from the Standard Process Company. In addition a daily teaspoon of high quality cod liver oil should be part of your daily regimen. [93]

Another serious consequence of vaccinations is its link to autism. Recent research into autism has indicated that vaccinations can bring on autism. See section in this book on causes and cures of illnesses.

Knee Surgery

According to researcher, Dr. Tom Mathieson, D.O. "Arthroscopic knee surgeries have been proven worthless" Surely this research would have put an end to these knee surgeries, right? Are you kidding? There are more performed now than ever (over 500,000 a year) because they make millions of dollars for doctors, surgery centers, and hospitals. And if you don't get good results, or even if you are crippled (yes, this simple surgery can cripple), it doesn't matter. The surgeon will simply tell you that you don't heal as well as most people." [94]

"For years I have stated that arthroscopic surgeries for arthritic knees were a sham. For years I have also stated that when it comes to knees, no one – either before or after all the scans, MRIs, and X-Rays – really knows what causes the knee pain. I also have stated that torn cartilage and even ligaments often have **nothing at all to do with the pain.** Studies reported in *the New England Journal of Medicine* (2008, Sept. 11; 359:1097 and 1108), showed that my statements are 100 percent correct.

"In these studies, 35% of the people whose knees were examined by MRI showed meniscus (knee cartilage) tear or destruction. Of these people, only **one-third** had any pain at all. And it gets even

---

[93] Ibid, pp. 3-4.
[94] Dr. West. *Health Alert. Vol. 25, No. 7.*

muddier for those people with both arthritis and cartilage tear or destruction. For these people, it was discovered that the cause of the pain is 'unclear.' But you can bet that most surgeons will get into that knee and begin to 'repair' the problem, whether they know what the real cause is or not.

Here is the problem. People do not know that surgeons do not know what is going on with their knees. So they subject themselves to invasive procedures, thinking that they will help. Most of the time these procedures do not help, and they can really, really cause damage. So keep this in mind if your knee is hurting. Arthroscopic surgery for the knee is no more effective than a **fake, sham surgery** where two holes are put into the knee, simulating the repair surgery (*New England Journal of Medicine, Vol. 25, No 7 July 11, 2002*). And whether you have cartilage tear or destruction or other damage that shows on your MRI, no one really knows what is causing your pain. And in most cases, the pain **has nothing to do with the findings on the MRI!**

What to Do:

First find a good therapist who handles knees. Often they are chiropractors or massage therapists. Deep tissue work is very effective. Active Release Technique (ART) is highly recommended. I have seen patients with severe arthritis, torn meniscus cartilage, and damaged tendons and ligaments, get completely better with deep tissue work, or ART. And then, despite all the dire findings on scans and MRIs, the patient gets 100% better – with no surgery at all." [95]

Marijuana

Marijuana is a street drug which is very popular with teenagers and young adults. It is considered to be harmless and non-addictive by those who use it. However, recent research showed that the use of this drug has long-lasting effects. It appears that the brain cells that are turned off by the drug results in a **spacey**, or ecstatic feeling for a short time and the desire to continue the desired feelings leads to its continued use. The real danger that was revealed by the recent study of its long range effects was the finding that even after a person stops taking the drug for a long period of time; the brain continues to react as though the drug was present at any given time without any ad-

[95] Dr. West. *Health Alert. Vol. 26, No. 1, Jan. 2009.*

vance warning. This can happen because the brain cells that produce the high feelings have been programmed to continue the reaction even after the drug is no longer used. This can continue to occur sporadically from time to time for an indefinite period of time. The message is clear: Stay away from all drugs, even those that appear to be harmless.

Milk

Cow's milk is a very dangerous food for humans. As pointed out in the *China Study* referred to above, milk is a leading cause of childhood type 1 diabetes, and is also linked to breast cancer, and many other diseases. Consider this fact, milk is one of the most mucus-forming foods; *Elmers Glue* is made from cow's milk. Fischer has this to say about cow's milk:

"Cow's milk usually comes to us pasteurized, homogenized, and frosty cold, very appetizing indeed. However, I remind you that man is the only creature in the world who continues *unnecessarily* to drink milk after being weaned. If you question the truth of that statement, you should know that the enzymes the human body requires to digest milk gradually disappear and are no longer available to the body after age 3. The calcium present in cow's milk is in a very heavy form, difficult for the human body to process and assimilate efficiently. In addition, this calcium is mixed up with the protein *casein* which is the principal amino acid in cheeses and milk curds. The calcium and casein in cow's milk are easily digested when they pass through the four stomachs of a baby calf, but they have a hard time making it through the human digestive tract. Cow's milk contains 300 times more casein than mother's milk." [96]

Dr. Dan Twogood, a certified kinesiologist and chiropractor studied the relationship between milk consumption and joint pains. Based on his six years of research, including studies of over three thousand patients, he came to the following conclusion: "Casein is the main cause of neck pain, back pain, and headaches." [97]

"To establish a patient's use of dairy products, I ask about each item separately and how often, in an average week, they consume each item: ice cream, sour cream, yogurt, cottage cheese, etc. The

[96] Op. cit. Fischer, pp.270-271.
[97] Dr. Dan Twogood. *No Milk*. P. 31.

average American uses dairy products regularly. When patients convey to me that they seldom use these products, more specific questions are required. Sometimes, just a spot check of a specific meal is revealing. 'What did you have for dinner last night? 'Pizza.'

Okay, they hardly ever have cheese, but they just happened to have some last night. It could happen. At this point, there is no need to doubt a patient's accounting of his or her dietary habits. When a sincere patient reports to me little or no use of dairy products in the diet, I usually say, 'Good, then it will be easy for you to avoid them.

Almost always, these patients return for subsequent visits and say, 'You know, I didn't realize how often I use dairy products until I tried to avoid them.' That's because that is the average American diet, the cause of average American health.

To avoid casein means not only avoid all milk products, but all foods made with milk. All of a sudden the chore becomes more difficult." [98]

Dr. Cousens, an M.D. and homeopathic physician, wrote the following comment about cow's milk: "The milk available today, even raw milk from organic cows is toxic, not pure. It loses prana, clogs the nadis; and could be high in pesticides, herbicides, antibiotics, hormones, radioactive iodine, and disease vectors including Mad Cow prions. This makes it an unacceptable choice for spiritual or healthful living. [99]

Monosodium-Glutamate (MSG)

An article was published in the Summer, 2004 edition of *Wise Traditions,* a publication of the Weston Price Foundation, which presents the dangers of MSG, as follows:

> For purposes of this paper we will report on the neurotoxins MSG (glutamic acid) which has been freed from protein, through a manufacturing process resulting in the formation of glutamic acid and aspartic acid, a breakdown product of the artificial sweetener aspartame. (About 40 percent of aspartame is aspartic acid.)

---

[98] Ibid, pp. 79-81.
[99] Gabriel Cousens. *Spiritual Nutrition.* Berkley, CA: N. Atlantic Books, 2005, p. 262.

In 1969, John W. Olney, M.D., a respected researcher at Washington University Medical School, published a paper on his findings, in which he described the hypothalamic lesions, stunted skeletal development, and obesity in maturing mice which had been given the food ingredient monosodium glutamate. He observed that the mice fed MSG became grotesquely obese.

Since 1969, many scientists have confirmed Dr. Olney's findings of damage to the hypothalamus from MSG with resulting obesity. As of May, 2004, you'll find 151 studies listed in addition to Dr. Olney's studies on the following website: www.pubmed.gov, a National Library of Medicine website.

When asked how the FDA can allow MSG to be used in food, FDA officials stated that one cannot compare the free glutamic acid in supplements to the free glutamic acid in food. Of course, this position is completely untenable since food products contain far more glutamic acid than supplements. Although there are a number of causes for obesity, there is no question in this writer's mind that the main cause for the obesity epidemic is the ever increasing use of MSG and aspartame – free glutamic acid and free aspartic acidin our food supply. MSG is most often found in food as a component of food ingredients with names that give consumers no clue to its presence. It was not used to any extent in this country until the late 1940s, and not widely used until the 1960s. Aspartame was approved by the FDA in 1981. Today most processed foods contain MSG and it is even found in personal care items and pharmaceuticals. According to the NutraSweet Company, aspartame is used in over 5,000 products. As the use of MSG and aspartame grows, the incidence of obesity appears to be growing.

Although there are a number of causes for obesity, there is no question in this writer's mind that the main cause for the obesity epidemic is the ever increasing use of MSG and aspartame. What can be done to stem the obesity epidemic? I would start by identifying the sources of MSG in processed food. MSG should be fully disclosed on processed food labels. Aspartame should be withdrawn from the market. There is no need for aspartame or the recently approved sweetener, neotame, described by some as a super aspartame. [100]

Non-Stick Cookware (Teflon)

Dr. Joseph Mercola, in his best-selling book *Take Control of Your Health,* presents evidence that non-stick cookware such as Teflon, can cause serious damage to vital organs such as the brain, prostate, liver, thymus and kidneys. The problem is something called perfluoroctanoic acid (PFOA) a synthetic chemical used in the production of Teflon and similar non-stick coatings. It's precisely this chemical that creates the slick surface. The reasons given by Dr. Mercola for avoiding this type of cookware are presented below:

Dupont which produces Teflon, and the companies who produce similar products, contend that PFOA is safe because it is used only in production and cannot be found in the final product. This is simply not true. According to a recent report in NaturalNews.com, PFOA is found in the bloodstream of 95 percent of Americans. Animals tested with PFOA were found to have tumors in at least four different organs. In April of 2000 a number of class action lawsuits were filed against Du-Pont, charging the company with exposing millions of Americans to health risks from pans containing PFOA. The suits even claimed that DuPont knew of the risks but failed to disclose them. One month later, a scientific advisory panel to the Environmental Protection Agency (EPA) advised that PFOA be labeled a "likely carcinogen." A voluntary action was implemented, which asks that manufacturers phase out 95% of production by 2010 and totally eliminate it by 2015. But this is only voluntary; no company is required by law to eliminate PFOA. However, at the same time that the agency was issuing these advisories, they were also suing DuPont for allegedly hiding health data about PFOA for 20 years. The company settled to the tune of $10.25 million. And finally, in May of 2006 DuPont acknowledged that they received a sub-poena from the U.S. Justice Department's Environmental Crimes Section requiring them to turn over documents about PFOA safety. There is absolutely no doubt that PFOA is un-safe.

[100] Jack Samuels. *MSG UPDATE, pp. 36-39.*

The Environmental Working Group, a nonprofit consumer safety organization, has found that non-stick pans begin producing dangerous toxins within just two minutes of heating. By five minutes, or 680 degrees, they release at least six toxic chemicals including two carcinogens, two global pollutants and a deadly chemical called MFA, which can kill human beings at very low doses. DuPont even has a word for symptoms of this exposure: they call it 'polymer fume fever.'

Thanks to the Web there are a variety of places to find out more about PFOA and other related chemicals (called PFCs). One of the best and most accurate is the site of the Environmental Working Group. You can access their PFOA/PFC information directly at www.ewg.org/reports/pfcworld.

Switching to stainless steel cookware is not absolutely safe. Contrary to popular belief, stainless steel cookware is not 100% safe. All stainless steel has alloys containing nickel, chromium, molybdenum, carbon and other metals. Plus, most stainless cookware is 'clad' or 'threeply,' meaning that it has an aluminum or copper base between layers of stainless steel. The fact is that both of these options are reactive and thereby increase the likelihood that metals will leach into your foods. Evidence continually points to aluminum exposure as a suspected factor in the development of Alzheimers.

The safest cookware is cast iron cookware and it can also be obtained with an enamel coating that is easy to clean and beautiful to look at. Advanced enamel coatings, unlike some ceramic material, is free of cadmium and lead. And while it is certainly heavier than other cookware, it's easier to handle and its weight actually helps improve your cooking by evenly distributing the heat and allowing you to cook at lower temperatures. [101]

Consumer Research rates cast iron cookware as the safest and most beneficial type of cookware to use. Some of its benefits are: (1) the iron of the pot leaches a small amount of iron into the food being cooked. This is of great value since most people today are lacking in the recommended amount of iron. (2)It diffuses heat evenly and

---

[101] Dr. Joseph Mercola. *Take Control of Your Health.*

without overheating which is excellent for frying or searing and for soups and stews which require a long steady cooking time. (3) Iron cookware can also develop a non-stick surface by the use of cooking oil that creates a permanent coating if the oil is not washed off with scouring. The pot can be cleaned by simply wiping the surface with a paper towel after each use.

Prescription Drugs

We have all been made aware of the fact that every drug has side-effects. The medical establishment would have us believe that the benefits offset the side effects. This just is not true. Medical researchers like Dr. David Williams present the facts in their health newsletters. Here is a sample of what Dr. Williams has to say about prescription drugs:

"A new wonder drug is rushed onto the market and five or ten years later its side effects become too widespread and dangerous to ignore. It's finally pulled from the market, but not before hundreds of thousands are permanently disabled or thousands die. The list keeps growing every month, but most of the time there are only a couple of short warnings and its back to business as usual for the pharmaceutical industry.

The most recent example is the medications for high blood pressure known as beta-blockers. Not only are beta-blockers widely used to treat high blood pressure but for the last decade or so they've been given routinely to patients prior to all types of non-cardiac surgeries to reduce blood pressure, heart rate, and strain on the heart. This now appears to have been a huge mistake. Giving beta-blockers to patients before undergoing surgery not only doubled their risk of having a stroke, but it also increased their risk of dying by 33 percent when compared to patients not taking the medication.

One of the authors, Dr. P.J. Devereaux noted: 'In the last decade, even if only ten percent of patients undergoing non-cardiac surgery were given beta-blockers, that means 100 million were given beta-blockers, and that means 800,000,000 people died unnecessarily and a lot of people suffered a major stroke because they were given beta-blockers.'

Beta-blockers aren't the only drugs that create their own problems. You've probably seen television ads where cancer patients undergoing chemotherapy have more energy after taking drugs that increase red blood production, to treat their anemia. Now studies show these ESAs (erythropoiesis-stimulating agents) actually speed the growth of tumors and shorten the life of cancer patients. Considering that these drugs have never been shown to improve the effectiveness of chemotherapy or the survival rate of patients, you would expect that the FDA would have stopped their use. Instead, they added a 'black box' warning to the drug label. Maybe that was because these drugs represent one of the highest US federal expenditures for cancer patients and bring the pharmaceutical companies over $10 billion annually.

We've become so accustomed to the widespread use of antibiotics that it may seem far-fetched to think they could increase the risk of something like cancer. The fact of the matter, however, is that studies show a direct correlation between antibiotics and invasive breast cancer. The researchers found that women who took antibiotics for more than 500 days, or had more than 25 prescriptions, over an average period of 17 years had more than twice the risk of breast cancer compared to women who had not taken any antibiotics."[102]

The few studies described above are just the tip of the iceberg. As mentioned earlier in this book, the fourth leading cause of death in America is the overuse and misuse of prescription drugs. There is even a new medical term, 'iatronic' which is used by doctors in reference to this new 'illness'. It means medically induced death.

Drugs for Prostate

Drugs for benign prostate enlargement have become a billion dollar business, although the results of taking these drugs is questionable. A recent study at the University of Southern California found that after taking the most popular prostate drug, Proscar, for one year, 30 percent of the men were found to have developed prosate tumors as compared to only one tumor found among men who received no drugs. Dr. Wright explains the reasons for this as follows:

"Proscar works by blocking the normal 'pathway' of testosterone. Ordinarily, some of your testosterone turns into a slightly different hormone, called DHT..and swollen prostates often contain

---

[102] Dr. David G. Williams. *Alternatives*. January 2009, pp. 155

high levels of DHT. So drug firms assumed DHT was causing the trouble. They developed powerful drugs like Proscar to suppress DHT production. The problem is: when your body can't make **DHT..Lots of Testosterone turns into ESTROGEN!** And a *little* estrogen, the female hormone, is normal in men but when a man's estrogen level gets too high…**The entire male edifice crumbles.**

Your erections wilt, your libido sinks, you can develop a form of diabetes, your heart risk rockets….*Is it really any wonder you're likely to get cancer too?*"[103]

Benign prostate swelling can be treated with common nutrients such as selenium, zinc, beta sitosterol, saw palmetto, and stinging nettle. You have a choice. Drugs are not the only answer.

Statin Drugs for Cholesterol

Statin drugs such as Crestor, Zocar and Lipitor became a billion dollar business for pharmaceutical companies because of the fact that they lower cholesterol. It was assumed that lower cholesterol levels reduce the risk of heart attacks although there was never any conclusive evidence supporting that view. In fact, the FDA requires these companies to place the following statement on their labels: "not shown to prevent heart disease or heart attacks." Studies also show that only 8 percent of people on statin drugs have heart disease to begin with. Long term research studies have shown that lower cholesterol levels have actually led to an increase in fatal heart attacks plus other life-threatening side effects such as a significant rise in diabetes among those taking the drugs. Other side effects from Statin drugs include memory loss, confusion, disorientation, irrational thinking, and other signs of dementia and senility. One of the chief causes of the harmful side effects is the fact that Statins do block cholesterol from being formed thus interfering with the body's normal control of how much is needed for each person's individual needs. Statins are dangerous because they impair the liver's ability to produce cholesterol which is a critical element for good health. Cholesterol is needed to metabolize Coenzyme Q10 which is an essential nutrient for the heart. Statins deplete Coenzyme Q10 thus leading to more heart attacks. In addition to the side effects mentioned above

---

[103] Dr. Jonathan Wright. *The Little Book of Big Health Secrets.* Nutrition and Healing, November, 2009, pp 14-17.

there is another factor to consider in regards to the use of statins. It appears that low cholesterol levels are more dangerous to health than high cholesterol levels. Geriatric journals have studied up to 150,000 people over 15 years. The studies have shown that people with lowered cholesterol have double the risk of death than those with high cholesterol, the lower the cholesterol the more dangerous. And in people over 65, lowered cholesterol is very dangerous—with a sharp increase in cancer. People with high cholesterol on the other hand are at a greatly reduced risk of getting cancer. It makes sense to avoid statins in spite of all the media and medical establishment support of these drugs.

A recent study, known as the JUPITER study, of the effects of a statin drug, Crestor, was hailed as the biggest medical news showing the benefits of statin drugs. This study made the front page in newspapers around the country. The participants in the study were individuals with normal cholesterol, but with high blood levels of CRP, a measure of the amount of inflammation present in the body. The results of the study showed that the treatment group (those who received Crestor) had fewer heart attacks and strokes, and fewer deaths from all causes compared to individuals given placebos. On the surface it would appear that there are wonderful benefits for those who take statin drugs. However, as is the case with most drugs there are dangerous side-effects to consider when taking any drug and on the other hand, there are other ways to reduce CRP with easy to take natural foods that can achieve he same or better results without the harmful effects of statin drugs. Let's look at the facts, as reported by Dr. David Williams, a noted health researcher, in his comments about this study:

"First of all, Crestor (the statin used in the study) did reduce the overall number of heart attacks compared to the placebo—but taking Crestor resulted in more fatal heart attacks. Taking Crestor also increased the incidence of diabetes among those taking the drug, which most reports failed to mention. This study also didn't address the findings of other studies which have been shown to increase the incidence of confusion, memory loss, inability to concentrate, impaired judgment, disorientation, irrational thinking, and other signs of dementia and senility. It has also been well documented that all statins are linked to severe liver and muscle damage, but that effect didn't show up in this study. A closer look reveals that this study's extensive screening process excluded individuals that earlier studies had shown would be more susceptible to these and other problems. The entire study was obviously well-manipulated to present statins in the most positive light. Clear objectivity apparently has no place in the marketing plan for Crestor.

One of the most interesting findings I see from this study wasn't even mentioned at all. The simple fact that any benefits provided by the statins could be linked to a reduction in inflammation just throws more water on the idea that cholesterol is the primary problem. Remember that the participants in this study had normal cholesterol levels. And this supports numerous other studies showing you can reduce your risk of heart attacks, stroke, and other cardiovascular diseases by strictly reducing inflammation.

For decades, I've written about the role of inflammation in the formation of disease in the heart and the arteries. Cholesterol has never been the culprit it's been made out to be, and research continues to support that fact. It's well known that *at least 50 percent of heart attack victims have normal cholesterol levels.* Inflammation triggered by either physical trauma—such as high blood pressure pounding on junctions of arteries—or by various chemical irritants, severe or chronic infections, et cetera, routinely cause cardiovascular damage, and the blockages eventually take their toll. Poor circulation, organ failure, heart attack, and stroke are the end results.

Reducing inflammation is one thing you should be consciously trying to achieve. Any effort you invest in this area will return healthwise at least a hundredfold. I'll show you several ways to reduce the burden of inflammation. The first step is to cut your exposure to toxins of all sorts. The most common of these is tobacco smoke. Smokers and inhalers of secondhand smoke, subject themselves to chronic inflammation of the airways, lungs, and blood vessels.

I would venture to say it's impossible these days to avoid all inflammatory toxins in our air and in our food and in our water supplies. That's why I think it has become important to periodically remove these toxins as best we can. Chelation is one option, but not available or practical for many people. That's why I like the herb **cilantro** so much. I call it the 'poor man's Chelation therapy.' Cilantro is also known as coriander or Chinese parsley. It has a powerful aroma and taste. It is rich in coriandrol which scientists believe may help protect against skin, liver, and breast cancer.

Along with short periods of fasting and the use of far-infrared saunas and clay, you have several easy, cost-effective ways to keep toxins and inflammation under control.

Exercise is one of the best ways to get rid of excess fat/weight. And when combined with a healthy diet, the reduction in CRP levels can be dramatic. CRP (inflammation) levels drop like a rock when someone loses excess fat. Low-fat diets have been shown to lower CRP levels by 50 percent in just four weeks and low-carbohydrate diets achieve even better results.

In the statin study mentioned earlier, Crestor reduced CRP levels by 37 percent over a period of two years. Simply adding 12 grams of fiber a day to the diet decreases CRP by 13.7 percent---*in just three weeks.* Other studies have found that for every increase of 10 grams of fiber intake a day, there was a 14 percent decrease in the risk of heart attack and a 24 percent reduction in death from cardiovascular disease. Psyllium husks are one of the best sources of fiber that cost less than $3 for a month's supply at your local health store. Psyllium has the added benefit of being able to help control blood sugar, and it helps feed the beneficial bacteria through a fermentation process in the lower bowel. You'll see even more benefit by adding either a daily probiotic supplement/and or fermented foods like real yogurt or unpasteurized sauerkraut to your diet.

There's also the problem of antibiotic use in animal feed, which can pass from the animal products to the consumer. Consuming antibiotic-laced foods destroys the beneficial bacteria in your bowel just like taking a prescription antibiotic would. Tyson Foods, the world's largest meat processor, just recently admitted that it injected chicken eggs with antibiotics before they hatched so they could label them as being 'raised without antibiotics.'" [104]

Another alternative to Statin drugs is the consumption of foods that are known to reduce the levels of harmful cholesterol-LDLs.

Pomegranate is one such food that has been found to reduce cholesterol, as reported in the following excerpt from the *Life Extension* magazine:

---

[104] Dr. David Williams. *Alternatives, Jan., 2009,* pp.145-148.

"There are *non-drug* approaches that have been documented to *reverse* clinical measurements of systemic atherosclerosis.

Scientific studies have demonstrated the ability of *pomegranate* and a natural superoxide dismutase (SOD) enhancing agent to *reverse* carotid ultrasound markers of atherosclerosis better than any prescription drug.

While some drugs, nutrients and hormones can slow the progression of *atherosclerosis,* very little has ever been shown to reverse existing artery disease.

Results of a recent study showed the following significant effects of pomegranate: 'In patients administered *pomegranate,* the paraoxonase-1 levels increased by **83%** after only one year.

Paraoxonase-1 is an antioxidant enzyme naturally produced in the body. It is believed to protect against the oxidation of **LDL**. Low levels of paraoxonase-1 predict increased severity of coronary heart disease.

The scientists involved in the study attributed the regression in carotid atherosclerotic lesion size in the **pomegranate** group to significantly reduced *oxidative stress* in both blood and atherosclerotic plaques, along with modestly lower *blood pressure* (beyond that of the antihypertensive drugs that were prescribed).

When looking at these incredible improvements in arterial health, the mere 'slowing of worsening progression' that Statin drugs are able to accomplish looks quite pathetic in comparison." [105]

Sugar and Synthetic Sweeteners (ASPARTAME)

There is a great deal of confusion about what kind of sugar is best to consume. When large numbers of people became aware of the dangers of white sugar, the food industry produced a number of sugar substitutes which are actually more dangerous to health than white sugar. For example, aspartame is known to lead to serious illnesses such as MS, Lupus and brain damage. It is beyond belief that this product is still being used especially in the most popular foods children consume such as cookies and ice cream. Let's look at the facts:

Aspartame is the most common sweetening additive in more

---

[105] *Life Extension Magazine*, Editors. Collector's edition, 2009, pp. 9-10.

than one hundred diet and sugar-free products, ending up in soft drinks, frozen desserts, and table-top sweeteners. It can also be found in such seemingly unlikely places as multivitamins, supplements, and pharmaceutical drugs. It contains three major components—methanol, phenylalanine, and aspartic acid. All three chemicals individually have been shown to either stimulate brain cells to death, upset hormone balances in the brain, or act as a nerve poison.

It took sixteen years for the FDA to finally approve the use of aspartame because many of the animal studies testing its safety had produced a disturbing pattern of brain tumors. In 1980 an FDA Board of Inquiry voted unanimously against approving aspartame for human consumption. A year later the commissioner of the FDA, Arthur Hull Hayes, Jr. overruled his agency's own scientists and approved aspartame for use in dry food products. He approved its use in carbonated beverages in 1983. Soon thereafter Hayes left the FDA and went to work for G. D. Searle & Company, the pharmaceutical company that manufacturers aspartame. (Searle has since become a part of Monsanto.)

Over the next two years, after aspartame was added to soft drinks, Professor J. W. Olney of the Washington School of Medicine found that the incidence of brain cancer among U.S. citizens increased by 10 percent on average, representing about 1500 new cases a year. For persons over age sixty-five, the increases in brain cancer rates were an astounding 60 percent or more. Olney conducted research which was published in the *New England Journal of Medicine* and elsewhere outlining how Aspartame may cause brain damage in children.

Warnings about the toxicity of aspartame were issued in 1991 by the National Institutes of Health, which catalogued 167 adverse effects: In 1992 the U.S. Air Defense issued a warning to its pilots not to fly after ingesting aspartame; and in 1994 the U. S. Department of Health and Human Services detailed eighty-eight documented symptoms of aspartame toxicity in humans, some of which can lead to death. Here is a partial list of diseases thought to be exacerbated or triggered by this additive: birth defects, brain tumors, epilepsy, multiple sclerosis, Parkinson's and Alzheimer's.

Yet this chemical toxin, once listed by the Pentagon as a prospective biochemical warfare weapon remains widespread as an additive throughout the U. S. food supply and that of seventy other nations. It has been banned in Japan and a few other countries. What is the secret to its survival? British toxins expert Paula Baille-Hamilton is blunt in her assessment. 'Few incentives are as powerful as cold, hard cash.' The manufacturers make so much money and exercise so much political influence that the regulatory system has been manipulated and compromised.

Other artificial sweeteners have been introduced after aspartame such as accsulfame K which is 200 times sweeter than sugar. It also causes serious illnesses such as leukemia, tumors and respiratory diseases.

A cruel irony underlying this saga is how these artificial swee-teners commonly taken to lose weight, actually become fat enhancers once absorbed by the body. An American Cancer Association study tracking eighty thousand women for six years concluded, "Amongst women who gained weight, artificial sweetener users gained more weight than those who did not use the products." One reason may be that the synthetic chemicals affect hormone levels, thus undermining our own natural weight control systems slowing metabolism and increasing appetite.

Using the FDA to suppress competition from natural sweetener alternatives to aspartame has been employed effectively to maintain market monopolies. A natural and virtually calorie-free sweetener and health remedy from South America, called Stevia, fell into a bureaucratic black hole when the FDA banned it, calling it "an un-safe food additive." This ban was enacted after a complaint was filed by a company the FDA refused to identify, charging that the stevia herb was being used in Celestial Seasonings tea without FDA ap-proval.

Arizona congressman Jon Kyle charged that the FDA was en-gaging in 'a restraint of trade to benefit the artificial sweetener industry,' and voiced suspicions the complaint had been filed by the makers of aspartame. Later Congress passed legislation dealing with dietary supplements and allowed stevia to be sold as one such sup-plement, but in a strange twist, manufacturers were still prohibited from making any claims that even imply stevia is a sweetener. It is common knowledge that stevia is three hundred times sweeter than sugar, and without the calories, but broadcasting this truth in either labeling or advertising is considered a crime. [106]

Because Stevia is not allowed to be labeled as a sweetener it cannot be used in diet sodas and other diet products that are able to claim they are sugar free. As a result the synthetic sweeteners such as Aspartame which are known to be harmful can continue without competition from natural sweeteners.

Saccharine which was banned years ago because it was the cause of many illnesses and even deaths, is now available again under the label of 'Sweet and Low.' Another popular artificial sweetener which should be avoided is 'Splenda,' which is made from Sucralose.

The following article about aspartame was sent to me by e-mail:

FDA IS SUING FOR COLLUSION WITH MONSANTO - (Article written by Nancy Markle):

If it says SUGAR FREE, on the label, DO NOT EVEN THINK ABOUT IT!!!

I have spent several days lecturing at the WORLD ENVIRONMENTAL CONFERENCE on ASPARTAME marketed as NutraSweet, Equal and Spoonful. In the keynote address by the EPA, it was announced that in the United States in 2001 there is an epidemic of multiple sclerosis and systemic lupus, that it was hard to understand what toxin was causing this to be rampant. I stood up and said that I was there to lecture on exactly that subject.

I will explain why Aspartame is so dangerous: When the temperature of this sweetener exceeds 86 degrees F, the wood alcohol in ASPARTAME converts to formaldehyde and then to formic acid, which in turn causes metabolic acidosis. (Formic acid is the poison found in the sting of fire ants).

The methanol toxicity mimics among other conditions Multiple Sclerosis. People were being diagnosed with having Multiple Sclerosis in error. The MS is not a death sentence, where methanol toxicity is. Systemic Lupus has become almost as rampant as MS, especially with Diet Coke and Diet Pepsi drinkers. The victim usually does not know

---

[106] Fitzgerald, op. cit., pp. 106-110.

that the aspartame is the culprit. He or she continues its use, aggravating the lupus to such a degree that it may become life-threatening. We have seen patients with systemic lupus become asymptomatic once taken off diet sodas. In the case of those diagnosed with MS, (when in reality, the disease is methanol toxicity), most of the symptoms disappear. We've seen many cases where vision returned and hearing improved markedly.

This also applies to cases of tinnitus. During a lecture I said If you are using ASPARTAME (NutraSweet, Equal, Spoonful, etc) and you suffer from fibromyalgia symptoms, spasms, shooting pains, numbness in your legs, cramps, vertigo, dizziness, headaches, tinnitus, joint pain, depression anxiety attacks, slurred speech, blurred vision, or memory loss--you probably have ASPARTAME DISEASE! [107]

High-Fructose Corn Syrup

An article in the December, 2008 issue of the *Life Extension Magazine* called attention to the dangers of high fructose corn syrup (HFCS) as follows: "Americans are being poisoned by a common additive present in a wide array of processed foods like soft drinks and salad dressings, cakes and cookies, breakfast cereals and brand-name breads. This common-place additive silently increases our risk of obesity, hypertension, and atherosclerosis. The name of this toxic additive is **high fructose corn syrup.** Excess fructose intake has been associated with adverse health effects such as metabolic syndrome, elevated triglyceride levels, hypertension, fatty liver disease, excess uric acid levels and elevated levels of advanced glycation end products (AGEs; linked with aging and complications of diabetes)." [108]

Trans-Fats (hydrogenated oils)

The extremely dangerous effects of consuming hydrogenated or partially hydrogenated oils has been so well documented that many leading cereal companies place the statement 'No Trans Fats' on their labels. This is no guarantee that there are zero trans fats in the product. The government allows the use of the 'zero' label if there is

---

[107] Nancy Markle. *Aspartame Disease. E-Mail, 2009.*
[108] *Life Extension Magazine, Dec., 2008, pp. 69-71.*

no more than a small percentage of the trans fats in the product. This small amount can add up to dangerous levels if several products with zero labels are used daily. One of the worst culprits is the artificial butter. When people became concerned about eating foods with saturated fats, food companies jumped on the band wagon and started to produce butter substitutes. By using a process of hydrogenation, oils were hardened to produce a buttery spread similar to real butter. Recent studies have shown that there is an increased risk of heart disease due to the trans fats. Other studies have shown an increase in weight due to eating foods with trans fats.

At the present time a wide variety of foods contain trans fats such as cookies and other baked goods. The reason food companies continue to use this harmful substance is because it adds to the shelf life of the products. The ordinary vegetable oils become rancid in time. Hydrogenation of oils adds to their shelf life. The best way to protect yourself and especially your children is to read labels on every commercial food product. If it mentions shortening or partially hydrogenated oil; **Do Not Buy It**!

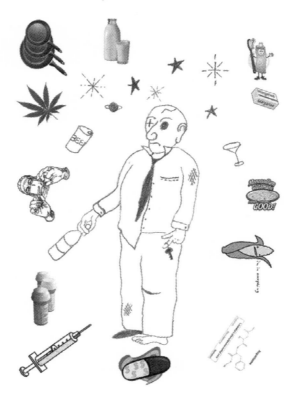

CHAPTER EIGHT

CAUSES & CURES OF ILLNESS

Acid and Alkaline Balance (pH)

In order to maintain the healthy balance in our bodies, usually referred to as *homeostasis,* we must be aware of the importance of the acid and alkaline effects of the foods we consume. It has been found that the alkaline/acid balance in our blood stream should be slightly alkaline. A neutral pH is 7, any measurement below 7 is acid, and any measurement above 7 is alkaline. The normal pH of blood is about 7.4 and must be kept at this level to remain healthy. In order to maintain the proper pH it is helpful to be aware of three important factors; one is to be aware of which foods have an alkaline reaction and which foods have an acid reaction. The second factor is to be aware of the need for an adequate level of HCL (hydrochloric acid) in the stomach in order to maintain proper pH balance. Lack of HCL leads to a lack of oxygen at the cellular level causing fermentation which results in low PH (acidity) at the cellular level. The lactic acid produced by fermentation lowers the cell pH and destroys the ability of DNA and RNA to control cell division. Cancer cells then begin to multiply. The lactic acid simultaneously causes severe local pain as it destroys cell enzymes. There are two ways to increase HCL. One is to take HCL tablets with each meal and the other method is to drink at least one quart of blended green leafy vegetables (green smoothie) each day. Victoria Boutenko, in her book, *Green For Life* describes how to make green smoothies. Felicia Kliment, in her book, *The Acid Alkaline Balance Diet* and Herman Aihara, in his book, *Acid & Alkaline,* provide us with a wealth of knowledge about the entire subject, including lists of foods that are either acid or alkaline. An excerpt from Aihara's book follows below:

Fruits and Acid Alkaline Balance... the organic acid (such as the acidity of an orange which you can taste) contains many elements such as potassium, calcium sodium, and magnesium. Organic acids, when oxidized, become carbon dioxide and water; the alkaline elements (K, Na, Ca, Mg) remain and neutralize body acid. In other words, strangely enough, *acid foods reduce body acids.* This is the reason that fruits and most vegetables are considered alkaline forming foods. Conversely, high protein foods and most grains, when metabolized, produce acid that must be neutralized; therefore they are generally acid forming foods.

Fat and Acid Alkaline Balance – Fat is considered one of the three major nutrients: namely carbohydrates, proteins, and fats. Fats are a source of linoleic acid and vitamins A and D. If animals are fed without fat, they will eventually die. However, if these animals are fed with a little amount of linoleic acid, they grow without trouble. In other words, the linoleic acid contained in fat is important. Since linoleic acid is contained in rice as well as in soy beans, we don't worry about its lack as long as we follow a basic diet of whole grains and vegetables, such as the macrobiotic natural food diet. Animal fat contains poisonous compounds. Even cod liver oil causes acidosis if it is consumed too much. The cause of baldness is consumption of too much fat.

Carbohydrates and Acid Alkaline Balance - Carbohydrates are the source of our energy. There are three types of carbohydrates. The simplest carbohydrates are the monosaccharides, of which the most important is glucose. Next are the disaccharides, which are made up of two monosaccharide molecules. The most important disaccharides are sucrose (ordinary cane sugar), lactose, and maltose. The third type of carbohydrates is polysaccharides, which have enormous molecules made of many monosaccharides. Since monosaccharides and disaccharides are absorbed quickly, the amount of glucose in the body cells increases to the point where an acidic condition is caused by overeating of candy or fruits. [109]

According to Dr. Theodore Baroody, Ph.D., author of *Alkalize or Die*: "Acid wastes literally attack the joints, tissues, muscles, organs, and glands causing minor to major dysfunction. In other words, you can develop digestion problems, weak bones, weight gain, fatigue, sluggishness, and kidney stones. When the small intestine is too acidic it can't properly digest foods. This can result in lowered immune function, fatigue, hormonal imbalances, and absorption problems! **To help your body regain pH balance, your bones will sacrifice one of its most alkaline minerals—Calcium! Less calcium in your bones means reduced ability to absorb other essential minerals. This causes bone density problems** that create fragile and porous bones! Too much acid creates an overproduction of insulin. This causes fat to be stored instead of being burned off. In order to remain healthy, cells must regularly expel all of the waste products they create. But if your blood becomes too acidic, the waste will cling to the walls of cells. This causes acidic fluoride that crystallizes and creates kidney stones. Physical and mental stress causes your body to produce more acidic waste—leading to acidosis."

Most people who consume the typical American diet have some degree of acidosis. The American diet is extremely acidic as you can see by the list of highly acidic foods below:

- Meat, including beef, pork, chicken and turkey
- Dairy such as milk, butter and cheese
- Grains such as rice, and barley
- Beverages such as coffee, tea, and soft drinks
- Fruit juices
- Simple carbohydrates such as **pasta and bread**

Acidity in the body is related to disease. Acid reflux is a painful condition that occurs when acidic stomach liquid backs up (refluxes) into the esophagus, causing irritation inflammation and damage to the lining of the esophagus.

High cholesterol occurs when the body produces excessive

---

[109] Herman Aihara. *Acid and Alkaline*. Oroville, CA: George Ohsawa Macrobiotic Foundation, 1985, pp. 11-12.

amounts of cholesterol to neutralize large amounts of acids in the blood stream before they damage living cells.

Fat is produced in the body to trap and neutralize acidic waste in the body. As Robert Young, PhD, author of The pH Miracle for Weight Loss, puts it, 'The body retains fat as a protection for the overproduction of acids produced by the typical American diet….Your fat is actually protecting your life.'

Inflammatory related diseases such as allergies, arthritis, fibromyalgia, psoriasis, and even stroke are related to low-grade metabolic acidosis.

It is very important to know your pH level so that you can take the necessary steps to correct any imbalance which will be indicated by a pH test. The most reliable type of test is a test of your urine the first thing in the morning.

Dr. Susan Brown, in her book, *The Acid-Alkaline Food Guide*, tells you how to do a pH test yourself:

"It is not difficult to estimate your metabolic pH. To do so you will need two items: pH test paper, also known as Hydrion paper, and your own first-morning urine. To obtain an accurate measurement, you should not have urinated for six hours prior to testing. To measure your pH, upon arising in the morning, simply wet the test paper with your urine, either by urinating directly on the test strip or by collecting urine in a cup and dipping the paper into the liquid. Then quickly place the paper on a tissue. Do not over saturate the test paper by holding it in the urine for an extended period of time, as may give a false reading. The pH paper will take on a color immediately and after five to ten seconds; you will be able to compare the color of the paper with the color chart that came with the test papers. This will give you a fairly accurate indication of your body's pH. In the beginning, it I recommended that you test your first-morning urine as many days a week as possible. After a week or two, you will know your average baseline pH measurement. If you are acidic, you will be able to watch your pH level rise as you make appropriate dietary and supplement changes. This may take several weeks. Once you have used the test paper to determine your body's pH, how can you interpret the reading? As you might recall, a pH of 7 is neutral, any reading below 7 is acid, and any reading above 7 is alkaline. Ideally you want your first-morning urine to have a pH between 6.5 and 7.5. This would indicate that your overall metabolic pH is mildly alkaline and that the small amounts of acid that build up from normal metabolism are being excreted. If your pH reading is below 6.5, it is likely that you are experiencing an excessive acid load. This acid load is probably caused by a diet high in acid-forming foods and low in base-forming foods. If you come up with an acidic reading, you will want to begin making food changes aimed at alkalizing your diet. In most cases, this will result in a pH that slowly climbs to a more healthy range. However, if you have a consistently low pH that does not respond to dietary changes or supplementation, this could be a sign of a disease state that requires medical attention." [110]

Michael Cutler, M.D. has this to say about the harmful effects of acidosis and what can be done to correct the problem: *"Tissue acidity has a long list of harmful effects upon the body if not neutralized or eliminated. For example,* the body's ability to absorb minerals and other nutrients decrease significantly in acid conditions. Additionally, the enzymatic processes that control the repair mechanisms for damaged DNA and other critical structures become weakened. And the liver cannot detoxify heavy metals from the body well when an acid pH predominates. Clearly, cancer cells proliferate wildly in acid conditions. Acid tissue pH causes fatigue that leads to depression and stress. If *your test results are acidic then* consider what you could do for yourself by increasing your intake of alkaline foods while reducing the intake of acid foods you eat. A good rule to follow is the 80/20 rule, where you eat 80% alkaline and 20% acid-forming foods. In order to simplify your selection of foods you can select foods by categories that include mostly acidic or mostly alkaline foods. For example, all fresh, green vegetables are alkaline producing while vegetables that have been processed in some way such as canned, pickled or preserved are acid forming. Whenever we cook, boil, freeze or otherwise alter foods, they become acid forming in the body. Most of the grains are acid forming except those that have been sprouted. The only alkaline grains are millet, spelt, and quinoa. Sweets, artificial sweeteners, sugar, chocolate, baked cakes and cookies are acid forming while natural sweeteners such as raw honey and stevia are alkaline. Watermelons and cucumbers are so alkalizing that when consumed they can neutralize the acidity of eating beef.

---

[110] Dr. Susan Brown and L. Trivieri, Jr. *The Acid Alkaline Food Guide.* Garden City, NY: Square One Publishers, 2006, pp. 44-48.

For this reason it is very useful to know which foods are the most acid and which ones are the most alkaline. [111]

A list providing this information is shown below:

MOST ALKALINE FORMING FOODS

All green vegetables, almonds, apples, apple cider, apricots, artichokes, asparagus, avocados, bananas beans, berries, borscht, broccoli, burdock root, cabbage, cantaloupe, cashews, cauliflower, chestnuts, cilantro, cinnamon currants, cumin, dill, eggplant, endive, fennel, flaxseed, garlic, ginger, grapes grapefruit, horseradish, kiwi, kohlrabi, kombu seaweed, lemons, limes, lotus root, mangos, melons, miso, muskmelon, mustard greens, nori seaweed, okra, onions, oranges, papayas, parsley, parsnips, peaches, pears, peppers, persimmon, pickles, pineapples, potatoes, pumpkin, radishes, rutabagas, sea salt, sea weeds, sprouts, squashes, string beans, thyme, turnips, yams, zucchini.

MOST ACID FORMING FOODS

Adzuki beans, American cheese, apple pie, aspartame, bacon, bagels, barley, beef, beer, biscuits, bison (buffalo), bran cereals, breads, brown sugar, brownies, burritos, Caesars salad dressing, carrot cake, cheddar cheese, (except soft cheeses) chicken, chicken noodle soup, chili, chips (all kinds), chocolate, cocoa, coffee, cola drinks, cookies, corn, corn syrup, cottonseed meal and oil, couscous, crabs, cranberries, croissants, croutons, cupcakes, donuts, eggs,, farina, filberts, fish, frankfurters, fried foods, fruit preserves, gouda cheese, grits, hamburgers, hard cheeses, hazelnuts, hot dogs, ice cream, iodized table salt, jams, jellies, kielbasa, linguini, liver, lobster, luncheon meats, malt, matzoh, mozzarella cheese, mussels, noodles, pancakes, pastas, peanut butter, pork, puddings, quiche, red wine vinegar, rice (white), ripe olives, root beer, sausages, soft drinks, soy nuts, spaghetti, sugar, Swiss cheese, swordfish, tofu, tortillas and chips, turkey, veal, white vinegar, waffles, walnuts, wheat, white bread, white rice cakes, wine, yeast, yogurt.

It is advisable to avoid highly acidic foods like pizza and cola drinks because they cause a number of problems. They are disruptive to the digestive system; pizza because of the white flour, overheated

---

[111] Dr. Michael Cutler's *Natural Health Answers.* Warrior, Alabama: self-published,

cheese and tomatoes; cola drinks because they are loaded with sugar or artificial sweeteners. All carbonated drinks disturb the water balance in the body because the liquid takes the place of natural water that is essential for health of the body. **Gatorade has a pH level of 2.95, more than 10,000 times more acidic than pH neutral water...** Cola drinks also eat away the enamel from our teeth which results in dental decay. The caffeine in cola drinks also causes dehydration (32 glasses of alkaline pH water are needed to balance one glass of Cola.)

You must stop drinking all soft drinks today! It is also very important to drink liquids to assist the kidneys in its job of removing excess acidic waste from the body, as explained by Dr. Vasey:

> There are two causes for acidification of the body's internal environment. One is the ingestion of excessive amounts of acids; the other is their insufficient elimination. Reducing the amount of acid through adequate diet and alkaline supplements has already been presented above. The organs for elimination are the kidneys and the skin. The skin and kidneys eliminate strong acids, such as uric acid, sulfuric acid, and phosphoric acid---the acids that primarily come from animal protein. The quantity of acids that the kidneys eliminate each day may not match the quantity consumed and produced by the body each day. Dietary reform that reduces the intake of acids helps, but it is also important to stimulate the kidneys to increase the amounts of acid they filter and void.

> A primary means of stimulating the work of the kidneys is to increase the amount of liquids you consume. An effective way of drinking enough liquid over the course of the day—and an easy way to remember to do so—is to have a drink after each time you urinate. Taking a drink immediately following urination, in a quantity equal to or greater than what was eliminated, causes the liquid level of the body to rise and this triggers a new elimination cycle automatically. The volume of liquid that thus travels through the body encourages the elimination of toxins, because it can easily dilute and transport numerous acids and salts without causing the urine to become overly concentrated.

> While an abundant supply of liquid encourages elimination, it

is also possible to increase the quantity of acids eliminated from the body by stimulating the kidneys' filtration capacities with diuretic (urination-producing) medicinal plants. These plants and herbs allow the kidneys to handle much larger quantities of toxins, and the body is therefore able to get rid of those toxins much more quickly. Many plants are available to assist the kidneys in draining acids from the body. The list below offers several recommendations:

Black currant: The leaves make a very pleasant-tasting tea. Make a tea by mixing 1 handful of leaves (11/2 oz) per quart of water, or 1 tablespoon per cup. Steep at least 10 minutes. Drink 3 cups daily before or between meals.

Artichoke: The leaves have an excellent diuretic effect and also stimulate liver function. They make a bitter-tasting drink. Drink 3 cups a day before meals.

Cherry stems: Save the stems when you eat cherries and put them aside to dry. Mix 1 handful of stems per quart of water and boil for 10 minutes. Drink 3 cups a day at a minimum.

Linden bark: It is excellent for draining acids from the body and also recommended for all forms of rheumatism, kidney stones, and gall stones. Make a decoction by mixing 11/2 oz of bark per quart of water. Boil until the liquid is reduced to of its volum e. Drink frequently during the day. Continue for several months.

Cranberry: This is a diuretic well known for its disinfectant effect on the urinary tract. It can be taken in capsules or as juice before meals. Be aware that most juices contain a very high level of sugar that places a strain on your pancreas and can lead to a spike in your blood sugar level.

Couch grass: It is an excellent cleansing plant. Its preferred use is in tablet form because of its flavor. Take 1—3 tablets with a little water 3 times a day.

Some additional plant medicines that have diuretic and anti-infective properties include: Goldenrod, ash, corn silk, elder, licorice, cat's whisker, and thistle. [112]

---

[112] Christopher Vasey, N.D. *The Acid-Alkaline Diet.* Rochester, Vermont: Healing Arts Press, 1999, pp. 163-169.

In addition to eating foods to maintain your PH at its normal alkaline level, it is helpful to use food combinations that will prevent acidosis from occurring. The value of selecting proper food combinations is explained in a cookbook, *Good Foods That Go Together,* which also contains over 1500 recipes. Some of the reasons for avoiding certain food combinations are:

The subject of gastro-chemistry may be barely touched upon here. It will be enough to remember that the digestion of starchy food begins in the mouth where such foods are attacked by an enzyme called ptyalin in the saliva. Hence thorough mastication of all starchy foods is advisable. Very little change takes place in this type of food while it remains in the stomach with other compatible varieties. It is passed on into the duodenum where the process of digestion is again taken up, still in an alkaline medium. To trace the digestion of protein to this point; no action takes place in the mouth except for the breaking up of fiber through mastication; but upon entering the stomach, gastric juice is secreted containing hydrochloric acid and pepsin. If both protein and carbohydrates are present, it is obvious that acid attacking the starchy food will start fermentation, while the presence of the starch will interfere with the protein digestion. The result is chaos - gas fermentation. Adherence to the laws of chemistry in choosing and grouping foods results in following the rules for compatible combinations. Healthy proteins (authors' opinion) include dark green, leafy vegetables, nuts, fresh fish such as salmon, tofu, and soft cheeses. Proteins are best raw but may be cooked and served with all kinds of vegetables, fats, acid fruits or gelatin. Carbohydrate foods include all sugars and molasses, honey, artichokes, pumpkins, winter squash; starches, i.e., all cereals and cereal products, potatoes, yams, sweet potatoes; sweet fruits such as dates, raisins, figs and bananas. These may be combined with fats and all vegetables. [113]

Acid Reflux (GERD), Heartburn

This condition is very common and may be caused simply by overeating, or by fast foods and lack of exercise. However, it is more likely due to an inadequate amount of stomach acid (HCL) and an underproduction of digestive pancreatic enzymes, as pointed out by

---

[113] Esther Smith. *Good Foods That Go Together.* New Canaan, Conn: Keats Publishing, 1975, Foreword.

Dr. Shallenberger in his health newsletter, *Real Cures, 12/08.* "Stomach acid is important for digestion but it also serves another critical purpose. It protects us from infections by killing infectious organisms such as bacteria, fungi, yeast and molds. When you have an insufficient amount of stomach acid, infections can develop in your stomach which hampers your digestion and then becomes a major cause of heartburn. The food mixed with stomach acid that is regurgitated into the esophagus can result in symptoms of discomfort, pain and/or vomiting. The problem is magnified when the typical medical treatment is used such as an antacid or a drug that decreases stomach acid production. The need of more stomach acid for proper digestion is thus weakened by the use of antacids such as Rolaids and Tums. Drugs such as Prilosec, Prevacid, Tagament, Pepcid, Nexium and Zantac can lead to an even more dangerous situation. They lead to bile reflux which is an acid reflux from the small intestine. Bile reflux is now known to be one of the major causes of esophageal cancer. Research also shows that by stopping the use of these drugs, the bile acid problem can be normalized in as little as 10 days.

Steps that can be taken to prevent or alleviate acid reflux are as follows:

1. Eliminate all antacids, both over the counter and prescription drugs.
2. Eliminate all alcohol, coffee, tea, caffeine, and carbonated drinks, including carbonated water.
3. Eat slowly, chew thoroughly and avoid eating for three hours before you go to bed.
4. Take supplements such as betaine hydrochloride tablets along with pancreatic enzymes before each meal. Also take aloe juice four times a day plus some cabbage juice extract.
5. Avoid drugs such as Aleve, Motrin and Celebrex taken for pain. Also avoid drugs for osteoporosis such as Fosamax and Actonel. Also avoid antibiotics which usually lead to Candida which is a major cause of heartburn.

Stay on the above regimen for six months and then gradually reduce the amount of supplements. You can then go back to a normal healthy lifestyle. You can have some tea, sweets and wine but use these foods and beverages with sensible moderation. Continue to avoid junk foods, MSG, artificial sweeteners, flavors, and colors.

Adrenal Exhaustion

The adrenal glands are an essential part of the endocrine system. They are involved with a number of physiological functions including energy metabolism, blood sugar metabolism regulation of blood flow and blood pressure, immune response and regulation of sodium, potassium and fluid concentrations. All these operations are essential to everyday function, so when a person's adrenals are run down, quality of life suffers. A person must therefore be certain to include the nutrients necessary for proper adrenal function.

A condition that causes many illnesses is the exhaustion or fatigue of the adrenal glands. The familiar fight or flight syndrome causes the adrenal glands to secrete large amounts of adrenalin and cortisol caused by the protracted everyday stresses of modern civilization. This is compounded by the additional stress of the typical American diet, which is high in sugar and processed foods, resulting in weakening the adrenal system to the point of exhaustion. The condition called 'burnout' is typical of adrenal exhaustion.

According to Dr. Junger, "Depletion of the adrenal system is rarely diagnosed by conventional doctors largely because most blood tests and other laboratory evaluations come back as normal despite the patient's experience of being constantly exhausted. This means they continue on without treatment as stress takes its toll on the body, when replenishing the adrenal function holistically is actually what is indicated." Dr. Junger offers the following list of questions to help you determine whether you have a problem with your adrenal function:

- Does it take you longer than average to recover from illnesses or injuries?
- Do you regularly have difficulty getting out of bed in the morning?
- Do you have a sense of ongoing fatigue that is not relieved by a good night's sleep?
- Do you feel light-headed when getting up from a sitting position?
- Do you have abnormally low blood pressure?
- Do you have a tendency to bruise easily?
- Do you have extreme sensitivity to colds or tend to feel cold in environments where others do not?

- Do you have chronic level of anxiety or have you ever had panic attacks?
- Do you have periods of depression or frequent crying jags (Also a hallmark of toxicity)?

Although some of these symptoms are similar to those of toxicity, as a group they are more specific to adrenal weakness. If you answered yes to two or more of these questions, it is important that you find a health-care practitioner who understands how to check your level of adrenal function and work with you to improve it. Embarking on a detox program would be counterproductive and even harmful as you will not have necessary energy to support the detox and intestinal rebuilding processes. Once you have rested and reactivated your adrenal glands, a detox program will be in order." [114]

The Standard Process Company provides supplements made from natural, mostly organically-grown foods and herbs that are designed for special health needs such as adrenal fatigue. They can be obtained at many chiropractor offices. They list the following Dietary causes of adrenal fatigue:

Excess consumption of Sugar: Includes honey, maple syrup, fructose dried fruit, fruit juice, sweet fruits and any kind of natural sugar.

Refined carbohydrates: includes all processed foods, bread and noodles. If grains are ground up they are processed and will metabolize in almost the same way as white sugar. White rice is also out. Thick whole oats are okay, but steel cut oats are not.

The refined grains have more surface area exposed to digestion so they digest more rapidly. They release their sugars quickly into the blood stream causing blood sugar to spike too high too fast. The body overreacts to this rapidly absorbed sugar releasing too much insulin. The release of too much insulin causes the blood sugar to go down too far. (Most everyone has experienced getting sleepy after a large meal of pasta, rice or some other carbohydrate or the drop in energy that follows a candy high. That's what happens after a large release of insulin).

The adrenals are constantly being assailed by the above reac-

---

[114] Dr. Alejandro Junger, MD. *Clean.* Harper Collins, Pp. 136-137.

tions. Processed foods and snacks are available all the time and they can be hard to resist. The adrenals are being called upon to produce more and more cortisol in response to the stress caused by sugar and processed food. Eventually they become exhausted. And so does the indulger.

So what can a person do? The obvious thing to do is to stop eating sugar and refined foods. A lot of people will do great just by modifying their diet alone. If you're really committed, you could give up grains all together. This is hard to do so minimizing grains is good. Eating boiled potatoes and sweet potatoes (not baked) can help you to feel full. Keep in mind it is stressful on the adrenals to go hungry, so it's important to eat when your body asks for food. Nutrients that support the adrenals should be added to your daily supplements. Vitamins from natural ingredients which support the adrenals are: The B vitamins, (B5 deficiency has been linked to adrenal fatigue) vitamin C and E, tyrosine, which is organic copper (an adrenal activator). Additionally Many amino acids are involved in the synthesizing of hormones and other important chemicals in the body. Wheat germ, buckwheat and oats - all contain amino acids. Selenium is another important nutrient to help strengthen the adrenals.

Ways to Manage Stress

Relieving stress can seem impossible. But it's how you handle the stress that will allow you to feel better and decrease cortisol levels.

Sleep - The best way to relieve stress is to ensure you get 8 hours of sleep per day. This allows time for cortisol levels to drop and give you deep, restful sleep. If needed take melatonin, a natural sleep regulator.

Exercise - Participate in regular 'moderate' exercise. An intense work- out may only complicate your adrenal issues.

Nutrition - Whole foods are important because they provide a wide variety of nutrients that are crucial during times of increased stress and adrenal fatigue. When the body is under stress your metabolism increases, thus creating a greater need for nutrients. Avoid sugar, high fructose syrup, and refined flour. Stick to high fiber foods (whole grains, fruits, and vegetables) and lean protein.

Supplements - Whole food supplements can provide additional support to help your adrenal glands stay healthy. Standard Processes adrenal products are made from whole foods.

Alzheimer's Disease

Alzheimer's is a neurological disorder that strikes the area of the brain primarily involved with thoughts, memory and language. It is characterized by abnormal clumps called amyloid plaques, as well as bundles of tangled nerves not found in the brains of normal older men and women. In this disease, nerve cells in parts of the brain that are critical to memory and thinking die. The medical establishment has not yet found a cure for the disease but continues to prescribe drugs to suppress some of the symptoms.

There is some evidence that inflammation in the brain may contribute to the development of Alzheimer's. Since inflammation is found in every diseased condition, it may be helpful to consume foods and herbs that are known to have anti-inflammatory properties such as 'curcumin' which holds promise for the prevention of Alzheimer's disease. Results of the massive China Study indicated that a plant based diet was helpful in curing and preventing most diseases including Alzheimer's. "Green smoothies", described elsewhere in this book, should be included in the diet as a preventative and possible cure of Alzheimer's disease. Another important factor to be aware of is the pH balance of the blood. The more acidic a body is, the more it holds onto heavy metals such as mercury. Heavy metals create a high oxidative stress that acidifies the body, making it even worse. The latest survey of all current Alzheimer's research has identified mercury as the prime suspect as a causative factor. A recent study indicates that **there may be a cure for this disease as indicated by the following report:**

"If you have a loved one with Alzheimer's disease, what you're about to read could be life changing. Researchers from the University of California, Irvine may have found a cure. That's right, a cure! And even better, this cure is remarkably inexpensive.

The cure is a nutrient that's been around for decades. In fact years ago, nutritionally-minded Abe Hoffer taught that this nutrient could cure mental illness. Now the California study shows some startling results in Alzheimer's mice. This nutrient actually restored their memory! Here's the story:

The scientists genetically engineered mice to get the equivalent of Alzheimer's disease. Yes, animals can get dementia just like humans, with beta amyloid plaque (Alzheimer's hallmark) in their brains.

The scientists added a vitamin to their drinking water beginning at four months of age. The researchers then tested the animals short –term and long-term memory during the next four months. They tested memory patterns known to be dependent on certain brain structures that are damaged by Alzheimer's.

The nutrient? It's the simple $2 nutrient niacinamide. Niacinamide is just an easy-to-tolerate form of Vitamin B3. And its ability to treat Alzheimer's is truly amazing.

The results of the study showed that oral niacinamide treatment prevents the cognitive deficits in mice with Alzheimer's, while improving the short-term spatial memory in non-demented control animals.

At the end of the study the Alzheimer's mice performed as well in memory testing as healthy mice. This suggests that the vitamin protected their brains from memory loss and restored memory that was already lost. 'Cognitively, they were cured. They performed as if they'd never developed the disease. The vitamin completely prevented cognitive decline associated with the disease, bringing them back to the level they'd be at if they didn't have the pathology. It actually improved behavior in non-demented animals, too,' said Dr. Green.

Dr. Frank LaFerla, the lead author of the study, said: 'This suggests that not only is it good for Alzheimer's disease, but if normal people take it some aspects of their memory might improve.'

How does niacinamide work? Neurons are constructed with microtubules. These are scaffolding within the cells that conduct information. When the microtubules breakdown, the cells die. The tubules are like highways inside the cells Dr. Green said that niacinamide is, 'making a wider more stable highway.' Alzheimer's disease breaks down the highway (tubules). But niacinamide prevents this from happening.

I've previously told you how the toxic metal mercury also destroys these microtubules, potentially causing Alzheimer's disease. So anything that can prevent the damage or reverse it is a huge discovery.

Dr. Green says that niacinamide has a very robust affect on neurons. It prevents the build-up of 'tau,' which are proteins along tracks inside neurons. In the early stages of the disease, these protein clumps impair the nerve-cell functions. But ultimately the tau proteins can stop the nerves from functioning and kill them. Dr. Green told the Alzheimer's Research Forum: 'It's absolutely dramatic. This [biomarker for Alzheimer's disease, the tau protein] is just wiped from the brain specifically.'

The dose the researchers gave the mice was 200 mg/kg per day. The UCI researchers have been recruiting patients for a human study. The participants in this study will take 1500 mg of niacinamide twice daily. From my perspective that's a very tolerable dose of a very inexpensive vitamin. As I mentioned earlier, Abe Hoffer showed years ago that vitamin B3 and other nutrients could cure or control schizophrenia. With the new understanding of its ability to protect microtubules, Hoffer's observations and work has reached even greater heights.

Niacinamide is an absolutely wonderful nutrient that has a lot more benefits than just treating Alzheimer's. If you have dementia of any kind, consider niacinamide, 1500 mg twice daily.

These incredible researchers have shown us, at least in a rodent model, that you can save and normalize Alzheimer's diseased neurons with vitamin B3. Considering that the pathology in humans is virtually identical to the disease in the experimental mice, if and when these results are duplicated in humans, niacinamide could be the Alzheimer's breakthrough of all time.

One final note: Be sure that you use niacinamide, and not its sister niacin. The latter is another form of B3 that will cause an uncomfortable prickly flush, and is often used for cholesterol problems. It sometimes irritates. Fortunately the niacinamide form does not produce the flush. And it does not have any significant irritating effects on the liver, even in high doses. You can find niacinamide at a health food store and on the internet." [115]

There are other treatments to consider which have demonstrated benefits for Alzheimer's patients. According to Dr. Jonathan Wright:

> Mainstream medicine is stumped when it comes to Alzheimer's. They don't understand why it strikes, how it erodes your mind, or how to get rid of it once it does. The only thing they do understand is how to overcharge you for useless pills and how to recommend a good nursing home.

---

[115] *Second Opinion Health Letter.* May, 2009, pp. 1-3.

But no matter what you've heard, just know that Alzheimer's is NOT a *death sentence* Natural treatments exist and fortunately, they're much, cheaper and much, much more effective than anything requiring a prescription. Scientists recently found what they once thought impossible...that you can actually 'regrow' and regenerate your brain before Alzheimer's strikes *at any age.*

So what is this mineral miracle that's been hiding under our noses the whole time? It's *lithium.* Now bear with me here. Most people think lithium's for loons. But that's high dose *lithium carbonate* —which is only available with a prescription and used to treat bi-polar disorder. Truth is lithium isn't a drug at all. It's a mineral—part of the same family of minerals that includes sodium and potassium. I'm talking about low-dose *lithium aspartate or lithium orotate*—completely safe mineral supplements you can pick up at many health food stores for about 26 cents a dose. So safe in fact, one healer has used them for 31 years without reporting a single side effect.

But even more astounding than the decade's long safety record of these two minerals is how powerful they really are. The FDA-approved Alzheimer's drug Nameda has been touted as the solution, but in reality, it blocks only ONE Alzheimer's pathway. Meanwhile *lithium aspartate and orolate* have been shown to BLOCK 6 MAJOR PATHWAYS in recent studies. Not to mention Nameda runs about $4.84 a day—almost 20 times what it costs you for your 26-cent-a-day lithium tablets.

But here's the worst part—one of Nameda's most common side effects is... *CONFUSION!?* That means that this drug that supposedly treats confusion is actually causing it! Unbelievable you say. Well, this is coming straight from the normally tight lipped FDA's own website. Now, you have to ask yourself: **'Why haven't I heard about this before?' If they can't patent it, they can't profit..so they don't want it!** You see, lithium aspartate and lithium orotate are mineral complexes. Which means they cannot be patented. And without a patent *Big Pharma* cannot profit.

Cognitive decline and memory loss need not be considered inevitable consequences of aging—rather, they are the natural result of a lifetime of oxidative and inflammatory injury to brain tissue. Support for the body's antioxidant and ant-inflammatory systems can be found in such substances as: blueberry extract, grapeseed extract, vinpocetine (a derivative of the periwinkle plant), pregnelone (derived from cholesterol) and a plant known as ashwagandha.

One of the major causes of injury to the brain cells is the lack of essential nutrients due to the inadequate and harmful foods and drinks consumed by most people. Among the foods that are particularly harmful are those that contain poor quality fat such as any item that contains hydrogenated oil or partially hydrogenated oil. Hydrogenated oils are found in such popular foods as potato and corn chips, crackers, cookies, cakes, and in most fried foods. Use natural beneficial oils such as virgin olive oil, flaxseed oil, coconut oil and sesame oil to improve your health and nourish your brain. Keep in mind the fact that fat is essential as an energy source for the heart and the brain. It's a nutritional source for the central nervous system, and it lines and protects every organ. For these reasons, the term essential fatty acids or EFAs is used when referring to these important fats. Since the brain cells contain a large amount of the essential omega-3 fat, a lack of this nutrient leads to a less efficient brain which can result in such brain diseases as dementia and Alzheimer's. [116]

Dr. Julian Whitaker provides evidence that there is a simple inexpensive food that can reinvigorate the damaged brain cells of an Alzheimer patient. He gives us an in-depth analysis of what the probable cause of Alzheimer's is and what can be done to prevent it, as follows:

"Unfortunately, in Alzheimer's and other neuro-degenerative diseases, neurons lose their ability to properly use glucose. Inefficient glucose metabolism in specific areas of the brain is an early feature of these disorders, present long before symptoms appear. Many experts believe that this due to insulin resistance—Alzheimer's is sometimes referred to as as 'type 3 diabetes.' Neurons deprived of energy obviously cannot function normally and they eventually die, contributing to the degenerative process.

---

[116] Dr. Jonathan Wright. *Nutrition & Healing Newsletter*, 2009.

Benefits of a Keytogenic Diet

Affected neurons can however use ketones for energy, and when they're made available, starving brain cells perk right up. When this fuel source is supplied on a consistence basis, remarkable things can happen.

Actually, the therapeutic effects of ketones for the brain are old news. Ketogenic diets have been used since the 1920s to effectively prevent or reduce seizures in patients with epilepsy, and a handful of studies suggest that such a diet would also improve other neurodegenerative conditions. However, the ketogenic diet requires eating lots of fat and almost no carbohydrates and is difficult to stick with over the long term. That's the beauty of coconut oil. When you supplement with unrefined coconut oil, it is converted into ketones, even if you don't change your diet. In other words, you can have your carbs and ketones, too. There is a medicine called Aricept which contains an active ingredient MCT which is derived from the natural fatty acids that are abundant in coconut oil. MCT oil, which is derived from coconut oil is used in conventional medicine to provide energy for premature infants and patients recovering from surgery, and those with malnutrition and absorption problems. It is used by athletes to improve performance and endurance and by dieters to control appetite and stimulate fat burning. Studies suggest that it also enhances heart and immune health.

Unrefined coconut oil has numerous benefits as well. Contrary to popular belief, it does not raise cholesterol. In fact, it is cardioprotective and contains compounds that support the liver, improve immune function, and have anti-microbial properties.

I am now recommending ketone therapy for all of my patients with Alzheimer's disease, Parkinson's disease, dementia, multiple sclerosis, and other neurodegenerative disorders. There is evidence to suggest that it may also be beneficial for individuals with Down syndrome, autism, and diabetes.

The most practical and economical way of raising ketone levels is with MCT/coconut oil combo. The recommended dose of MCT for neurodegenerative disorders is 20 g per meal (21/2 tablespoons). As a preventative you can mix MCT with coconut oil and add it to your meals on a regular basis, starting with 1-2 teaspoons per meal. It can be added to cereals, used in cooking, and in salad dressings and as a spread. Because coconut oil contains no omega-3 essential fatty acids, a minimum of 2g of fish oil should also be taken daily. It is best taken three times a day preferably at mealtimes. It hardens in a refrigerator, so keep it at room temperature." [117]

Another approach to curing Alzheimer's is offered by Dr. Frank Shallenberger, as follows:

What if I told you there's a treatment for Alzheimer's disease that's proven, inexpensive and safe? What if I told you this treatment is something you can do without the help of your doctor? And what if I told you it might also help you lose weight? Sound too good to be true? Well it's not. It's very real and it works wonders for my Alzheimer's patients.

In fact, the journal *Neurotherapeutics* recently reviewed the treatment and found it to be amazingly effective. The article pinpoints how a simple change in diet can significantly improve memory and mental function in patients with Alzheimer's. It all has to do with ketones.

Ketones are a class of molecules that are produced from fat. Eating carbohydrates suppresses ketone formation because it suppresses fat metabolism. The more carbohydrates you eat, the less ketone you will make. For people without diabetes, ketone production is a normal part of metabolism. The reason that this is so important is because ketones are an important food for the brain. Injured or impaired brain cells cannot metabolize glucose well resulting in many serious illnesses. These brain cells, even if they can't use glucose well, can still metabolize ketones effectively. So, a diet low enough in carbohydrates to induce the formation of ketones can correct all kinds of abnormal brain function from seizures to ADD to depression to bipolar to Alzheimer's. These facts are sup-ported by research studies.

The ketones alleviate the symptoms of Alzheimer's because the brains of Alzheimer's patients cannot use glucose efficiently. This is the major reason they function well. By raising the ketone levels in the blood, we simply give the brain cells of an Alzheimer's patient the energy fuel that they so desperately need. In effect, when all we feed them is glucose, they effectively starve. So how do you increase the blood ketone levels of

---

[117] Dr. Whitaker's *Health & Healing.* October, 2009, pp-1-3

your loved ones with Alzheimer's? Actually it's one of the easier things to do. Just decrease their carbohydrate-intake enough.

Here's How I Have My Patient's Do It

First, buy some Ketostix from your local pharmacy. These are urine dipsticks, and they're readily available. When you place a Ketostix indicator in urine, it will turn purple as the ketones in the blood increase.

Then put them on a diet that completely eliminates the high-carbohydrate foods. This includes fruit, root vegetables (such as potatoes, carrots, beets, etc.), legumes (beans, soy, peas, lentils, etc.), grains (bread, corn, rice, chips, rolls, etc.), and all sugars.

Once they've started the diet, start checking the urine every morning. In about two to three days, the Ketostix should be turning a good strong purple color, indicating that the body is producing a lot of ketones.

Stay on the diet for another two to three days just to make sure the ketone level nice and steady. Then start adding in known amounts of carbohydrates every day until ketone formation is suppressed and the Ketostix stops turning purple. Once the Ketostix stops turning purple then you can calculate how many carbohydrates the patient can eat daily. All you have to do to calculate the carb limit is to take 80% of the carbs they ate to stop ketone production. That's the maximum number of carbs the Alzheimer patient can eat each day in order to maintain an effective blood ketone level. [118]

An article in the *Life Extension Magazine--March, 2009,* presents a review of the latest research which provides evidence of what causes Alzheimer's plus natural treatments for Alzheimer's which can help to prevent and may in some cases reverse the ill effects of the disease. Excerpts from the article are presented below:

According to growing research, there is just no question that oxidative stress leads to aging brain cells, resulting in decreased availability of natural antioxidants such as glutathione and increased destruction of vital lipid molecules in cell membranes - all of which impair cells ability to communicate effectively.

---

[118] Dr. Frank Shallenberger, MD. *Real Cures, Vol. 8, No 12, Dec 2007* pp. 1-6.

Not only is the central nervous system especially vulnerable to oxidative stress in general, but it becomes more progressively so with advancing age, as structural changes in cells accumulate. Inflammation adds insult to oxidative injury in the nervous system. Even by middle age, there is an increase in the production of inflammatory proteins. The interactions of inflammation and free radicals perpetuate a cycle of cell damage and dysfunction.

The ability of many plant food components to reduce or block the effects of the oxidation-inflammation-oxidation cycle has captured the attention of researchers. The beneficial way these plant compounds affect behavioral and neuronal aspects of aging has stimulated intense research into this area of dementia prevention. Phenols are plant molecules which have potent antioxidant capabilities; people with a high consumption of these molecules have lower rates of neurodegenerative disorders including Alzheimer's disease. Grape skins and seeds are especially rich in a group of polyphenols known as *proanthocyanidins,* which are proving to have astonishing anti-aging effects in the brain. The exciting and dramatic research on grapeseed extract and cognition is in Alzheimer's disease, where it has long been known that moderate red wine consumption is protective. Researchers at Mt. Sinai in New York fed mice a concentrated grapeseed extract and found that it resulted in a significant reduction in the deposits of the damaging *amyloid-beta* proteins associated with Alzheimer's disease, and a concomitant reduction in cognitive deterioration.

Other researchers at Tufts University found that the blueberry polyphnol molecules can cross the vital brain barrier, and hence that they exert their potent neuroprotection directly within the brain. In late 2008, neuroscientists at the University of South Florida discovered that blueberry extracts actually prevent the final steps in formation of the dangerous amyloid-beta proteins in Alzheimer's disease. They concluded that these findings could tip the scales away from formation of these destructive proteins in those at risk for Alzheimer's disease.

To support its many vital functions, the brain receives a huge proportion of total blood flow. One cause of cognitive decline with age is the gradual diminution of blood flow to vital areas, along with a decreased responsiveness to moment-by-moment needs, much of which results from oxidant damage to vessels. A little known compound called *vinpocetine* derived from the common periwinkle plant, has shown great promise in improving cerebral blood flow and restoring lost cognitive abilities. As early as 1987, geriatricians showed that vinpocetine could produce a significant improvement in elderly patients with chronic cerebral dysfunction. In 2003, a Bulgarian research group summarized evidence that vinpocetine can actually protect brain tissue from the effects of cerebrovascular disease, the silent blood vessel damage that precedes a stroke. They showed that vinpocetine passes rapidly across the brain barrier, and that it is selectively accumulated in parts of the brain most closely related to cognitive function. A 2005 clinical study in Hungary clinched the effects of vinpocetine on blood flow. In this elegant study, patients with multiple past strokes showed significant improvement in blood flow after three months of supplementation compared with the *placebo* recipients—and on cognitive tests, placebo patients deteriorated significantly while supplemented recipients had no change at three months. This study dramatically demonstrated both the cause and the effect of neuroprotection by vinpocetine. *There is increasing evidence that vinpocetine improves the quality of life in chronic cerebrovascular patients.*

Numerous herbs from ancient India are reputed to promote physical and mental health and among the most promising of these for promoting cognitive health is a plant known as ashwagandha. Indian researchers found that ashwagandha extracts increased concentrations of antioxidants in animal brains after supplementation. These researchers concluded that their findings explained the anti-stress, immuno-modulatory, cognition-facilitating, anti-inflammatory and anti-aging effects reported by other researchers in animal and clinical studies. In 2007, further support for the use of ashwagandha extracts in Alzheimer's disease was provided by the discovery that the extracts are among the most potent inhibitors of *acetylcholinesterase,* an enzyme that breaks down the vital memory-related neurotransmitter acetylcholine. Drugs like Aricept are used to block acetylcholine breakdown as does ashwagandha, except that the drug has side-effects and ashwagandha does not have any.

Pregnenolone, which is made from cholesterol, is another natural substance that is intimately connected with cognitive performance. It directly influences the release of the crucial neurotransmitter acetylcholine in regions of the brain linked with memory, learning, cognition, and sleep-wake cycles. With aging, individuals experience a dramatic decline in the production of pregnenolone. Administration of pregnenolone reverses the decline in new nerve growth that commonly occurs in disorders like Alzheimer's disease. Pregnenolone particularly enhances nerve cell growth in the hippocampus, the brain region responsible for memory, which undergoes marked deterioration in Alzheimer patients. Supp lemental pregnenolone may thus support youthful cognition and health by contributing to optimal hormone levels, supporting acetylcholine activity, and promoting cell growth in the brain's memory center.

It is now apparent that many traditional spices, in addition to their adding interest to our food, can provide vital anti-inflammatory and anti-oxidant functions. Four of these in particular deserve special mention for their powerful effects on learning and memory.

Curcumin is the yellow pigment in the popular Indian curry spice, turmeric, which provides the popular flavor of most Indian dishes. It has very powerful anti-inflammatory effects which research shows have benefits for Alzheimer patients.

Ginger is useful for digestion but we focus on it here for its ability to regulate platelet aggregation, which contributes not only to cardiovascular disease but also to cerebrovascular disease risk. Experimental studies demonstrated that ginger extract could protect cells from the inflammatory action of the Alzheimer's disease-related protein amyloid-beta. By its blood pressure-lowering effects, ginger can protect against the chronic brain injury caused by hypertension.

Rosemary is an herb that has a distinguished record as a protectant through its antioxidant constituent, carnosic acid. Rosemary extract blocks damaging lipid peroxidation, the destruction of brain cells' fatty membranes that impairs cognitive performance. Rosemary also protects cell nuclei from DNA damage that results from both oxidative stress and ultraviolet light—such damage is at the root of many cancers, but short of cancer it can impair a cell's ability to function normally.

Hops value may be primarily in its ability to promote relaxation and sleep. In one study, the combination of hops with valerian compared equally with a Vallium-like, sleep-inducing drug, and had none of the hang-over effects seen with the drug. Hops is also effective in the improvement of memory which may be of help in cases of Alzheimer' disease.

Alkaline Water although not an herb, is of such importance to the body's ability to maintain its normal pH balance that it is included here as another source of help for Alzheimer patients. Asian medicine says that **many adult diseases can be treated by alkalizing the bloodstream.** [119]

Fluoridation of Water is a major factor in the cause of Alzheimer's disease according to Dr. Douglas. Here's what he has to say about *'Slashing your risk of Alzheimer's overnight:*

People who warned against FLUORIDATION used to be ridiculed, but guess what? In Scandinavia, in fact all of Europe and nearly every other medically advanced nation, they have now banned the practice. Know why? Because fluoride makes your body absorb extra aluminum. And where does the aluminum go? To your brain. And what metal show's up alarmingly in the brains of Alzheimer's victims? You guessed it. (Hmm….maybe our health authorities have been drinking too much tap water. [120]

Detoxification programs that eliminate heavy metals, such as chelation therapy, will help to filter out the aluminum from your blood stream.

Autism

Autism is a debilitating disorder suffered by 1 in 150 children, making it more common than childhood cancer, diabetes and AIDS combined, according to the Centers for Disease Control and Prevention. Recently England and Ireland reported that autism is affecting

---

[119] *Life Extension Magazine.* Editors. March, 2009,
[120] *Dr. Douglas Report, Summer, 2009,* pp. 8-9.

one in 58 individuals. Loretta Schwarts-Nobel describes autism as follows:

Autism locks children into a world of their own. As the National Autistic Society explains, its symptoms can include 'a lack of speech, repetitive behaviors, little or no social inter-action, withdrawal from parental and sibling contact, jerky body motions of specific limbs, head banging, hand flapping, and weird individual obsessions like eating cardboard containers or breaking certain specific objects.

Many parents, doctors and scientists now believe that the increase in autism is directly linked to the number of scheduled vaccinations babies received. During the 1990s, the vaccinations each child was mandated to have were doubled from about 20 to almost forty. Many of these vaccines contained a mercury additive called thimersol, a dangerous, highly toxic preservative that stops contamination of vaccines and preserves shelf life at very low cost to drug manufacturers. It costs states about $2 million for each child with autism for the first eighteen years of life…. Despite drug company studies from seventy years ago that concluded mercury-containing serum was not fit for cattle or dogs not one of the federal agencies that is supposed to protect us had taken the time to total up how much thimersol and mercury had been added to the average child's intake with the new increased immunization schedule. The simple fact was that all of our children were now getting about 120 times the mercury exposure allowed by the EPA, while medical journals continued to tell parents that there wasn't any connection between thimersol and autism. As Robert Kennedy, Jr. points out in *Deadly Immunity* history suggests otherwise. Eli Lilly, the first pharmaceutical company to use thimersol, knew from the start that its products could cause damage or even death in both animals and humans….Medical research reported in medical journals found the following reactions to the pertussis vaccine: "Vaccine-induced brain injuries appear to be on a continuum from milder forms such as ADD or ADHD and learning disabilities, to autism-spectrum and seizure disorders, to severe mental retardation, all the way to death. On this continuum, and often coinciding with brain dysfunction, is immune system dysfunction ranging from development of severe allergies and asthma to intestinal bowel disorders, rheumatoid arthritis, and diabetes.

According to Dr. Hugh Fundenberg, one of the most quoted biologists of our time,' it isn't just children who are at risk...if an adult receives too many consecutive flu shots containing thimersol, his or her chance of developing Alzheimer's disease is ten times greater than if he or she had one or two, or no shots at all...the reason is 'the gradual mercury and aluminum buildup in the brain causes eventual cognitive dysfunction.

Medical research reported in medical journals found the following reactions to the pertussis vaccine: "Vaccine-induced brain injuries appear to be on a continuum from milder forms such as ADD or ADHD and learning disabilities, to autism-spectrum and seizure disorders, to severe mental retardation, all the way to death. On this continuum, and often coinciding with brain dysfunction, is immune system dysfunction ranging from development of severe allergies and asthma to intestinal bowel disorders, rheumatoid arthritis, and diabetes. [121]

Bernard Rimland, considered to be the father of autism research and the founder of the Autism Society of America found that mercury in vaccines was the primary culprit in the epidemic increase in autism cases - from 1 in 10,000 infants in 1990 to 1 in 150 today.

Actress Jenny McCarthy noticed signs of autism in her child, Evan, shortly after he had been given vaccination shots. Medical examinations confirmed that Evan did have autism. Jenny took steps to help her child offset the effects of autism which led to his recovery. Here's what she had to say about it: "We believe that what helped Evan recover was a gluten-free, casein-free diet, vitamin supplementation, detox of metals, and anti-fungals for yeast overgrowth that plagued his intestines. Once these neurological functions were recovered, speech therapy and applied behavior analysis helped him quickly learn the skills he could not learn while he was frozen in

---

[121] Nobel, op. cit., pp. 85-95.

autism. After we implemented these therapies for one year, the state re-evaluated Evan for further services. They spent 5 minutes with him and said, 'What happened? We've never seen a recovery like this.'

Evans is now 5 years old and what might surprise a lot of you is that we've never been contacted by any member of the CDC, the American Academy of Pediatrics, or any other health authority to evaluate and understand how Evan recovered from autism. When Evan meets doctors and neurologists, to this day they tell us he was misdiagnosed—that he never had autism to begin with.

We think our health authorities don't want to open this can of worms, so they don't even look or listen. Many parents of recovered children will tell you they didn't treat their children for autism; they treated them for vaccine injury. Many people aren't aware of the fact in the 1980s our children received only 10 vaccines by age 5, whereas today they are given 36 immunizations most of them by age 2. With billions of pharmaceutical dollars, could it be that the vaccine program is becoming more of a profit engine than a means of protection?" [122]

In addition to the steps that Jenny took to help her child there are other procedures that have proven to be effective such as the use of a detox agent called Zeolite and an allergy treatment called NAET.

Cancer Cures and Prevention

Cancer is the number two killer in America. It is greatly feared and a tremendous cause of pain and suffering not only from the disease itself but also from the treatments used by conventional medicine such as drugs, chemotherapy and surgery, not to mention the tremendous financial cost to the patients. There are a number of treatments that are available that are known to cure, prevent and/or reverse cancer. These alternative treatments are, for the most part, relatively inexpensive making use of natural foods and herbs.

As mentioned earlier in this book, it is essential for optimum health to avoid milk and to reduce the amount of animal protein in the diet to a minimum amount. (See the China Study)

It is also very important to restore the beneficial bacteria in the

---

[122] *The Day I Heard My Son Had Autism.* Jenny McCarthy. Google 1/15/09.

body which has probably been weakened by toxins and by treatments such as flu shots, vaccinations and chelation therapy.

Vitamin C and Cancer

A common vitamin, vitamin C, has been found to cure cancer when taken in accordance with the specific needs of each patient. Details of this treatment are presented in the book, *The Cancer Breakthrough,* by Dr. Steve Hickey. Dr. Hickey describes how important it is to maintain a specific amount of vitamin C in the blood stream for an extended period of time in order for it to destroy cancer cells. This requires the infusion of a certain amount of vitamin C (determined by a physician skilled in this protocol) to be given intravenously by a slow drip method (for a minimum of several hours, several times a week. Additional supplements, such as selenium, are also prescribed in accordance with the needs of each patient.

Another respected vitamin C expert, Dr. Thomas Levy in his book *Curing the Incurable* has this to say about vitamin C: "There is no condition of ill health that I am aware of, that doesn't respond positively to properly administered vitamin C treatment. I've studied most of the research and I've successfully employed vitamin C therapies well over a thousand times. I have personally witnessed many vitamin C miracles… cataracts and periodontal diseases are actually a symptom of vitamin deficiency."

Dr. Levy points out that the medical establishment has failed to make full use of the many benefits of vitamin C therapy such as:

1. Documented evidence that vitamin C cures both acute polio and acute hepatitis.
2. Properly dosed vitamin C can reverse and almost always cure other significant medical conditions such as cancer and heart disease.
3. Properly dosed vitamin C can replace the reliance on vaccinations as a preventative of viral diseases.
4. Vitamin C is the ideal agent for helping in the destruction of most bacteria, fungi, and other microbial agents that continue to afflict mankind.
5. Vitamin C reduces tooth cavity. It is vastly more desirable for reducing dental decay than ingested forms of fluoride. Fluoride will always be toxic when enough of it accumulates in the body.

6. Vitamin C can eliminate aluminum from the body. [123]

A number of other treatments that are known to cure cancer are described in detail in the following pages.

Essiac (Flor-Essence)

A Canadian nurse, Rene Caisse, came across a cure for cancer which was made from natural herbs. The cure was given to her by an Ojibwa Indian medicine man. She made it available at no charge to terminally ill cancer patients who in 95 percent of the cases were cured. She named the cure Essiac which was her last name spelled backwards. People who were cured spread the news to their family and friends and before long there were thousands of people from all over Canada coming to her home seeking the cure.

Several medical doctors whose patients were cured came to visit her and observe what she was doing. They were amazed with the fact that the cure consisted of simple herbs taken as a tea. There was a special way in which the tea was prepared with a specific amount of each herb in the formula. Some leading cancer specialists made her offers of substantial amounts of money if she would give them the formula so that they could test the ingredients in a laboratory and then make it available as a medically approved medicine to their patients. Rene was leery of these offers as she knew from her experience as a head nurse at a hospital in Toronto that the conventional medical authorities were committed to their methods of treating cancer and if they could make the herbal formula available as a medicine they would charge exorbitantly high prices for it. She continued to turn down the offers even though she could have retired as a very wealthy woman had she accepted the offers. The following excerpt from the book *The Essiac Report* tells what Rene went through at the hands of the medical authorities:

> A number of doctors, whose patients had made remarkable recoveries although their cases were considered hopeless, sent a petition to the Department of National Health and Welfare in Ottawa asking that Rene be given facilities to do independent research on a scale worthy of her discovery. The Petition included the following statement: To the best of our knowledge, she has not been given a case to treat until everything

---

[123] Dr. Thomas Levy. *Curing the Incurable.* Pp. 17-29.

in medical and surgical science has been tried without effect and even then she was able to show remarkably beneficial results on those cases at that late stage. We would be interested to see her given an opportunity to prove her work in a large way. To the best of our knowledge she has treated all cases free of any charge.

The Department of Health and Welfare was less than impressed. They promptly sent two investigating doctors empowered with the proper documents to have Rene arrested. When they arrived and found that she was working with nine of the most eminent doctors in Toronto and heard their opinions, they did not arrest her.

By 1938 Rene's support had grown enormously. Another petition was circulated. This time it garnered 55,000 signatures! They were demanding in no uncertain terms that Rene be allowed to, in effect, practice medicine without a license. Imagine if you will the wrath Rene was about to incur from a Medical Establishment firmly entrenched in their faith in the wonders of modern medicine. A Medical Establishment that legally held the power to crush anyone who had the audacity to practice the art of healing not in accordance with the precepts of the ordained faith. A bill was created in the legislature, the Kirby Bill, by supporters of the Medical Establishment to protect the public from 'unorthodox' cancer treatments, Rene's treatment being of course the main target. Rene was told to turn over her formula to the authorities or else be subject to heavy penalties including a jail sentence.

Rene became increasingly worried that it was only a matter of time before she would be prosecuted and imprisoned under the Kirby Bill. She closed her clinic in 1942. She continued to treat desperate cancer patients who sought her out where she was living but the numbers were small and she felt thwarted. In 1959, a major breakthrough occurred. Although 70, she was about to begin the most important phase in the development of Essiac.

A highly respected medical doctor in the United States, Dr. Charles Brusch, learned of the curative powers of Essiac and he contacted Caisse in 1959. He invited her to come to America and make use of his clinic to further her work with Essiac. Under Dr. Brusch's supervision cancer patients were treated with Essiac with uniformly excellent results. The original formula was also improved upon by Dr. Brusch and his colleagues. However, in a short time, the American Medical Establishment pressured medical doctors to stop sending patients to the Brusch Clinic for treatment of cancer with the result that Caisse realized her efforts in the United States would be restricted just as they had been in Canada. She returned to her home in Canada where she died in December, 1978.

Her efforts were not in vain, however. Dr. Brusch continued using Essiac for his cancer patients with impressive results. He actually cured himself of cancer using Essiac in 1984. He realized that it would be next to impossible to get Essiac approved as a drug so he gave up trying to get the approval of Medical authorities. A major breakthrough occurred in 1984. A very popular radio talk show host and producer, Elaine Alexander, contacted Dr. Brusch and offered to do a series of radio shows featuring the Essiac cure with the understanding that he would be willing to take part in the show as an authority on Essiac. The people who listened to the radio show were so convinced of the benefits of Essiac that they demanded to know where they could obtain the product. The huge response convinced Elaine Alexander that she should find a way to make the formula available to the public. She got the support of Dr. Brusch who had the formula and they searched for a company to manufacture the product. They found a company in Canada called Flora which produced a variety of supplements using natural herbs which was highly respected for the quality of its products. An agreement was reached to produce the Essiac formula in a liquid form and sell it to the public under the name of Flor-Essence. At first it was sold only in Canada but as it grew in popularity, it was eventually made available in the United States. In order to avoid any conflicts with the medical doctors the product was labeled as a toxic cleanser without any reference to its curative power for cancer. It can now be obtained in many health food stores or by contacting the Flora Company. [124]

Flaxseed (Linseed) Oil Cure for Cancer

Flaxseed oil has already been mentioned above as having been of benefit for cardiovascular problems such as high blood pressure. It has also been found to be a cure for cancer when used in combination with cottage cheese. This simple combination of two ordinary foods has been used in Europe for many years to help cure cancers, as reported in the book *Cancer Free: Your Guide to Gentle, Non-toxic Healing*. The author, Bill Henderson, has been publishing books and newsletters about cancer treatment and helping people deal with cancer since 1998. His mission to help everyone possible was born from watching his wife Marjorie, go through conventional cancer treatment, which destroyed her body in the process of killing her. The following excerpt from his book provides convincing evidence of the effectiveness of this cure:

> In my research, starting in 1998, I had run across Dr. Johanna Budwig's name several times. I always glossed over it when I heard her 'formula' - a little flaxseed oil mixed with cottage cheese. Thanks to one of my faithful readers, I learned that this substance **uniquely** kills cancer cells by the billions and makes every other cell in our body healthier - **at the same time.** Since that time, I have read many articles and books on this subject. It seems that there is nothing like it in the world. The cottage cheese is the perfect carrier for the oil. Once the flaxseed oil, with its high concentration of Omega 3 oil, gets to the cell wall (membrane), it surrounds it with magnets which 'suck in' oxygen. This action of the cells has been recognized since 1931 as the very best way to make healthy cells healthier and kill cancer cells.

> Dr. Dan C. Roehm, an oncologist and cardiologist made the following statement based on his own observations of patients in his practice: 'This diet is far and away the **most successful anti-cancer diet in the world.** What she (Dr Johanna Budwig) has demonstrated to my initial disbelief but lately, to my **complete satisfaction** in my practice is:

---

[124] Richard Thomas. *The Essiac Report.* Los Angeles: Alternative Treatment Information Network, 1993.

CANCER IS EASILY CURABLE. The treatment results in an immediate response; the cancer cell is weak and vulnerable; the precise biochemical point was identified by her in **1951** and is specifically correctable, in the (test tube) as well as **in vivo (real).** I wish that all my patients had a PhD in Biochemistry and Quantum Physics to enable them to see how, with **such consummate** skill, this diet was put together.

In 1967, Dr. Budwig broadcast the following sentence during an interview over the South German Radio Network describing her treatment of patients with failed operations and x-ray (radiation therapy): 'Even in these cases it is possible to restore health in **a few months** at most, I would truly say **90% of the time.'** This has never been contradicted, but this knowledge has been a long time reaching this side of the ocean, hasn't it? Cancer treatment can be **very simple and very successful** once you know how. The cancer interests don't want you to know this. May the miscreants who have kept you from knowing of this simple information for so long be forgiven? Here's another quote from a noted doctor, Robert Willner, MD., PhD.: 'A top European cancer specialist, Dr. Johanna Budwig, has discovered a **totally natural formula** that not only protects against the development of cancer but people all over the world who have been diagnosed with incurable cancer and **sent home to die** have been actually cured and now lead normal, healthy lives.' [125]

The basic linseed oil and cottage cheese formula is prepared by mixing 1 or 2 tablespoons of organic flaxseed oil with 8 to 16 ounces of low fat cottage cheese. Place the mixture in a blender and blend to a smooth consistency. Remove the mixture from the blender and place it in the refrigerator for about 30 minutes. It is then ready to eat. You can add any kind of fruit or vegetable to the basic formula to suit your taste. It is recommended that this be eaten every morning for breakfast. Not only does this help to cure cancer but it can be used to help prevent cancer also. In the book *How to Fight Cancer and Win* which is based on documented facts for the successful treatment and prevention of cancer, the author, William Fischer has

---

[125] Bill Henderson. *Cancer-Free: Your Guide to Gentle, Non-Toxic Healing.* Internet: Booklocker. Com, 2007, pp. 100-101.

this to say about the Budwig formula: "I personally take as a dietary supplement 1 or 2 tablespoons of cold-pressed, unrefined virgin linseed oil mixed with   to one cup of low-fat cottage cheese every day. Because of all the very strong evidence, it seems to me that this is the very best preventative medicine in the world to ward off the degenerative diseases." [126]

Prostate Cancer Metastasis and Citrus.

One of the problems associated with prostate cancer has been metastasis, in many cases caused by biopsies and by surgery. One reason why cancer is so lethal is its tendency to *metastasize* to essential organs throughout the body. A special form of fruit pectin derived from the pulp and peel of citrus fruits called **modified citrus pectin** (MCP) has demonstrated unique properties in blocking cell aggregation, adhesion, and metastasis. Clinical research shows that MCP helps limit disease progression in men with advanced prostate cancer. In addition to its cancer-inhibiting effects, modified citrus pectin shows promise in chelating toxic heavy metals that can be so damaging to overall health. Some of the advantages of taking modified citrus pectin are presented in an article in the March, 2009 *Life Extension Magazine* as follows:

"Compelling research suggests that modified citrus pectin may help block the growth and metastasis of solid tumors such as breast, colon, and prostate cancers. Intriguing clinical studies suggest that supplementation with MCP stabilizes disease progression and lessens PSA doubling times in men with prostate cancer. Modified citrus pectin may represent a safe, non-toxic method of chelating toxic metals—without the need for intravenous infusions. Supplementation with MCP has been shown to increase excretion of dangerous metals such as mercury, arsenic, lead, and cadmium—without removing essential minerals like calcium, magnesium, and zinc from the body. MCP is considered safe and well tolerated. Dosages range from 6 to 30 grams per day in divided dosages; A typical dose is 5 grams three times a day."

---

[126] William Fischer . *How to Fight Cancer and Win*. Baltimore: Agora Health Books, 2001, p. 167.

Wheat Grass Cure for Cancer

A cure for cancer was developed in the 1950s by a remarkable woman, Ann Wigmore. She had been diagnosed with colon cancer and instinctively began chewing on common lawn grass and credited the juice with healing her cancer. She came up with the idea of growing sprouts from wheat seeds (berries) and then when the sprouts were about 5 inches tall, she cut them and put them in a blender making wheatgrass juice.

Wigmore founded the Hippocrates Health Institute in Florida which makes use of wheatgrass juice as the centerpiece of its cures for serious illnesses and diseases. It became famous for its cures and people started to come from all parts of the world, including many famous celebrities such as Paul Newman, Dick Gregory and Coretta Scott King. Hippocrates has a staff of 85 healers and support personnel.

Randall Fitzgerald describes his experience at Hippocrates: "During my three-week stay in the program, I encountered people of all ages battling a range of deadly diseases - cancer, multiple sclerosis, Parkinson's, leukemia, diabetes. A Los Angles real estate investor in his late fifties arrived with severe MS symptoms. I watched him the first week shuffle along slowly and stiffly on wobbly legs like someone trying to keep his balance on a storm-tossed ship. After two weeks on the diet he marched around with renewed vitality, showing no obvious symptoms of the disease.

The idea of pure food as medicine is taken quite literally here, and wheatgrass juice is the food drink of choice. Less than two ounces of wheatgrass juice is said to be nutritional equivalent to consuming nearly three pounds of fresh vegetables and 103 vitamins and minerals. Wheatgrass contains nature's richest source of chlorophyll and acts as a potent immune system booster, body-organ cleanser and toxin neutralizer The Hippocrates program utilizes a mix of components that act synergistically with the wheatgrass. These include sprouted seeds and grains, raw un-cooked vegetables, daily exercise, periodic fasting, colon cleansings to remove toxic waste accumulations, taking supplements derived only from naturally occurring whole foods, and the cultivation of positive attitudes." [127]

---

[127] Fitzgerald, op. cit., pp.230-233.

In the 1960s Wigmore left Florida and moved to Boston where she planned on retiring. People who learned of her cure for cancer came to her home and she accepted a few patients at a time. She took people into her home who were very ill, mostly cancer patients. She believed that it was necessary to detoxify the body before any cure could take place. She placed the patients on a fast and on a series of colonic irrigations. She then had them drink small quantities of wheatgrass juice which was made fresh each time it was served. Many people provided testimonials about their recovery from various kinds of cancer by consuming wheat grass juice but mainstream medicine ignored this evidence. The benefits of wheat grass include its abundant, easily-absorbed nutrients plus its ability to deacidify and detoxify the body, as described by Dr. Vasey:

"Wheat sprouts contain more alkaline minerals than any other sprouts or green vegetables; more than one hundred different nutrients, including almost all the minerals and trace elements, and the entire range of vitamins from the B group. The iron content of wheat sprouts, essential for good tissue oxygenation, is higher than spinach, which is considered to be one of the best sources for this mineral.

Wheat sprouts are the highest in chlorophyll of any plant source. Chlorophyll, which gives plants their green color, has a molecular structure that is almost identical to that of blood hemoglobin, which is indispensable for transporting oxygen into the cells. The similarity of chlorophyll to hemoglobin has led to the description of chlorophyll as the 'blood' of the plant.

Chlorophyll plays an important role in deacidifying the body by oxygenating the tissues, enabling the tissues to oxidize many more weak and volatile acids than normal and eliminate them via respiration. But chlorophyll also has the property of breaking down carbon dioxide (which is acidic) and dissolving the deposits of strong acids, such as kidney stones. Furthermore, chlorophyll has diuretic and purifying properties that facilitate the elimination of acids.

Other plants that produce very valuable sprouts are *kamut, barley grass and alfalfa*. Kamut is a very ancient wheat variety that has never been hybridized. Its grains are three times fatter than those of wheat, and their nutrient content, especially that of several alkaline minerals, is significantly higher. This richness is present in the juice of young sprouts. Kamut juice is 90 percent higher in potassium, 148 percent higher in calcium, and 50 percent higher in iron than wheat juice; furthermore, the pH of this juice and the powder made from it is the most alkaline of all the green foods, which contributes to excellent deacidification of the body. Barley grass has been recognized by researchers as the most nutritious plant in existence; it contains the most minerals, including a high concentration of alkaline minerals. Its vitamin B1 content (thiamine) is four times higher than that of wheat flour and thirty times higher than that of milk. Young barley grass is also the best natural source of the anti-oxidant superoxide dismutase (SOD), which prevents acidification of the tissues.

Alfafa (also known as lucerne) is not a cereal grain like wheat, kamut, and barley, but a legume like peanuts or soy. It is used as a forage plant for livestock because of its high protein content, up to 55 percent of its total weight, and its high content of minerals such as calcium, iron, zinc, copper, and selenium, all alkaline minerals.

Green-food powder - is available in capsules or as a powder to be mixed with water, making a drink with a distinctive but pleasant taste. These green drinks are useful because plant juices do not hold up for very long. Drinking it regularly every day provides the body with a host of alkaline minerals for deacidification purposes, but also with other nutrients, enzymes in particular, that fight against acidification indirectly by making metabolism more efficient and thus reducing the production of acids by the body. (see Green Smoothies)

Melatonin and Cancer

Researchers consider melatonin to be one of the most promising 'new' cancer therapy agents. The incidence of breast cancer is about five times higher in people who live in industrialized countries where excess light interferes with the natural day-night rhythms, and where working the night shift is common. People with low levels of melatonin are at significantly higher risk of many different kinds of cancer, including breast, endometrial, and colorectal. Cells from these and other kinds of cancers slow down or even stop growing in response to melatonin alone.

Melatonin strengthens your immune system through a number of different avenues. It does all this as a modulator, not a stimulator - it helps you launch a stronger defense against any challenge, including cancer, while also fighting excessive inflammation, to keep your immune system from becoming over-reactive and self-defeating.

Antibiotics and Cancer

According to a report by Dr. Williams, "a recent study linked antibiotic use to an increased risk of developing cancer. A Finnish study analyzed the health history of over 3,000,000 individuals. It tracked their antibiotic use for a two-year period and then the incidence of cancer for the next six years following the antibiotic use. Those with no antibiotic prescriptions were the reference group and their risk of cancer was not increased. In the group having 2 to 5 prescriptions, the relative risk of cancer increased 27 percent and those having over 6 prescriptions had an increase of 37 percent. The most common sites for the cancers were endocrine glands, prostate, lung, breast, and colon.

Other studies have found similar results. Scientists at the University of Washington, working with the National Cancer Institute, studied the association between antibiotics and invasive breast cancer. "They discovered that women who took antibiotics for more than 500 days, or had more than 25 prescriptions, over an average of 17 years had more than twice the risk of breast cancer compared to women who had not taken any antibiotics. Even women who had between one and 25 prescriptions over a period of 17 years have an increased risk of about one and a half times that of women who took no antibiotics."

When you consider that breast cancer is the second leading cause of death of women in this country, it seems strange that these well-run studies haven't been better publicized. We're constantly being told about the new antibiotic resistant-resistant bugs and the need for the development of new, stronger antibiotics. You would think that women, in particular, would want to know that antibiotics may be doubling their risk of dying from breast cancer. We've become so accustomed to the widespread use of antibiotics that it may seem far-etched to think they could increase the risk of something like cancer. The fact of the matter, however, is that 80 percent of our immune system is directly dependent on the balance of bacterial flora in our lower intestinal tract. Any imbalance in the beneficial bacteria can lead to overgrowth in pathogenic bacteria and impair the function of our immune system. Antibiotics destroy all bacteria, both good and bad. It shouldn't come as any surprise when we learn their overuse is contributing to the development of all types of diseases, not just cancer." [128]

The above mentioned treatments for cancer are just a few of the alternative treatments available. Important things to keep in mind for both the cure and prevention of cancer are to eat foods in their whole raw state as much as possible. Drinking raw green smoothies is an easy, enjoyable way to gain the benefits of consuming fresh, raw green leafy vegetables. The benefits of a low protein diet have already been described elsewhere in this book but bear repeating since this is a vital factor. Avoid the protein in milk, casein, as much as possible. It promotes rapid cellular growth as required by a baby calf but can also increase the growth of cancer cells in humans.

Candida is usually caused by the frequent use of antibiotics for a number of reasons, as explained by David Webster:

Today it is known that when lacobacteria, such as Bifidus, predominate in the colon, putrefactive types are unable to live in large numbers. Putrefactive bacteria in the colon produces toxins which, when absorbed into the blood stream, cause slow poisoning of the entire system.

Our colon health depends primarily on three factors: (1) existence of a slightly acidic pH; (2) maintenance of a predominantly acidophilus colon flora and (3) regular elimination. Factors such as antibiotics and other drugs, diet, stress, and exposure to microorganisms in food and environment are all major factors in determining the condition and population of colon flora.

Chronic constipation and diarrhea are often eliminated when the colon is restored and maintained at a slightly acidic pH. The presence of a putrefactive alkaline producing flora may be indicated by dry, dark brown and solidly formed feces, having a putrid odor, as well as by one that is semi-fluid. A stool that floats in water is soft but firm and amber in color with little or no odor is a sign of a healthy colon flora.

With the destruction of beneficial acidophilous bacteria, the acidic pH of the colon changes to one of alkalinity. This sets up perfect conditions for Candida overgrowth. When in the minority, Candida inhabits the human body without harm. When the immune system is weakened by any cause, an opportunity arises for Candida

---

[128] David Williams, MD. *Alternatives*. Jan 2009. Pp 150-151

to multiply rapidly, creating and releasing highly toxic substances into the system. Candida of fungal variety can penetrate the mucosa (lining) of the colon, allowing minute particles of undigested protein to enter the system and trigger allergic reactions.

As long as Candida predominates in the colon, symptoms will continue to reoccur in other parts of the body. In humans, Candida affects both males and females and may be transmitted by sexual contact. At this time, many health professionals report a world-wide epidemic of Candida is occurring. It is possible to destroy Candida with known anti-fungal remedies. Following this, immediate replacement of acidophilous and its acid production in the colon (and vagina in women) is essential to assist in preventing a relapse.

Today the need for an effective post-antibiotic approach to implant acidophilous is essential. This will reestablish the normal colon flora so often depleted or destroyed by a course of antibiotics and prevent Candida albicans and other harmful organisms from becoming predominant in the colon.

All animal proteins (including eggs), consumed to excess, without a balance of foods to stimulate acidophilous, lead to overgrowth of gas-forming proteolytic types of bacteria, a decrease in acidophilous and may contribute to a change in stool to alkaline. Milk, cheese and a high casein diet have been found to promote the growth of unfavorable saprophytic bacteria. When an excess of fats/oils are consumed, a flora is developed that can produce estrogens from the excess bile acids present in the colon. These estrogens can circulate in the bloodstream and contribute to many health problems.

When the colon is out of balance, it is necessary to first, clear toxins that have accumulated. Then acidify the colon so acidophilous will be able to establish and grow there. Next a human strain of viable acidophilous must be implanted rectally into the colon. Finally, acidophilous must be provided with proper food to help it multiply, thrive and take hold.

Another powerful anti-carcinogenic substance which is inexpensive and easily available is the chlorophyll found in dark green leafy vegetables such as collard greens, kale, spinach, and cilantro. Dr. Slaga has this to say about chlorophyll:

"Because of the abundance of chlorophyll in the food supply, it has been getting a lot of attention for its potential in preventing cancer. Chlorophyll, the water-soluble green pigment in plants, and chlorophyllin, its water soluble derivative, has been shown to possess strong antimutagen activity against a wide range of human carcinogens. In several experimental models, chlorophyllin has been shown to inhibit the induction of liver, skin, esophageal and stomach cancer." (see section on green smoothies) [129]

Cardiovascular Diseases

Blood Pressure

One of the best ways to maintain normal blood pressure, in addition to exercise and a low fat diet, is to consume foods which reduce inflammation such as flaxseeds which are rich in linolenic acid. Dr. A. Weil has this to say about the value of linolenic acid:

> "Linolenic acid which is contained in flaxseed oil, legumes, nuts and citrus fruits, may be the principal dietary polyunsaturated fatty acid related to blood pressure. Flaxseed oil is a very good source of omega 3 which is usually not found in most oils.

> Elements needed for the efficient processing of the essential fatty acids include vitamins A as beta carotene, C, B3, B6, and zinc. Pumpkin seed oil, soybean oil, and walnut oil contain linolenic and linoleic acids that are essential oils for the body.

> These oils rid the body of dangerous arterial plaque and gradually rebuild the cell and tissue damage caused by fatty degeneration of harmful oils." [130]

> The high fiber content and alkalinity of celery and Bok Choy are known to lower blood pressure.

Cholesterol and Nutrients - Resveratrol

"Thanks to new research on animals, there's exciting evidence that a powerful nutrient, Resveratrol, can lower your cholesterol, even better than drugs. It can also lower your triglycerides and reduce the risk of heart attacks.

---

[129] Slaga, op. cit., p. 102.
[130] Andrew Weil, M.D. *Spontaneous Healing.* New York: Ballantine Books, 1995, p. 12.

Statin drugs can lower cholesterol levels in the body by inhibiting the cholesterol-making enzyme of the body. This impairs the natural function of the enzyme system and causes serious side-effects. Resveratrol, on the other hand, turns down the amount of the enzyme naturally without impairing the enzyme as drugs do. This is very important when you consider the fact that this cholesterol-making enzyme is of critical importance in your brain and that it also makes CoQ10, an essential heart nutrient." [131]

Vitamin K2 for Cardiovascular Health

"Taking supplemental K2 has already been shown to be associated with significantly reduced cardiovascular risk. (It must be K2, not just the regular vitamin K). New studies show that a vitamin K2 deficiency also allows varicose veins to develop, through the same kind of mechanism that happens in your arteries. When vitamin K2 levels are low, a compound known as MGP doesn't get activated, and as a result, the smooth muscle cells in your vein's walls get plastered with the calcium that was meant for your bones.

Studies show it's very common to be silently, subclinically deficient in vitamin K2. That means you have substantial amounts of incompletely carboxylated MGP in your circulation, and as a result you're taking calcium from your bones and slathering it onto the interior walls of your arteries and veins.

The discomfort and appearance of varicose veins are an outward indication of an inward problem. As your veins begin to look and feel better, know that you're healing the rest of your body as well. Other ways to promote healthy blood flow is to include fish oil, ginko biloba, and vitamin E." [132]

Felder, a cardiologist, refers to a breakthrough study which found that when consumed together in the specific quantities detailed below; the following foods reduce the risk of cardiovascular disease by 76% all by protecting the endothelium (the lining of blood vessels):

1. Garlic – 1 clove a day – Garlic inhibits cholesterol production in the liver. It lowers the bad form of cholesterol (LDL)

---

[131] *Second Opinion Health Newsletter, October, 2008,* p. 3.
[132] *Second Opinion, Feb., 2008, p. 5.*

2. Red Wine – 5 ounces a day – lowers LDL and raises HDL.

3. Fruits & vegetables – 4 cups of fruit and veggies daily – lowers blood pressure, and inflammation.

4. Wild caught, cold-water fish like salmon, mackerel and herring, 3 five-ounce servings per week. The omega3 in these fish prevent blood clots, lower triglycerides, raise HDL, reduce inflammation and prevent fatal heart arrhythmias.

5. Nuts—almond and other nuts that have proven heart protective mono-unsaturated fats. Use 2 oz. of nuts daily. They also lower blood pressure by their minerals – about 170mg of potassium and 60mg of magnesium per ounce.

6. Chocolate – eat 2 ounces of dark chocolate, minimum of 60% cocoa.

7. Supplements – fish oil, niacin, coenzymeQ10, grape seed extract and policosonol.

8. Exercise and fish oil together: 3 grams of fish oil daily plus one hour of aerobic exercise.

Dr. Julian Whitaker, M.D. offers some new insights into the causes and cures for heart disease as follows:

Way back in 1983—long before angioplasty became the revenue-generating darling of cardiology—the Coronary Artery Study (CASS) was published. This definitive clinical trial was expected to confirm the benefits of bypass surgery in patients with significant heart disease.

Instead, CASS showed that bypass was a bust. Rates of heart attack and death from heart disease were no lower in patients who had surgery than they were in a similar group without surgery. The death rate in the patients who did not have bypass surgery was a surprisingly low 1.6 per cent per year. The chance that any surgery will improve on a death rate this low is virtually nil. It boils down to one indisputable fact. You cannot save the life of someone who is not going to die.

When you weigh the certain pain and cost of surgery against the slim chance of benefit, it's an easy call. Yet today, bypass, angioplasty, and other heart procedures continue to be foisted upon more and more folks who don't need them. If hard science and patient benefit were central factors here, these procedures would be a rarity. But invasive surgery has nothing to do with science. It has nothing to do with saving lives or improving quality of life. It has to do with money. Period!" [133]

Another factor associated with heart attacks is each person's personality type. In 1974, cardiologists, Meyer Friedman and Ray Rosenman reported on their research in *Type A Behavior and Your Heart,* indicating that personality type is a critical factor which determines a person's likelihood of a heart attack. Other researchers at the Mount Zion Medical Center in San Francisco have been able to detect by behavior pattern alone the man likely to have a heart attack (Type A) and the man unlikely to have a heart attack (Type B). Dr. Harold Bloomfield describes the differences between the Type A and Type B personalities as follows:

Type A consists of those feelings and their respective motor expressions displayed by an individual possessing an exaggerated drive, ambition, aggressiveness, competiveness, and above all,, sense of time urgency—even at supposed times of leisure. Most people have some or all of these attributes, but the person likely to be stricken with a heart attack possesses them to an unusually high degree. He appears to walk, talk, and even eat to the pace of a stop watch. In contrast, the easygoing Type B personality is much less likely to suffer from a heart attack. In one study, Type A men showed eight times the narrowing of the coronary arteries due to build-up of fatty plaques than did a similar group of Type B men. 'Hard facts from dozens of retrospective studies by investigators worldwide,' writes Dr. Rosenman, 'have shown that the majority of coronary patients under the age of 60 are Type A.'…Under chronic tension, the hypothalamus releases hormones that discharge cholesterol, increase clotting elements in the blood, and even produce an abnormal blood sugar state—all of which contribute to the development of heart disease. Suggestions for how to shift from Type A to Type B behavior are: 'Remind yourself daily that *being* is more important than *having;'* 'Learn to hold opinions loosely'; 'Become more intimate with your friends'; 'Stop and start to really take in the wonders of the universe'; Slow down'; Stop interrupting and start listening.' Enroll

---

[133] Dr, Julian Whitaker *Health and Healing Newsletter, Vol.17, No.2, pp. 2-3*

in a program of Transcendental Meditation (TM).

Psychological research indicates that the TM program naturally changes the Type A individual into a happier, more relaxed and more flexible person. (See section in this book on Meditation.)

EDTA Chelation Therapy

EDTA is a powerful, yet ultra safe amino acid called ethylene-diamine tetra-acetic acid or EDTA for short. It is very similar in composition to common vinegar. Dr. Michael Cutler provides the following benefits of Chelation therapy:

> Research shows EDTA is effective in removing heavy metals and toxins from the 75,000 miles of your arteries, veins, and capillaries leaving them squeaky clean for healthy blood to flow throughout your entire body! And **clinical and scientific studies have proven that EDTA is up to 82% effective at eliminating plaque from your arteries!**

> Until recently, getting the full benefits of Chelation therapy was uncomfortable, time-consuming, and expensive. You had to drive to the nearest Chelation clinic....get poked with an I.V. needle and wait for several for at least three hours while EDTA was pumped into your body through the I.V. When it was over you got a bill for up to 300 dollars and instructions to return for at least nine more treatments.

> The high price and inconvenience of I.V. Chelation therapy put it out of reach for many Americans. But now, those days are gone for good—thanks to the miracle of oral Chelation!

> Dr. Garry Gordon, known as the 'father' of I.V. Chelation—and the medical doctor who established the Chelation protocol over 30 years ago—has presented research proving oral Chelation to be a safe and effective method for getting all of the benefits from EDTA. According to the *Journal of Laboratory and Clinical Medicine,* taking oral EDTA every day works just as well over time as the painful, time-consuming I.V. Chelation therapy! And studies show that oral Chelation has the benefits of I.V. chelation without any

negative side-effects. [134]

Vitamins C and E plus Lysine

In the book *Vitamin C Cures*, Dr. Hickey presents a wealth of evidence that points to the healing powers of Vitamin C among which are its ability to help avoid and also cure atherosclerosis. He also points out the importance of including an amino acid, Lysine and vitamin E. When taken together with vitamin C they act as a powerful way to avoid heart attacks and also as a way to cure or reverse heart disease .Here is what he has to say:

"The evidence indicates atherosclerosis is caused by prolonged, low level deficiency of vitamin C and other antioxidants in the diet. Most heart diseases and strokes are therefore a form of scurvy. In addition vitamin E, in a specific form, has been reported as an effective treatment for heart disease.

Lysine may help generally to prevent cholesterol build up in the artery wall. Lysine acts on cholesterol to prevent plaque formation and help heal existing damage.

This suggests that suitable antioxidant supplements can both reverse and prevent atherosclerosis." [135]

Diabetes

Diabetes (*diabetes mellitus)* is the third leading cause of death in the United States. It is associated with arteriosclerosis. It results from a lack of sufficient insulin being produced by the pancreas. Without insulin the body cannot utilize glucose, thus creating a high level of glucose in the blood and a low level of glucose absorption by the tissues. It is divided into two categories: type I, called insulin-dependent or juvenile diabetes, and type II in which the onset of diabetes occurs during adulthood.

The ideal thing is to prevent the occurrence of diabetes. Once a person has type I diabetes, it requires insulin shot therapy under the directions of a doctor. Prevention of diabetes requires following a healthy lifestyle that includes a healthy diet, an adequate amount of exercise and freedom from stress. Prevention includes the avoidance of all types of refined foods such as white sugar, artificial sugars, and

---

[134] True Health Special Report, pp.3-5.
[135] Hickey, op. cit., pp. 162-163.

white flour, which unfortunately are found in most popular foods such as rolls, breads, cakes, cookies, candies, ice cream, sodas, fruit drinks and many other products. These products are properly referred to as 'junk foods'.

Obesity is common among type II diabetics. A weight reduction program is usually all that is required to control this type of diabetes. Diet (avoid junk foods) and exercise are the key factors which can help you avoid the need for any medication.

Dr. Brownstein has the following suggestions on how to prevent and or cure diabetes:

"Newer treatments for diabetes that address the underlying causes, rather merely manage the symptoms, involve methods that work with your healing system. These treatments include eating a proper diet, getting adequate exercise, practicing stress management techniques, drinking plenty of water, taking natural medications and addressing the deeper emotional, mental, and spiritual factors that may be driving this unhealthy condition. Natural herbs that can help decrease as well as stabilize blood sugar include cinnamon, 125 mg per day. It appears to be more effective if combined with biotin, 8 milligrams twice daily. Ginseng has also been found to reduce blood sugar. Ginseng can be combined with queen crepe myrtle, 550 mg, one to six times daily, for even better effectiveness. An herb from India, *gymnema sylvestre,* 400 milligrams twice daily has been used for centuries to reduce blood sugar and this has been supported in a study by Baskaran in 1990. It can be combined with other herbs for better results, including bitter melon, 400 milligrams, as reported by Ahmad, in 1999 and 200 mg of fenugreek, studied by Gupta in 1998, both twice daily. It may take 2-3 months to obtain benefits. These strategies are obviously more effective if they are instituted in the early stages of the illness. Insulin may be required until these other other methods are well established, but a large number of patients have successfully weaned themselves from insulin dependence in a relatively short period of time. If diabetes happens to run in your family, focus on incorporating preventative strategies before the illness has a chance to surface in your body." [136]

---

[136] Art Brownstein, M.D. *Extraordinary Healing.* Emmaus, PA: Rodale Press, 2005, pp. 341-42.

Dr. James Balch makes the following recommendations:

A high-carbohydrate, high fiber diet reduces the need for insulin and also lowers he fat levels in the blood. Olive oil may help adult-onset diabetes. Fiber will reduce blood sugar surges. Use oat and rice bran crackers with nut butters or cheese. High at levels are linked to heart disease.

Spirulina helps produce a stable blood sugar level. Go on a spirulina diet consisting of raw fruits and vegetables as well as fresh juices. This diet will help to reduce sugar in the urine. Foods that normalized blood sugar include berries, brewer's yeast, cheese, egg yolks, fish, garlic sauerkraut, soybeans and vegetables. A low protein diet consisting of less than 40 grams of protein each day is recommended for diabetic nephropathy (kidney disease). It is important to get protein from a vegetable source.

Avoid fish oil capsules, large amounts of PABA, white flour products, and salt. Consumption of these products results in an elevation of blood sugar. Do not take large doses of cysteine. Be careful not to take exceedingly large doses of vitamins B1 and C. Excessive amounts may inactivate insulin. They may, however, be taken in normal amounts.

Type II diabetics should avoid large amounts of niacin, but niacinamide for type I diabetics slows down destruction of beta cells in the pancreas and enhances their regeneration. You may also wish to try the following herbs: buchu leaves, dandelion root, goldenseal, and uva ursi. In addition huckleberry helps to promote insulin production and a tea made of ginseng is believed to lower the blood sugar level. [137]

Another herb that has been found to have benefits for diabetics is the **Astragalus.** It is known to be effective to fight colds and strengthen the immune system. It's been used for thousands of years in eastern cultures for all sorts of health benefits. Dr. Nan Fuchs provides us with an excellent report on how this herb can help diabetics. She also includes a number of other herbs that, when taken together, have remarkable healing benefits:

---

[137] James Balch, M.D. *Prescription for Nutritional Healing.* Garden City, NY: Avery Publishing Group, 1990, pp. 154-156.

A landmark study found that astragalus has the ability to balance your blood sugar. Not just lower it. *Balance it.* That means if your blood sugar is too high, it drops it. If your blood sugar is too low, it raises it. That's important. Because many other remedies can lower your blood sugar too far or too fast. This can cause the opposite problem--not enough blood sugar. Astragalus protects against that. And that's just the tip of the iceberg for this amazing herb:

- In one study, researchers found that astragalus prevented the onset of blood sugar problems in healthy subjects.
- In another study, astragalus scavenged free radicals and protected against nerve damage caused by high blood sugar.
- In still another study, astragalus guarded against kidney damage brought on by high blood sugar.

And that's not all. Researchers took a group of animals with high blood sugar and gave them astragalus. After just 12 weeks, the astragalus-treated animals had lower blood sugar, higher insulin levels, and less peripheral nerve damage.

Astragalus also boosts glutathione levels in your nerves. Glutathione, as you may know, is one of the most powerful anti-oxidants in your body. It controls other antioxidants such as vitamins C and E. In fact, studies show that your glutathione level is one of the best predictors of your overall health.

Fibromyalgia (FM)

Fibromyalgia is the name for a syndrome or condition that is not classified as a disease since the cause has not yet been determined by medical doctors. It affects about five million Americans. It is difficult to diagnose FM since the symptoms are similar to other conditions such as severe fatigue, insomnia, arthritis, and pain in different parts of the body. A distinguishing aspect of FM is the extremely painful tenderness at certain points in the body. The usual medical treatment is to use powerful pain killer drugs to ease the pain which does nothing to cure the condition. According to Dr. Marcus Laux:

FM tends to first appear after a significant stressor that's often, but not always, a physical trauma - especially one to the head or neck. One study showed that 22 percent of people who suffered whiplash in a car accident developed FM during the ensuing year. It also commonly occurs after viral infections such as a nasty bout with shingles or the flu. But because it doesn't appear until months after the initial stressor, the basic causes are largely overlooked.

A professor of biochemistry, Dr. Martin Pall, PhD, unearthed what could be the cellular mechanism that drives the whole fibromyalgia scenario. He has gone on to devise a treatment protocol that can dismantle that mechanism, making it possible for your body to push FM out of your life for good. When you experience a major stress, inflammation increases a molecule called inductible nitric oxide (iNO). Inflammation is a normal part of the healing process, but it's supposed to subside once you're healed. If FM has you down, however, your inflammation doesn't subside. It starts a biochemical loop that keeps the iNO coming and keeps your pain and inflammation churning. By addressing only your symptoms, conventional medicine compounds your pain with the side effects of prescribed medications.

Dr. Pall, together with other doctors, such as Dr. Jacob Teitelbaum, came up with a new way to treat FM. There are powerful agents that have proven in clinical trials, to benefit FM patients. Some of the therapeutic agents are:

Antioxidants: There are several sources of antioxidants. An excellent combination is one that includes vitamins A, C, E, and selenium. Other antioxidants rich in polyphenols such as cacao are very good for FM. Believe it or not, dark chocolate (85 percent or higher) can help FM by increasing levels of the neurotransmitters serotonin and dopamine which relieves pain and fatigue. Water-based plants such as algae and kelp contain different polyphenols which are very potent. A brown algae known as *Echlonia Cava* is particularly good for FM. It reduces pain and stiffness, and improves sleep.

SAMe: Supports optimal immune function and maintains cell membranes. Its been shown in clinical trials to reduce pain, fatigue and stiffness in FM. Recommended dose is two 400 mg tablets daily on an empty stomach.

Vitamin D3: Deficient levels of vitamin D have been associated with FM and other chronic pain syndromes. Begin with

3000-10,000 IU daily then back down to 1000-3000 IU. Sunlight and cod liver oil are excellent sources of vitamin D3.

Herbal blend: In my experience, the combination of Chinese skullcap and acacia is the Rolls Royce of pain relievers. Together these two are typically used to provide joint comfort but because of their mechanism they can provide relief anywhere in your body.

D-Ribose: This simple sugar corrects faltering mitochondrial metabolism. It's reported to reduce pain and improve energy, sleep, and sense of well-being. Dose: 1 scoop, 2-3 times daily.

Melatonin: Your own natural 'sleep hormone' is a powerful antioxidant that improves sleep and reduces pain and fatigue in FM patients. Take 1 to 3 mg as a sublingual pill before bed.

Tryptophan or 5-HTP: Both are precursors of serotonin in the brain. They help rebalance FM's distorted stress-hormone pattern, normalize pain-modulating systems in the brainstem, and reduce the number of tender points, pain severity, stiffness, fatigue, depression, and sleep disturbances. Recommended dose: 500 mg of tryptophan or 100 mg of 5-HTP before bed.

Drs. Pall and Teitelbaum have each developed programs to go with their views on fibromyalgia. For more information about these programs contact Pro Health (*immunesupport.com* or call 800-366-6056) [138]

Flu and the Common Cold

The section in this book (below) which deals with the harmful effects of flu shots should provide enough evidence that it is better to use natural curative herbs and teas to ward off and help to cure the flu rather than submit to flu shots. Some proven beneficial things to take during flu season are:

Garlic - Take several cloves a day (preferably raw) to boost your immune system.

Green Tea - combats viruses. Drink several glasses a day.

Tea Tree Oil - stimulates the immune system and fights infections. Inhaling the vapors of tea tree oil is a pre-

---

[138] Dr. Marcus Laux. *Naturally Well Today, Dec, 2007, pp. 1-4.*

ventative to use against viruses.

Ginger - made into a tea is especially good for stomach flu.

Miso Soup - provides beneficial bacteria for the digestive system. Add shitake mushrooms and garlic for a potent beverage to fight the flu.

Oscillococcinum - is a homeopathic remedy for the flu made from duck livers. It can be obtained at health food stores. When taken at the first symptoms of the flu –chills, fever and aches-it can stop the flu from taking effect. It is very effective at the onset of the flu.

Echinacea - is one of the most potent flu fighters around. It is especially potent when taken together with goldenseal a natural anti- biotic. It can be taken as a tea or for more potency take 10 drops of the tincture several times a day. Do not take goldenseal for more than seven days as it will weaken the friendly bacteria just as synthetic antibiotics do.

Colds

Apple Cider Vinegar and Honey - stir a teaspoon of honey and a teaspoon of apple cider vinegar in a glass of warm water. Use as a tea or as a gargle. Take frequently during the day.

Vitamins A, C, and E - act together as a potent antibiotic. Vitamin C can be taken every one to two hours apart for one or two days to kill the infection.

Decongestant Vapors - Add 5 to 10 drops of eucalyptus oil to one quart of boiling water and pour into a large pot. Drape a large towel over your head and inhale the vapors.

Acupressure - use one hand to apply pressure to the fold between your forefinger and your thumb on the other hand and massage for at least one minute. Then change to the other hand and repeat. This alleviates sniffles and cold symptoms.

Rest - Get plenty of sleep and naps during the day.

Water - Drink at least 6 glasses of pure water each day to flush away toxins in your system.

Free Radicals and Illness

The free radical theory states that the body's natural immune system is seriously impaired by free radicals which lead to serious illnesses. Free radicals are chemical units that, instead of having an even number of electrons, as is the rule, have an odd number. The odd number of electrons makes free radicals highly unstable and therefore reactive, because the solitary electron is making every effort to find another electron with which it can bond in order to stabilize. This quest is non-selective; the free radical attacks any molecule it comes in contact with in order to steal an electron. But when it steals this electron, it transforms the other molecule into a free radical, as the latter now has an odd number of electrons. The theft of an electron alters or destroys its structure; it then becomes destructive.

The harmful activity of free radicals leads to the destruction of cells, DNA, proteins and various other useful substances creates acid wastes, such as uric acid, phosphoric acid, and sulfuric acid, thus causing the pH balance of the body to become too acidic. Free radicals are actually an oxygen derivative, and their destructiveness is the result of oxidizing the substances with which they come into contact with.

Several vitamins have an antioxidant effect, such as vitamins A, E, C, the flavonoids (vitamin P), and certain trace elements like selenium and zinc. But there are plants that contain even more antioxidants. The antioxidant proanthocyanidin (OPC), for example, which is forty times stronger than flavonoids, can be found in grape seeds and in various small fruits including all of the berries. The catechin extracted from green tea is 200 times stronger than vitamin E, and the OPC extract from pine bark is 50 times stronger than vitamin E and 20 times stronger than vitamin C.

A very good review of the damage caused by free radicals appeared in the following article in the July Issue of the *Journal of Health and Longevity:*

Mainstream infectious disease medicine practiced today is based on the 'germ theory put forward by Louis Pasteur (1822-1895). His theory viewed the body as a sterile machine that will operate properly unless a foreign substance is introduced. Therefore, it is thought that when specific microbes enter the body, they will produce a specific disease. In an attempt to correct the imbalance, antibiotics and other medicines are used to destroy these organisms. No microbes, no disease. It was believed that health is restored only if there are no germs present that might cause disease.

In contrast, the famous French physiologist Claude Bernard (1813-1878) focused on the importance of the body's internal environment. In contradiction to the then current doctrine of Pasteur, he taught that microbes (e.g., bacteria, viruses) could not produce disease unless the body's internal environment was unbalanced and susceptible for the development of disease. Bernard's theory was that the whole must be sick before any germ can make us ill.

Renowned microbiologist, Rene Debous agreed with this basic principle, saying: Most microbial diseases are caused by organisms present in the body of a normal individual. They become the cause of disease when a disturbance arises which upsets the equilibrium of the body. Debous, like Bernard, thought it was not the presence of bacteria or viruses that cause disease; it is the imbalance of the body's normal functions that fails to hold the microbes in check. Even today, more and more doctors and researchers know that microbes are always present. Some of these are harmless and others have harmful potential. Some of these microbes are absolutely necessary to allow the body to function properly; they are only able to cause disease if the body is in a weakened or upset state. If a significant dose of the microbe is contacted, those with strong immune function may completely resist infectious manifestations or develop only mild infectious symptoms.

Furthermore, an improperly balanced bodily environment may lead to a compromised immune system and more serious disease. Degenerative diseases result largely from an unstable condition of the internal environment. Once the body is in a weakened state, the tissues can be secondarily affected by disease causing microbes that lead to chronic failure of bodily tissues or organ systems. Pasteur himself condemned his own theory on his death bed saying: *Bernard is right. The microbe is nothing. 'The environment is all important.'*

Even more importantly, in 1954 Dr. Denham Harman described

his free radical theory of aging and disease. He stated: 'Aging is caused by free radical reactions which may be caused by the environment, from disease and intrinsic reactions within the aging process.' At that time, Dr. Harman's work was, for the most part, ignored by the entrenched medical establishment. They were still convinced that disease must come from outside of man as represented by Louis Pasteur's germ theory.

Today, scientists agree that aerobically respiring (alive) cells produce two kinds of radicals, the good which need to be nourished—and the bad, that can cause irreparable destruction. The trouble is that the body can't fight the bad when it is compromised by any number of outside contaminants. Your body has antioxidant enzymes such as superoxide dismutase, catalese and glutathione peroxidase that moderate the harmful effects of free radicals. But when bombarded by environmental sources of free radicals, such as smoke, alcohol, air pollution, etc. these natural enzymes are not enough to defend against the onslaught of natural and environmental free radicals.

And if that is not enough, here is what Dr. James Balch, M.D. has to say about our oxygen supply: "Oxygen is the source of our 'life energy,' but there is a problem. We aren't getting enough of it. The oxygen-producing forests are being destroyed. Modern industrial technology is polluting the air, further depleting the Earth's oxygen supply. In the past few hundred years, the oxygen content of our atmosphere has decreased by almost 50 percent.'

It is common medical knowledge that most diseases will not thrive in an oxygen-rich environment. That has been proven in the case of cancer. If there is enough oxygen in the cells, cancer and other degenerative diseases cannot exist. Dr. Balch goes on to say:

'As antibiotics in the last fifty years of the twentieth century helped cure many infectious diseases, so antioxidants will affect a cure of many supposedly incurable diseases in the twenty-first century and slow the aging process dramatically." [139]

A list of natural foods and herbs that can help destroy free radical damage follows below:

---

[139] James Balch. *Journal of Health and Longevity, Vol.3, Issue 7.* 2008 Henderson, New York, pp. 1-2.

Curcuminoids are one of the richest sources of phytonutrients such as turmeric which helps destroy cancer cells. It is found in the popular Indian spice curcumin. Curcumin is the yellow pigment in turmeric which has many other benefits as well.

Vitamins obtained from fresh fruits and vegetables as well as in natural supplements, particularly Vitamins C, E, and B complex; and Beta Carotene which is a natural source of Vitamin E.

Lycopene is a power antioxidant which is found in foods that have red pigment such as tomatoes, beets, watermelon and in natural supplements. It is an aid in the prevention of prostate cancer.

Grapeseed Extract An anti-inflammatory bioflavonoid has many benefits such as: the improvement of circulation which benefits vision and reduces varicose veins and allergies; helps to heal ulcers; reduces blood pressure and cholesterol levels; and has been found to reduce symptoms of multiple sclerosis and emphysema. It can be obtained in fruits such as grapes, plums, cherries and blueberries.

Rutin is a bioflavonoid which offers protection against ulcers, cataracts, hemorrhoids, bruises and high cholesterol.

Glutathione is a powerful antioxidant to be taken intravenously for Parkinson's disease.

Vitamins A C and E taken together are powerful antioxidants.

CoenzymeQ10 (CoQ10) is a potent antioxidant. It supports muscle function and energy levels. It is an essential for heart health.

To review, free radicals are atoms with unpaired electrons that can cause damage in a normal metabolic process known as oxidation. Although the destructive effects of free radical activity have been heavily implicated in cancer, we don't usually hear about free radicals. We hear about carcinogens. Carcinogens are toxic substances that enter the body and cause free radical formation that in turn mutates normal cells into cancer cells. In earlier chapters we talked about a number of carcinogens and the importance of avoiding them: pesticides on our produce; nitrosamines in food; bromates in baked goods; food dyes and colorings; DEPC, a chemical that in a laboratory kills microbes but in our body combines with ammonia to harmful effect; and a list of chemicals used in food. These include glycerides, monosodium glutamate (MSG), propylgalate, sodium citrate, sulfating agents, and disodium phosphate; DDT shows up in imported foods that still use this deadly pesticide; and radioactive substances from nuclear plants and mining can be found in our water." [140]

Pain and Inflammation

Joints

Joints require a fluid called synovial fluid to cushion the bones as they move in their sockets. Lack of synovial fluid causes pain and eventually can lead to severe injury to the joint. This subject is dealt with more fully in this book in the chapter on exercise, where the benefits of Tai Chi are described. This section deals with problems associated with inflammation of the joints and what can be done to alleviate inflammation.

Inflammation occurs naturally in the body at sites which have been injured by falls; lack of lubrication at joints or when the body has any kind of infection or trauma. The inflammation usually subsides when the injury is on the way to being healed. However, when injured parts of the body do not heal quickly, the inflammation continues on to the point where it becomes chronic causing pain and in the case of joints may result in serious disabilities. Before resorting to medicines or surgery to relieve the painful condition, it is better to make use of natural methods which relieve tension and inflammation. There are a number of natural foods and herbs which are known to reduce inflammation as follows:

Anti-Inflamatory Foods and Supplements

Omega 3 fatty acids contained in fish oils and flaxseed oil help maintain proper fluidity of cellular membranes and work as a natural anti-inflammatory agent providing protection against heart disease and diabetes.

Turmeric, ginger, and boswellia serrata are also excellent anti-inflammatory agents which should be added to your daily diet.

One of the most effective ways to reduce inflammation of the joints is to take the following supplements together: red yeast rice and tart red

---

[140] Null, op. cit., pp. 118-119.

cherry extract.

In addition to the anti-inflammatory agents mentioned above there are a number of supplements which, when taken together, are known to bring about welcome relief to very painful, disabling joint problems, as follows: Hyaluronic acid, MSM, glucosamine sulfate, boswellia, and chondroiton. It is very important to take these supplements together at the same time twice a day morning and evening.

Chronic inflammation, regardless of the location in the body, causes tissue destruction and failure and weakens the immune system--which lessens your capacity to overcome additional health threats. Chronic inflammation causes ongoing damage to the site of any inflammation. Studies have shown a significant link between inflammation and the risk of cancer. Numerous studies have identified the role of inflammation in the formation of disease in the veins and arteries. Extensive research also shows that you can reduce your risk of heart attacks, stroke, and other cardiovascular diseases strictly by reducing inflammation. An article in the *Life Extension Magazine,* June, 2009, pointed out the danger of consuming fried foods such as potato chips. Foods exposed to high heat during cooking contain acrylamides: toxic chemicals linked to sharply increased states of inflammation. There are many things that can be done to reduce and/or eliminate inflammation as recommended by Dr. Williams and others, such as:

Avoid environmental toxins such as tobacco smoke (both firsthand and secondhand). Avoid working around wood-fired BBQ pits, and avoid pesticides.

Detoxify by drip Chelation or by taking the herb cilantro along with periodic short fasts.

Get rid of excess fat/weight by exercise and low-fat and low-carbohydrate diets.

Increase your intake of fiber-rich foods such as psyllium husks.

Take probiotic supplements and eat fermented foods like real yogurt and unpasteurized sauerkraut.

Consume natural anti-inflammatory supplements such as; Vitamins C and D, folic acid, niacin, turmeric, ginger, quercetin, tart cherries, cherry juice and pomegranate juice.

Avoid statin drugs; they all have serious side-effects. [141]

Additional supplements which I have found to be helpful are red yeast rice and white willow.

Insomnia and sleep disorders

One of the leading causes of insomnia is an excessive amount of Beta brainwaves. The Beta is the predominant frequency when we are fully awake. The problem is an overactive mind that does not get relief from stress during the day and gets little or no relief at night because of faulty sleep patterns. It is associated with excessive **mental chatter.** These brain waves are present with stress, paranoia, worry, fear, anxiety, depression, irritability and moodiness. Too much time in the Beta state weakens the immune system.

The condition can be improved by spending more time in the Alpha state through changing our sleep patterns and by practicing meditation. The alpha state is the first layer of our subconscious mind. The Alpha state is where meditation and relaxation begins. Practices like Chi Gong and Tai Chi also increase the ALPHA BRAIN WAVES. TM (transcendental meditation) has been proven to be very effective in improving the quality of sleep and reducing or eliminating insomnia.

It is estimated that about one-third of the adult population suffers from a sleep disorder. Pharmaceutical companies have found a gold mine in tranquilizers and sleeping pills. Studies show that over 11 million people have been using tranquilizers every day, for at least a year or more. These drugs can cause dizziness, memory loss, decreased mental function, confusion, loss of coordination, and auto accidents. Some of the causes of insomnia are lack of exercise, hypoglycemia, lengthy airplane trips, overeating late in the day, sleeping late in the morning and during the day and poor health. Dr. David Williams makes the following suggestions for eliminating insomnia:

Exercise-You must exercise on a regular basis, and you should do it on a regular basis. Exercises such as walking, jogging, swimming, bicycling are excellent choices.

Kava Kava - this herbal extract improves the sleep patterns by lengthening the sleep cycle, without any of the harmful side effects that drugs have.

---

[141]Dr. Williams. *Alternatives. Jan. 2009, Vol. 12, No.19.*

Gaba - an amino acid which provides relief by taking 200 milligrams four times a day. Reduce the amount if you experience any uncomfortable reactions. Gaba soothes and stabilizes mood disorders. Addicted persons lack Gaba.

L-tryptophan - a natural product that increases the level of serotonin in the brain which is the substance that normally makes us sleepy. Foods with high L-tryptophan content are: wheat germ, oat flakes, eggs, cottage cheese, pork, anchovies, almonds, Swiss and Parmesan cheeses. L-tryptophan can be purchased in health food stores and should be taken together with vitamins B6 (50-100mg) and niacinamide (100-200mg).

Melatonin - a hormone created in the body is a great aid for insomnia and jet lag. The reasons for an insufficient amount of melatonin are: the taking of anti-inflammatory products like aspirin and ibuprofen. Beta blockers and calcium channel blockers used to treat high blood pressure inhibit the formation of melatonin. Sleep aids and drugs that treat anxiety problems also stop melatonin formation. It can be dramatically increased by meditation. I don't recommended taking it as a supplement on a continuing basis since it is a hormone. It is fine to use it for a day or two to overcome or prevent jet lag or shift changes at work, or for a couple of weeks to reset your biological clock to correct insomnia. Certain foods are high in melatonin such as rice, bananas, barley, ginger and corn.[142]

In addition to the above recommendations, I can tell you of two things that I have personally found to be very helpful as aids to a good night's sleep. One is a breathing technique, which is described in my chapter on breathing, known as the rebirthing technique. It simply consists of lying on your back and counting to the count of four as you breathe in and to the same number of counts as you breathe out. You repeat this sequence 20 times. In addition to the extra oxygen you inhale during this procedure, you also relieve your mind of its usual chatter while focusing on the counting of your breaths. The second thing which I have found that brings on a very sound sleep, is taking a capsule of an herb called Maca, which is known for its aphrodisiac properties, about one hour before retiring.

---

[142] Williams, op. cit.

Obesity

One of the most rapidly increasing ailments is that of obesity. The large numbers of people, including young children, who are obese, has reached epidemic proportions according to leading health authorities. Sixty-one percent of American adults are overweight, meaning that they weigh 30 pounds more than they should.

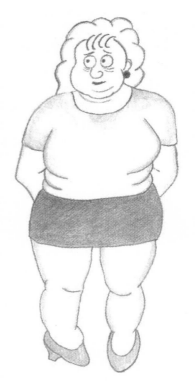

While diabetes is one of the major risks in being overweight, there are many other conditions that you can avoid by staying within a healthy weight range according to Earl Mindell, as he states below:

"Men who are 20 percent over their desirable weight have a 20 percent increased likelihood of dying from all causes, are 10 percent more likely to die from stroke, have 40 percent greater risk of gallbladder disease, and have double the risk of developing diabetes. At 25 to 35 percent over ideal weight, the risk for a man aged 19 to 35 dying from all causes is 170 percent, At 40   percent above desirable weight, the likelihood of dying from diabetes complications skyrockets 400 percent, and the risk of dying from stroke rises 75 percent. Overweight men are more likely to develop colorectal cancer, while heavy women are at increased risk of uterine and ovarian cancer. Women who are *abdominally* obese are at greater risk of breast cancer.

Ninety-five percent of people who do manage to lose weight end up gaining it back again because over time they revert back to their customary diet which consists for the most part of processed, low-nutrition, fat-filled junk food instead of an organic, whole food diet which can keep the weight at a normal level if accompanied by an effective exercise program.[143]

---

[143] Mindell, *Prescription Alternatives*.pp.350-351.

The obvious causes of obesity are poor diet and lack of sufficient exercise. Genetic causes appear to be a primary factor since it is common to find overweight parents with overweight children. However, it may be the lifestyle and diet of such families that contribute to the obesity rather than the genetic predisposition to such a condition.

Aside from the need for more exercise, other factors that are known to contribute to obesity are a low rate of metabolism; overconsumption of sugar in the form of white sugar and corn syrup; lack of sufficient fiber; lack of good fats such as flaxseed oil and fish oils rich in EFAs (essential fatty acids); overconsumption of refined flour products (breads, cakes, pastas, cereals and cookies); and hyperinsulinism. Hyperinsulinism is probably one of the most important factors in causing obesity, as Dr. Atkins pointed out many years ago:

If your blood-sugar levels go sharply up, as they do soon after you eat carbohydrates, your body makes an instant decision. How much of that pure energy is it going to use for immediate need and how much it will store for future requirements?

The instrument of its decision is insulin, because insulin governs the processing of blood sugar.

Insulin is manufactured in a part of your pancreas called the islets of Langerhans. As the sugar in your blood goes up insulin rushes forth and converts a portion of that glucose to glycogen, a starch stored in the muscles and the liver and readily available for energy use. If all the glycogen storage areas are filled, and there is still more glucose in the body beyond that which the body needs to function, insulin will convert the excess to fatty tissue called triglyceride, which we carry in our bodies as the main constituent of adipose tissue - the fat that puts on weight. That's why insulin has been called the 'fat-producing hormone.'

It's easy to see that there's a relationship between the kinds of food you eat and the amount of insulin in your bloodstream. Refined carbohydrates such as sugar, white flour, white rice, and potato starch speedily convert to glucose that requires a lot of insulin. As an overweight person becomes fatter, the insulin problem expands too. Numerous studies have shown that the obese (and diabetic) individual is extremely unresponsive to the action of insulin. That's where you will see the term 'insulin resistance.' Carbohydrates are triggering the release of large quantities of the hormone, but the body is incapable of utilizing it efficiently. The body responds by putting out yet more insulin. Consequently overweight and high insulin levels are almost synonymous.

What appears to happen is that the insulin receptors on the surface of the body's cells are blocked from carrying out their function, which in turn prevents insulin from stimulating the transfer of glucose to the cells for energy use. It's one reason why overweight people are tired much of the time. Because insulin is not effective in converting glucose into energy, it transfers more and more into stored fat. You'd like to slim down but your body is, in fact, becoming a fat-producing machine. The next step in this tragic process is indeed diabetes, a disease that's epidemic *among* the overweight.

Mediated by high insulin levels, your body has become intent on saving fat. And in so doing, the excess insulin prevents weight loss either directly or indirectly by giving you a constant sensation of hunger that can be satiated only by constant overeating.

To lose weight, you're going to need to restrict your carbohydrate consumption and burn your fat off. Once you've been fat for some time, you're in a metabolic trap. This trap can be lifted and the fat burned off by a process called Benign Dietary Ketosis (BDK). The term 'ketosis,' when it applies to the benign diet-induced type of obesity is really a shortening of the term ketpsis/lipolysis which is commonly referred to as 'ketosis,' and why the die is called the 'ketogenic diet.'

The Atkin's weight-loss diet is simple and overwhelmingly effective. Being in ketosis simply means that you're burning your fat stores and using them as the source of fuel they were meant to be. When your body is releasing ketones—which it will be in your breath and in your urine—that is chemical proof that you're consuming your own stored fat. The more ketones you release, the more fat you have dissolved. BDK is the physiological method of weight loss—the exact opposite of the process that got you fat to begin with. It can be your life raft, gaining you not only slimness but health, putting you at a good healthy distance from the obese person's perils of diabetes, heart disease, and stroke.

Ketosis is the reversal of the biologic pathways that are involved in obesity. As you gain weight, your pancreas releases more insulin.

In a normally functioning body, fatty acids and ketones are readily librated from adipose tissue and converted into fuel but in the overweight person the high insulin levels prevent this from happening. With very little carbohydrate in your diet, your insulin levels will become normal and you will lose weight. [144]

Because of space limitations the complete Atkin's Diet program cannot be included in this book. For those who desire more information you can easily obtain a copy of Dr Atkin's most recent book, *Dr. Atkins' New Diet Revolution.*

The above presentation of why people on the Atkin's diet lose weight provides an excellent understanding of the role insulin and ketones play in the process. This method does require strict attention to the amount of carbohydrates a person consumes and the need to count calories. A simplified method of doing this has been offered by Dr. Frank Shallenberger in his suggested cure for Alzheimer's disease. (See section on Alzheimer's disease above).

Another factor to be aware of is the importance of knowing about the dangers of eating a high-protein diet. This is one of the chief weaknesses of the Atkin's Diet. He recommended eating large amounts of animal protein and animal fat. It is now known that these kinds of food contribute to heart disease and liver problems. His diet can be followed safely simply by using other forms of protein such as nuts and dark green leafy vegetables as described in the Nutrition section of this book under Green Smoothies.

In the book, *Make the Connection,* an exercise and fitness program is described which is simple to follow and which has proven to be very effective in weight control and an improved state of well being. Oprah Winfrey went through the program that was developed by Bob Greene and was able to take off weight and achieved a heightened state of well-being. She joined Greene as a co-author of the book.

---

[144] Dr.Atkins. *New Diet Revolution.* New York

The basic program consists of ten steps which are designed to accommodate different levels of ability on the part of the participants as described below:

1. Exercise aerobically, 5 to 7 days each week in the morning.
2. Exercise at a zone level of seven or eight.
3. Exercise for 20 to 60 minutes each session.
4. Eat a low fat, balanced diet each day.
5. Eat 3 meals and 2 snacks each day.
6. Limit or eliminate alcohol.
7. Stop eating 2 to 3 hours before bedtime.
8. Drink 6 to 8 glasses of water each day.
9. Have at least 2 servings of fruit and 3 servings of vegetables each day.
10. Renew your commitment to healthy living each day. [145]

Parkinson's Disease

This is a very serious disease which is caused by a lack of sufficient dopamine due to the degeneration of neurons which manufacture dopamine in the brain. Adding dopamine containing foods is of some help but has not been able to arrest the disease because it is impossible to digest a sufficient quantity from foods alone. The usual medical treatment is the use of drugs which mimic or replace dopamine. They relieve symptoms in some cases but are not able to cure the disease and do have harmful side effects with continued use.

The Whitaker Wellness Institute reports very good results with their treatment for patients with Parkinson's as follows:

Although there's a lot that medical science does not know about Parkinson's, we do know that free radical damage contributes to its progressive nature. That's why we use glutathione. It's a powerful natural antioxidant, and patients with Parkinson's have dangerously low levels of glutathione in the affected area of the brain. Boosting stores of this protective antioxidant not only guards against further damage, it also enhances the function of *surviving* neurons.

Unfortunately, oral glutathione has a hard time crossing the

---

[145] Bob Greene and Oprah Winfrey. *Make the Connection.* New York: Hyperion, 1996.

brain barrier, so supplements aren't very helpful. When glutathione is infused intravenously, however, it hits its target. Most patients see dramatic improvements after just a handful of treatments—and many perk up after their first infusion.

Our patients with Parkinson's disease are also treated with hyperbaric oxygen therapy. HBOT is highly beneficial for stroke, multiple sclerosis, and brain injuries. It floods the brain with oxygen, slows neuronal degeneration, mobilizes rejuvenating stem cells, and enhances angiogenesis (the growth of new blood vessels that nurture damaged areas). It is the combination of these two treatments, working synergistically, that provides such remarkable results.

Parkinson's is a serious condition that requires serious intervention. CoenzymeQ10, vitamin E, fish oil, curcumin, creatine, and vitamin D, along with vitamin C and N-acetyl-cysteine are known to be of help for patients with Parkinson's Disease.

Stomach Acid (HCL) and Digestive Disorders

Hydrochloric Acid (HCL) in the stomach is needed in proper amounts in order to properly digest food. An inadequate amount of HCL is the cause of many problems such as: heart problems, heartburn, indigestion, gum and tooth disease, colitis, nausea, osteoporosis, pneumonia, and vomiting, plus many other maladies. Lack of acid causes foods to ferment producing acid and gases which irritate the stomach and frequently causes food and acid to be pushed up into the esophagus resulting in a condition called hiatal hernia. Medical treatments such as drugs or antacids do not cure the problem. The only cure is to restore the HCL in a natural form to the stomach. Two proven, safe ways to maintain HCL are:

Take 2 Zypan tablets after each meal. (This product is produced by the Standard Process Corporation.)

Drink one quart of Green Smoothies each day. This drink consists of freshly blended raw, dark green leafy vegetables, plus one or two cups of spring water and fresh fruit such as bananas or berries to suit your taste.

(For further information see the Green Smoothie section in this book in the chapter on Nutrition.)

CHAPTER NINE

ALTERNATIVE HEALTH CARE

Acupuncture

Acupuncture is an ancient Chinese therapy used by practitioners trained in its application. Very fine needles are inserted at meridian points in the circulatory and nerve systems of the body. It is usually associated with pain relief, and it certainly is a safe, effective way to combat pain caused by all kinds of different conditions. It has been used for control of pain during certain operations. It has been used for thousands of years to restore, promote and maintain good health.

According to ancient theories, a subtle form of energy flows throughout the body along specific pathways. These pathways are known as meridians. **If your energy flows smoothly, your cells and organs are nourished and you will experience good health.** When the energy isn't flowing smoothly, a person might experience a disease (disease). This can be in the form of aches, pains, emotional disturbances, fatigue, or a combination thereof. Energy blockages can be caused by physical and emotional situations. Negative stress contributes to the improper flow of energy. When we are stressed, our brain releases molecules called neuropeptides, which affect the release of hormones causing us to feel ill. Acupuncture releases blockages and helps restore the normal flow of energy.

Central to the concepts behind acupuncture is the idea of the body as self-healing-that as living beings we are all naturally full of vitality and are being rebalanced and regenerated from within. This should not be difficult to understand. Cuts heal "on their own"; food is broken down, digested and absorbed into our body; plus many other functions without any conscious interference. In other words, there is a great source within the body that continually maintains order and our general well-being.

Acupuncture sees the body as a self-rectifying dynamic whole, a network of interacting energies. Their even distribution and flow maintains health, but any interruption, depletion or stagnation leads to disease. Acupuncture is a system of Chinese medicine which seeks to aid these natural processes, helping the body to correct itself by a realignment or redirection of energy, which the Chinese call **Qi** (pronounced chee).

The concept of Qi is difficult to define. It is often translated as breath, life force, vitality, energy or simply as that which makes us alive. If there is no Qi, there is no life. A wilting plant is lacking in Qi; a feeble person and a weak voice both show a lack of Qi; strong, energetic people have plenty of Qi. There is a lot of Qi in quiet strength. In illness, the Qi is depleted, causing tiredness and depression: or it may be disturbed, causing irritability and over-reaction.

Along with the idea of Qi, acupuncture recognizes a subtle energy system by which Qi is circulated through the body in a network of channels or 'meridians'. Among these meridians or channels lie the acupuncture points, and when an acupuncture needle is inserted it is the Qi that is affected. This interlacing network of meridians is the crux of traditional acupuncture. It is similar in some ways to the blood circulation and nervous system but is invisible to the eye. By needling the points, the Qi can be 'tapped' or affected to influence the state of health.

Although the flow of energy through the meridians is invisible, recent scientific studies conducted by Dr. R. Becker, M.D. and Maria Reichmanis, a biophysicist proved that energy does indeed flow along pathways similar to those used in meridian theory.

From an understanding of the body as an energetic and vibrating whole comes a new approach to health and disease. Modern Western medicine tends to be divisive, often looking at one part without seeing its relation to the whole. Acupuncture draws together all the diverse signs and symptoms of ill health to form a basic pattern of disharmony. This pattern will include the mental /emotional state as much as physical symptoms. These signs and symptoms are not regarded as problems in themselves to be 'eliminated', but as warning signs, pointers to imbalance in the patient. These imbalances can be corrected by inserting fine needles into specific acupuncture points on relevant meridians.

Acupuncture, then, stimulates the body's own self-healing powers and as there is a return to normal, the symptoms disappear of their own accord. Nothing can ever replace the patient's own efforts to discover and remedy the causes of their illness. Acupuncture is not a panacea for all ills. But until we learn to live wisely, of our own accord, there is a need for help to restore the balance, without upsetting it. Acupuncture is grounded in the theory of traditional Chinese medicine with its practical and subtle understanding of health.

With health understood, disease is put in its proper context-health must be restored, rather than disease removed. There are many other beneficial applications of acupuncture besides those mentioned above. A master acupuncturist, Stacey Hachenberg, provides us with a few of its many benefits as follows:

1. Stroke Recovery: See results after just one session.

   In a recent British study, researchers found that one year after a stroke, patients who underwent acupuncture therapy were more likely to be living independently in their own homes than patients who did not use acupuncture. Those findings were echoed in a Norwegian study: 20 patients received traditional rehabilitation, while another21 underwent the regular plan plus 30-minute acupuncture sessions three or four times a week. After six weeks of treatment, the acupuncture group scored better than the control on all three stroke recovery assessments, and their scores continued to improve (and surpass controls) over the following year. I've treated a lot of stroke patients in my practice and I've seen some amazing recoveries. The most important thing is to get started quickly—the sooner you get acupuncture after a stroke, the better.

2. Partnering up on fertility

   When a couple is having difficulty conceiving, it may be caused by a problem with either partner. Fortunately acupuncture can help in either case. Studies have shown that acupuncture can help boost the number of normally shaped sperm in semen (abnormally shaped sperm are a common cause of male infertility). And research suggests that acupuncture can help normalize ovulation and balance hormone levels, even increasing egg production in women undergoing IVF treatment.

Of course, infertility is often huge emotional ride as well, and the stress can be destructive and hinder the ability to conceive even further. Acupuncture can help with that, too, and help relieve the physical manifestations of stress that can undermine all other efforts.

3. Relief - Period

For many of the same reasons that acupuncture can help with female infertility, it can also help with all sorts of menopausal issues. Research shows that acupuncture can help regulate estrogen and progesterone levels, as well as lesser-known but still important sex hormones like follicle stimulating hormone (FSH), luteinizing hormone (LH) and estradiol. Imbalances and irregularities in these substances can contribute to all sorts of female problems---and acupuncture can help relieve them.

For example, one study showed that acupuncture relieved dysmenorrheal (doctor-speak for a dysfunctional menstrual cycle, whether it involves serious cramps, irregular periods, and /or mid-cycle bleeding) in 90 percent of subjects. Others showed that acupuncture reduced the number of hot flashes in menopausal women by about 50 percent.

Acupuncture can also help with PMS symptoms; in one study, treatment using specific acupuncture points effectively reduced PMS symptoms in nearly 80 percent of subjects compared to those using 'placebo' points.

And in addition to its impact on female hormones, acupuncture also affects the production and utilization of neurotransmitters like serotonin that influence mood---so it can also help relieve the emotional manifestations of these hormonal imbalances.

4. Settle your stomach

Gastrointestinal problems are some of the most difficult for conventional medicine to treat---and also some of the most common. Whether you're plagued with constipation, irritable bowel syndrome, or more serious conditions like ulcerative colitis or Crohn's disease, acupuncture may be able to help.

Animal and human studies have suggested that acupuncture can influence gastric acid secretion and help regulate the contractions on the intestines, helping relieve both diarrhea and constipation. Specifically, animal studies have shown that acupuncture can reduce blood levels of a hormone called 5-hydroxytrytamine or 5-HT, which has been linked to irritable bowel syndrome, and that it can help improve symptoms of colitis by regulating proteins that prevent the death of cells in the lining of the colon.

5. Ease Cancer Treatment side effects

For cancer patients, the 'cure' can seem worse than the disease - chemo-therapy and radiation treatments can leave you exhausted, weak, and depressed, with nausea and vomiting, headaches, pain, and uncomfortable skin reactions. Acupuncture can help address any or all of these side effects, without adding to the list of pharmaceuticals already in your system.

For many of the same reasons that acupuncture helps with digestive problems, it can be very effective against nausea and vomiting brought on by chemotherapy. It's also been proven useful for cancer pain and for reducing anxiety in cancer patients. Acupuncture isn't a cure for cancer but it can certainly improve your quality of life while you deal with it.

The above list of benefits of acupuncture is just a partial list. Acupuncture has many additional benefits such as relieving migraines, insomnia, and anxiety. From acupuncture theory we know that the Chi channels are distributed throughout the entire body. These channels are closely related to the internal organs and are also related and connected to each other. All these channels have terminals at the hands, feet or head. Because of this we can apply acupressure or reflexology to these points to stimulate the circulation by massaging the feet, hands and ears.

Acupressure

Dr. Mark Stengler presents the following information about acupressure: "Acupressure has been used long before acupuncture in China, Japan and India. Simply, it was pressing on tender spots to relieve local pain and discomfort. But practitioners in acupressure and acupuncture have identified specific points of the body that contribute to pain and to healing. Chinese medicine has relied on acupressure for over 4,000 years. Today, it remains a major treatment at Chinese hospitals. Its popularity has been growing steadily throughout the world.

The traditional Chinese system of medicine focuses on the concept that the life-giving energy called 'Qi' circulates throughout the body in 12 main channels. Each channel represents a certain organ system such as kidney, lung and large intestine. The points that connect are located bilaterally—that is on both sides of the body. It is believed that when there is a blockage of Qi circulation in the channels, then disease or illness arises. Here are four easy steps for self treatment:

1. **Make sure you are relaxed.**
2. **Locate the desired point to which you are going to apply pressure.** Press on the point using your thumb or fingers. Some points may be very tender, indicating a blockage. Chronic conditions will need more treatments. Press the acupressure point and hold for 10 to 15 seconds. This can be repeated 5 to 10 times.
3. **Make sure to breathe while you stimulate the acupressure.** Slow, deep, relaxed breaths are best.
4. **Relax in a quiet atmosphere after a treatment.** Drink a glass of water to help detoxify your body.

Pressure points for some common problems are:

Constipation – between the webbing of the thumb and index finger. Press this spot on both hands.

Eyestrain – located one-half inch below the center of the lower eye ridge (you can feel an indentation), relieves burning, aching and dry eyes.

Headache – located below the base of the skull in the space between the two vertical neck muscles.

Liver – located on top of the foot in the hollow between the big toe and second toe.

Sinusitis – located on the lower, outer corner of each nostril. This pressure point is also useful for sneezing and nasal symptoms. The point between the webbing of the thumb and index finger also relieves nasal symptoms due to allergies [146]

---

[146] Op. cit. Stengler, *Natural Healing.* Bottom Line, pp. 45-49.

Emotional Freedom Technique (EFT)

There is another form of healing called 'Emotional Freedom Technique' which makes use of acupuncture, chi gong, and acupressure, plus the use of a phrase that is focused on a positive thought. An article in *Natural Awakenings* describes what it is and how it works, as follows:

This technique was developed in its present form by Gary Craig who drew upon the work of Dr. Roger Callahan who found that all negative emotion is present as the result of imbalances in the body's subtle energy systems. In addition to our well-known biological systems such as the circulatory, musculoskeletal, and nervous systems we also have an energy system that is linked both to our physical and emotional well-being. EFT rapidly restores emotional balance and resolves the physical expressions of these imbalances. EFT accomplishes this through tapping acupressure points (or meridians) with one's fingers rather than applying needles as in traditional acupuncture while using a setup phrase. The phrase is targeted specifically at the issue being worked on in that session.

Our cultural tradition is to have a specialist or specific treatment for each item we struggle with and the self-help schedule can just become too much. EFT is one strategy that can be applied to everything with remarkable results. EFT works on specific issues and with a few rounds of tapping results in a noticeable improvement. Let's use the fear of public speaking, a nearly universal fear, as an example. Many people take for granted that this is a natural fear and have to 'just get through' the handful of speeches they'll make in their lives, and avoid situations that provoke their fear. If EFT were used, the fear would be broken up into the individual parts that produce the intensity and tap on each one, such as past memories, where the speaker was ridiculed or embarrassed, the nausea before going up to speak, and so on. In one tapping session a discomfort level of 10 can be reduced to zero, and this may take only a few minutes, rarely more than an hour. EFT is one of the most economical choices for self-improvement. The basic manual written by Gary Craig is available as a free download on his website (www. emofree.com) and teaches everything you need to know to successfully apply EFT to yourself. [147]

---

[147] *Natural Awakenings, March/April, 2009, "EFT"* by Carla Burkle.

As you can see by the above information, there are many benefits to be had by making use of the services of acupuncturists, reflexologists, and masseurs. For those who are interested in making use of the reflexology **technique** by doing it yourself it can be done by making use of the charts which illustrate where the various points are located. By applying pressure with your fingers or knuckles to these points you will be able to experience the benefits as described above. I have been doing this for myself for many years, and also for my own family, and I can vouch for the fact that it really works. As I mentioned above the book by Dr. Yang contains all the information you will need in order to make use of this knowledge. There are many other books available on this subject so you should have no difficulty in finding all the information that you could want.

Chelation (EDTA)

- EDTA chelation may be one of the most effective, least expensive, and safest treatments for heart disease ever developed, yet it is practiced by perhaps only 2,000 physicians in the United States.

- EDTA chelation is not typically covered by medical insurance, even though insurance companies would save billions of dollars each year if they did.

- Although they save far more lives than conventional treatments for heart disease and other chronic degenerative diseases at a fraction of the cost, physicians who practice and promote EDTA chelation for these uses have been harassed, vilified, smeared, and, in some cases, driven from their profession by powerful medical societies and government agencies that practice and promote conventional medical treatments.

What Is EDTA Chelation?

EDTA chelation is a therapy by which repeated administrations of a weak synthetic amino acid (EDTA, ethylenediamine tetra-acetic acid) gradually reduce atherosclerotic plaque and other mineral deposits throughout the cardiovascular system by literally dissolving them away.

EDTA chelation has frequently been compared to a "Roto-Rooter" in the cardiovascular system, because it removes plaque and returns the arterial system to a smooth, healthy, pre-atherosclerotic state. A better metaphor might be "Liquid-Plumr," because, where Roto-Rooter violently scrapes deposits off the interior surfaces of your plumbing with a rapidly rotating blade, Liquid-Plumr simply dissolves them away.

Roto-Rooter is a far better metaphor for conventional medical treatments for heart disease, all of which are closely tied to the concept of the cardiovascular system as plumbing. When a pipe/artery gets clogged, simply ream it out or flatten the deposits (angioplasty). If that doesn't work, just cut away the bad section(s) and replace it (them) with a new piece of pipe (coronary artery bypass graft, or CABG). It's the same basic strategy older cities use for replacing their century-old water mains. And we know how successful that is!

It is commonplace for physicians who regularly prescribe EDTA chelation to encounter heart disease patients who have failed all the standard treatments but who make remarkable even unbelievable recoveries once given EDTA. Other patients, on waiting lists for CABG surgery, found they did not need the surgery following a series of EDTA chelation treatments.

CABG, known affectionately in the medical profession as "cabbage," is the most frequently performed surgery in the United States. At up to $50,000 per procedure, that indeed amounts to a lot of "cabbage," not only for cardiac surgeons but also for hospitals. As we shall see, these figures provide a powerful incentive for physicians to reject an effective, but inexpensive and unpatentable treatment like EDTA chelation.

Despite the danger and costs associated with these procedures, they are often only temporary fixes. Restenosis of treated coronary arteries occurs within 6 months in as many as one in three cases. By contrast, EDTA chelation permanently removes blood vessel obstructions throughout the body without dangerous and expensive surgery. How well does EDTA chelation work? Virtually every study that has looked at the efficacy of EDTA chelation in vascular disease has demonstrated significant improvements. Here is a brief sampling of a few of the major results:

A 1993 meta-analysis of 19 studies of 22,765 patients receiving EDTA chelation therapy for vascular disease found measurable improvement in 87%.

In a study of 2,870 patients with various degrees of degenerative diseases, especially vascular disease, almost 90% of the patients showed excellent improvement, as measured by walking distance, ECG, and Doppler changes.

A small, blinded, crossover study of patients with peripheral vascular disease found significant improvements in walking distance and ankle/brachial blood flow.

In 30 patients with carotid artery stenosis, there was a 30% improvement in blood flow after EDTA treatment.

Using retinal photographs in patients with macular degeneration, one researcher demonstrated significant improvement following EDTA treatment.

EDTA chelation treatment was evaluated in patients with carotid and coronary disease using technetium 99 isotope techniques. Significant improvement in arterial blood flow and ejection fraction (a measure of heart pumping ability) was reported.

When 65 patients on the waiting list for CABG surgery for a mean of 6 months were treated with EDTA chelation therapy, the symptoms in 89% (58) improved so much they were able to cancel their surgery. In the same study, of 27 patients recommended for limb amputation due to poor peripheral circulation, EDTA chelation resulted in saving 24 limbs.

EDTA exerts its beneficial effects on the body because this molecule is extremely proficient at chemically bonding with mineral and metal ions. This bonding process, known as chelation, is a natural and essential physiologic process that goes on constantly in the body. EDTA's chelating abilities make it ideal for many tasks.

Because EDTA is so effective at removing unwanted minerals and metals from the blood, it has been the standard "FDA-approved" treatment for lead, mercury, aluminum and cadmium poisoning for more than 50 years. EDTA normalizes the distribution of most metallic elements in the body.

Because it is so safe and effective, EDTA is also used widely as a stabilizer for packaged food. Minute amounts of EDTA (33-800 PPM) added to food help to preserve flavor and color and to retard spoilage and rancidity. (Read your food labels.)

Because EDTA inhibits blood clotting so well, it is routinely added to blood samples that are drawn for testing purposes.

EDTA improves calcium and cholesterol metabolism by eliminating metallic catalysts that can damage cell membranes by producing oxygen free radicals.

Thanks to these and probably other effects of EDTA, it has been reported to have a wide variety of benefits such as: increased energy, lower blood pressure, improvements in vision, mental functions, and skin conditions.

Chiropractic

Chiropractic procedures relieve and prevent most of the illnesses of the body by restoring the flow of energy to every area of the body. Everyone is subject to dislocations (subluxations) of the spinal vertebrae due to such frequent occurrences as poor posture, falls, missteps, accidents which cause whiplash, lifting improperly, and procedures used during the delivery of newborn infants. As a result, one or more of the vertebrae may be shifted out of their normal position and cause pressure against the nerves that go through every vertebra to various parts of the body. When nerve flow is curtailed the parts of the body involved will begin to lose their ability to function properly and if left uncorrected may lead to serious illnesses.

Besides the external causes of subluxations mentioned above there are internal causes that lead to subluxations such as a lack of essential minerals which is the major cause of osteoporosis. Dr. CJ Mertz, who is the president of *Chiropractic USA,* in his book *The World's Best Kept Health Secret Revealed,* sums up the benefits of chiropractic as follows:

So what exactly is subluxation?

It's actually pretty simple. Your brain, spinal cord and spinal nerves are responsible for controlling everything in your body. All of your muscles, organs, tissues and cells are controlled by your nervous system. Your spinal cord is protected by 24 moveable bones, or vertebrae. In between each vertebra there is a pair of nerves branching off the spinal cord extending to different parts of your body.

A subluxation occurs when spinal bones, or vertebrae, become misaligned. This could cause potentially dangerous pressure on the nerves. It can also make it difficult or impossible for the nerves to function normally.

So what causes subluxation? There are many situations in life that could cause subluxation. Things as common as car accidents, sport injuries, slips and falls, poor posture, childhood falls, gravity, the birthing process and even the stresses of life itself.

How do people know if they have subluxations? A doctor of chiropractic can properly examine and check you for subluxation. Medical doctors are rarely trained in detecting or correcting subluxations, just like chiropractors are rarely trained in performing surgery. Chiropractors focus on keeping your nervous system functioning as optimally as possible, so you can live and enjoy life to the fullest extent.

Chiropractic's core philosophy is based upon checking for and eliminating nervous system interference allowing brain messages to communicate clearly with the cells and body parts intended.

Bodies have been designed to experience a lifetime of wellness. Without clear messages from the brain, the cells and body parts can become misinformed or lack communication. The result can be a chemical imbalance. Remember, your body cells and body parts create natural body chemicals according to instructions from the brain. Clear communication through the spinal cord allows the body the best opportunity for healing and sustaining optimal health. [148]

Homeopathic

Homeopathy is a natural method of healing the body. It makes use of highly diluted herbs, minerals, and organic extracts. Everything is natural and most homeopathic remedies have no side effects. Conventional medicines, on the other hand, are concentrated doses of chemicals, with a long list of side effects that are often worse than the illness itself. Where prescription drugs normally must be taken for long periods of time, and at great cost to you, homeopathic remedies are often taken

---

[148] Dr. Cj Mertz, et al. *The World's Best Kept Health Secret Revealed.* Minnesota: Chiropractic Press, 2006, pp. 8-14.

just once. Sometimes just one tiny pill is required, and that pill often costs less than small pocket change.

Many profit-hungry drug company medicines are new and have not been tested for long-term effects. Homeopathic remedies have been in use for more than 200 years. Their safety record is well-established.

Homeopathy is the second most widely used system of medicine in the world. It's safe, surprisingly cheap, and effective. In the United States, where the influence of big drug companies has its strongest grip, the average person is unaware of its many benefits.

Unlike so many prescription drugs, homeopathic remedies are not addictive. Relief is experienced with just one dose, as long as the remedy you take is the right one for you. Even babies and pregnant women can use homeopathy without the dangerous threat of side-effects.

Homeopathic remedies work in harmony with your immune system by correcting the underlying causes of illness, whereas conventional medicine usually suppresses symptoms and weakens the immune system. For example, cough medicine is prescribed in order to suppress your natural reflex to cough, which is your body's attempt to clear your lungs. Homeopathic remedies can clear the problem that causes your coughing.

Kinesiology

Dr. George Goodheart of Denver, Michigan studied muscle testing techniques extensively in his clinical practice and made the breakthrough discovery that the strength or weakness of every muscle was connected to the health or pathology of a specific corresponding body organ. He further determined that each individual muscle was associated with an acupuncture meridian and correlated his work with that of the physician, Felix Mann on the medical significance of the acupuncture meridian.

By 1976, Goodheart's book on applied kinesiology had reached its twelfth edition; he began to teach the technique to his colleagues. His work was rapidly picked up by others, which led to the formation of the International College of Kinesiology.

The most striking finding of kinesiology was the clear demonstration that muscles instantly become weak when the body is exposed to harmful stimuli. For instance, if a patient with hypoglycemia put sugar on his tongue, on muscle testing, the deltoid muscle (the one usually used as an indicator) instantly went weak. It also was discovered that substances which were therapeutic to the body made the muscles instantly become strong.

Thousands of practitioners began to use the method and data rapidly accumulated showing kinesiology to be an important and reliable diagnostic technique which could accurately monitor a patient's response to treatment. The technique found widespread acceptance among professionals from many disciplines, and although it never caught on in mainstream medicine, it was used extensively by holistically oriented physicians.

Researchers, Dr. Goodheart and a psychiatrist, Dr. John Diamond, continued to conduct large-scale tests to find out the reliability of the technique when applied to a wide variety of applications. They found that the muscle test was always accurate in any type of test. For example, when it was applied to responses to questions which the respondents may or may not have had any knowledge of, the results would be the same. One such test was conducted with a large audience. An apple which had been sprayed with pesticides was held up in front of the audience. All of the people were told to look at the apple and then given the muscle test. Everyone went weak. Then an apple which had been grown organically was held up. As everyone looked at this apple everyone went strong. No one had any knowledge of which apple was which. In the foreword of the book, *Power Versus Force,* the following observations were made by the editor:

In the late seventies, Dr. John Diamond refined this technique into a new discipline which he called Behavioral Kinesiology. Dr. Diamond's startling discovery was that indicator muscles would strengthen or weaken in the presence of positive or negative *emotional and intellectual stimuli, as well as physical stimuli.* A smile will make you test strong. The statement, 'I hate you,' will make you test weak.

A striking aspect of Diamond's research was the uniformity of responses among his subjects. Diamond's results were predictable, repeatable, and universal. This was so even where there was no rational link between stimulus and response. For totally undetermined reasons certain abstract symbols caused all subjects to test weak, while other 'neutral' pictures caused all subjects to test strong. Music, such as classical and most 'rock and roll' caused a universally strong response, while the 'hard' or 'metal rock produced a universally weak response.

There was one other phenomenon which Diamond noted which has extraordinary implications. Subjects while listening to tapes of known falsehoods—Lyndon Johnson perpetrating the Tonkin Gulf Hoax; Edward Kennedy stonewalling the Chappaquiddic incident—universally tested weak. While listening to recordings of demonstrably true statements, they universally tested strong. This was the starting point of the author of *Power Versus Force,* Dr. David Hawkins, the well-known psychiatrist and physician. Dr. Hawkins began research on the kinesiological response to truth and falsehood in 1975.

It has been established that test subjects did not need any conscious acquaintance with the substance (or issue) being tested. In double-blind studies-and in mass demonstrations involving entire lecture audiences—subjects universally tested weak in response to unmarked envelopes containing artificial sweetener, and strong to identical placebo envelopes. The same naïve response appeared in testing intellectual values. One element of this phenomenon is the binary nature of the response. Hawkins found that the questions must be phrased so that the answer is very clearly yes or no.

As Dr. Hawkins' research continued his most fertile discovery was a means of calibrating a scale of relative truth by which intellectual positions, statements or ideologies could be rated on a range of one to one thousand. One can ask, 'This item-book, philosophy, teacher-calibrates at 200(Y/N?); at 250(Y/N?),' and so on, until the point of common weak response determines the calibration. The enormous implication of the calibrations was that for the first time in human history ideological validity could be appraised as an innate quality in *any* subject.

Through 20 years of similar calibrations, Hawkins was able to analyze the full spectrum of the levels of human consciousness. This anatomy produces a profile of the entire human condition, allowing a comprehensive analysis of the emotional and spiritual development of individuals, societies, and the race in general.

The research reflected in this volume has taken Dr. Diamond's technique several steps further through the discovery that this kinesiological response reflects a capacity of the human organism to differentiate not only positive from negative stimuli, but also anabolic (life-enhancing) from carbolic (Life-consuming) and, most dramatically, true from false.

Moreover, we found that this testable phenomenon can be used to calibrate human levels of consciousness so that an arbitrary logarithmic scale of whole numbers emerges, stratifying the relative power of levels of consciousness in all areas of human experience. Exhaustive investigation has resulted in a calibrated scale in which the log of whole numbers from 1 to 1,000 calibrates the degree of power of all possible levels of human awareness. The millions of calibrations which confirmed this discovery further disclosed a remarkable distinction between power and force and their respective qualities. By the use of the kinesiological testing procedure described below, unlimited information about any subject, past or present, is universally available. [149]

The test itself is simple, rapid, and relatively foolproof. It requires two persons. One acts as the test subject by holding out one arm laterally, parallel to the ground. The second person then presses down with two fingers on the wrist of the extended arm and says, 'resist.' The subject then resists the downward pressure with all his strength. That is all there is to it.

A statement may be made by either party. While the subject holds it in mind, his arms strength is tested by the tester's downward pressure. If the statement is negative or false or reflects a calibration below 200 the test subject will 'go weak.' If the answer is yes or calibrates over 200, he will 'go strong.' [150]

Massage

In the book, *QIGONG FOR HEALTH,* Dr. Yang devotes a lengthy chapter to massage and rubbing in which he shows illustrations of all the acupuncture points in the feet, hands and ears plus illustrations of how and where to use your hands to apply pressure

[149] David Hawkins, M.D., PhD. *Power vs Force: An Anatomy of Consciousness.* Sedona, AZ: Veritas Publishing, 2004, pp. 2-10.
[150] Ibid, pp.43-44.

effectively. Dr. Yang presents an overview of the effectiveness of massage and acupressure as follows:

People have always instinctively rubbed sore muscles and other painful areas to ease their pain and to help the sore muscles recover more quickly. Long ago it was found that this kind of rubbing can also cure a number of disorders such as headaches, joint pain, and an uneasy stomach, and that simple rubbing can even strengthen weakened organs.

The therapeutic effects of massage are known worldwide. The Japanese have used acupressure which is derived from Chinese massage, for centuries. The Greek upper classes have used a form of massage—slapping the skin with switches—to cure various disorders. However, the Chinese have systematized massage to agree with the theory of Qi circulation.

There are three general Chinese massage treatments. The first is massaging the muscle: the second, massaging the cavities, or acupuncture points; and the third, massaging the nerve and channel endings. Each category of massage has its own specific uses, but generally a mixture of the three is used.

Muscle massage is used to relieve soreness and bruises. The masseuse follows the direction of the muscle fiber using rubbing, pressing, sliding, grasping, slapping, and shaking techniques. The result is an increase in the circulation of blood and Qi on the skin and in the muscle area. It also helps to spread accumulated acid, which collects in the muscles due to hard exercise, or blood (in the case of bruises), or stagnant Qi, allowing the circulation to disperse them more quickly. Commonly this type of massage is used to help a person overcome a feeling of weakness or tiredness.

The second category is massaging the acupuncture points. These same points are used in Japanese acupressure, with the addition of a few other points. The principle of massaging the acupuncture points is the same as in acupuncture theory: to stimulate the channels by stimulating cavities that can be reached easily by rubbing or pressing with the hands, rather than needles. In acupressure, some non-channel points are used to stimulate minor Qi channels to help circulate energy locally.

The third category of massage is to rub or press the endings of the nerves and Qi channels. These channels are located on the hands, feet, and ears. You can easily rub the zones that correspond to the different organs, or that are effective for specific symptoms or illnesses. This form of massage is known in the West as reflexology. Theoretically, if the channel endings are rubbed, the Qi will be stimulated to a higher level, which increases the circulation and benefits the related organ or cures the illness. [151]

Meditation

The popular method of practicing meditation is based on the Buddhist tradition of sitting in the lotus position and clearing your mind of your usual thoughts to the point where you can focus on one thing or thought only. This way of meditation is incorporated into Rajah Yoga and also practiced in other forms of Yoga. A feature of meditation, in addition to mind control, is the use of breathing exercises to enhance the health benefits of the practice.

The popular Chinese healing method known as Chi Gong, in addition to its physical exercises, emphasizes the importance of deep controlled breathing and the conscious control of vital energy 'Qi' throughout the channels and meridians in the body. One of the leading teachers of Chi Gong, Dr. Yang, describes the techniques of breathing and its relation to meditation as follows:

The first and most important step for effective meditation is proper breathing. There are two basic methods in use in Chinese meditation: Daoist and Buddhist.

Daoist breathing, also known as Reverse Breathing is used to prepare the Qi for circulation, and its proper development is crucial. If you are coming to meditation seriously for the first time, you should not attempt to circulate Qi from the very start. The primary goal of the beginner must be to train the muscles around the Dan Tian or lower abdomen so that the Daoist method of breathing is easy and natural. The training of the muscles is achieved through the pre-

---

[151] Yang, op. cit., pp. 119-120.

liminary practice of reverse breathing. Once your muscles have been trained and your mind sufficiently calmed, you may then attempt to circulate the Qi.

In Daoist breathing the normal movement of the abdomen is reversed during inhalation and exhalation. Instead of expanding when inhaling, the Daoist contracts, and vice versa. Never hold your breath or force the process. Inhale through the nose slowly, keeping the flow smooth and easy, and contract the Dan Tian or lower abdomen. This is best done by pressing your rectum against the floor or mattress while lying on your back. As the air flows in, lift the lower abdomen up behind the navel. When the lungs are filled, exhale gently.

Inhalation is considered Yin and exhalation is considered Yang. They must operate together like the Yin-Yang symbol, one becoming the other smoothly and effortlessly in a fluid circular motion. As exhalation occurs, slowly push out the Dan Tian or lower abdomen. The area of the Dan Tian is where the Qi is generated and accumulated in order to start Small Circulation. Because of this, the muscles around the Dan Tian must be trained so that they can sufficiently contract and expand while you inhale and exhale. At first, expanding the lower abdomen while exhaling may be difficult; but with practice the muscles learn to expand more and more until the entire lower abdomen expands upon exhalation from the navel to the pubic bone. Do not force the Dan Tian to expand, but work gently until success is achieved.

This whole process of Daoist breathing is a form of deep breathing, not because the breathing is heavy, but because it works the lungs to near capacity. While many people who engage in strenuous exercise breathe hard, they do not necessarily breathe deeply. Deep breathing causes the internal organs to vibrate in rhythm with the breath, which stimulates and exercises them. Many forms of strenuous exercise only condition the external muscles while doing very little for the vital organs.

In the Buddhist breathing method, the movement of the abdomen is the opposite of the Daoist. When you inhale, expand your lower abdomen, as you exhale, contract it. This kind of breathing is called Normal Breathing. It is the same kind of breathing a singer practices. Both methods use the same principle of Qi generation. The main difference is that the coordination of the abdominal motion and the breathing is opposite. In fact, many meditators can use either method, and can switch very easily.

Once you can breathe adequately according to the Daoist and Buddhist methods, you can take up sitting meditation to begin the process of Qi circulation. The first goal is to achieve a calm mind while concentrating on deep breathing. You create a type of hypnotic state to do this. You should stay at this stage until you can expand and withdraw your Dan Tian while breathing with no conscious effort, and without your attention wandering.

Some beginning meditators say they cannot feel the Qi flow, while others say they feel it is stopped at a particular point. The response to both of these comments is to continue doing the cycle. At first, it will be mostly your imagination and not much Qi, but with perseverance the flow will become stronger and more perceptible. Remember, the Qi is always flowing or you would not be alive. Since Qi follows the mind, keeping your attention moving will keep the Qi flowing through the channels and gradually open the constrictions.

Transcendental Meditation (TM)

A method of meditation that can be done easily by anyone is known as Transcendental Meditation (TM). The TM technique was introduced to the United States by Maharishi Mahesh Yogi in 1958 and rapidly became a very popular form of meditation because of its many benefits. Reports of outstanding improvements in both physical and mental health led to numerous research studies which scientifically verified the many benefits of TM, some of which are listed below:

- Increased strength and efficiency of brain functioning
- Improved cardiovascular efficiency
- Improved resistance to disease
- EEG brain wave patterns show an increased state of alertness at the same time the brain is in the restful state of deep sleep.
- Development of full potential of thinking, understanding, and feeling is enhanced leading to growth of awareness.
- Stress, brought on by fears and anxieties, is reduced or eliminated entirely.

- TM helps prevent mental illness and also provides beneficial therapy for the mentally ill.
- Drug use is reduced dramatically by the practice of TM.
- TM provides the deepest state of rest, deeper than sleep.

The potential for the growth of individual consciousness is enormous and, on the basis of the growth of awareness through the TM program, the growth of achievement and fulfillment is virtually unlimited.

The practice of TM requires four 2 hour sessions of training by a qualified instructor. It is practiced twice a day, about 15--20 minutes each morning and again in the evening. You sit in a comfortable position wherever you wish.

The actual process is described fully in the book, *TM: Discovering Inner Energy and Overcoming Stress,* as follows:

"The technique of TM consists of giving the attention an inward turn by easily thinking a single thought. In this way, the mind remains active but is left undirected. Theoretically it should be possible to initiate the process of TM by repeatedly experiencing any thought, emotion, sensation or perception. However, thought, as opposed to other possible experiences, constitutes the ideal vehicle for facilitating the inward shift of attention. But what is the nature of thought? Studies of memory and attention have shown that much of a person's thinking activity amounts to mentally repeating the sounds of various words. Modern psychology's recognition of the importance of thought as sub-vocalized sound echoes a number of ancient traditions which hold that sound, especially on the subtle level of thought, is a powerful vehicle for influencing consciousness.

Sound as entertained in thought provides a most effective vehicle for disengaging the mind from the everyday thinking process and turning the attention toward increasingly quiet mental activity. The thought sounds used in TM are called 'mantras.' Mantra is a Sanskrit term which designates 'a thought the effects of which are known' not on the level of meaning - in fact, the mantras taught for use in TM have no denotative meaning - but on the level of vibratory effect, analogous to sound quality. MANTRAS ARE SPECIALLY SELECTED FOR EACH INDIVIDUAL WHO RECEIVES INSTRUCTION IN TM. Once learned, the mantra is confidential and is used for only one purpose; to affect the spontaneous process of reducing mental activity during the practice of TM.

Because TM permits the meditator to experience quiet levels of mind where the influence of each thought is especially profound, the selection of the correct mantra for each individual is of critical importance. Maharishi and the thousands of trained teachers of TM rely on an ancient tradition through which many generations have fathomed the full depth of the mind. This tradition provides a systematic procedure for selecting the most suitable sounds for use in TM by particular individuals. Such procedure has been maintained since 5000 B.C., r earlier, the time of mankind's most ancient teachings, the Vedas.

Learning TM consists not only of learning the right mantra but also how to use it correctly. To insure correctness in every aspect of these fundamentals, personal instruction in the technique by a qualified instructor is necessary. The technique cannot be learned secondhand from a book or from another meditator. Extensive preparation is required to qualify a teacher to guide a novice through all possible variations of personal experience. Nor is it feasible to select a mantra for oneself, by chance, by consultation of ancient texts or by intuition. What seems to be an appropriate mantra on the surface level of intellectual understanding may unfortunately turn out to have inappropriate effects." [152]

NAET Cure for Allergies

The letters NAET stand for Nambudripad's Allergy Elimination Technique. This technique has been used to identify and to eliminate allergies and sensitivities to a wide variety of substances. A major cause of illnesses, which is largely overlooked, is the widespread prevalence of allergies. Many serious illnesses are actually due to allergies which are overlooked and as a result are treated with various medications which have little or no effect on the underlying cause of the condition but, as is usually the case, cause serious side-effects. In recent years, there has been a breakthrough in the methods of testing for allergies and in the treatments for allergies. The successes of the new treatments are so outstanding that they will be given a thorough review in this chapter.

---

[152] Denise Denniston. *The Transcendental Meditation TM BOOK.* Allen Park, MI: Versemonger Press, 1975, pp. 17-18.

The breakthrough in the knowledge of allergies is largely due to one person Dr. Devi Nambudripad, an Indian physician. She is a trained acupuncturist in addition to her medical training. In her book, *Goodbye to Illness,* she states:

It is important to recognize that allergies, like people, do not exist in a vacuum. They are part of a complex interrelation between the allergen and the central nervous system. The central nervous system controls the proper function of the various organs and systems in the body. Each of these systems is capable of ignoring or reacting to a given stimulus. This happens in concert with all the other systems causing either a massive shut down of the human machine, or producing weakness and malfunction of any single part of the total system.

One reaction which has undergone intensive observation is asthma. Strangely, asthma sufferers do not experience attacks when they are frightened. In such situations it is believed the body prepares for 'fight or flight.' The theory states that in this hyper-chemical state the allergens are completely ignored. The adjustment has been made as though a switch was suddenly thrown. I utilized this idea when I developed NAET as a treatment to permanently eliminate allergies.

Every time a patient is tested for an allergen, the central system is alerted to the presence of an approaching danger. When the patient is then treated for the allergen, an intentional hyper-chemical state or a temporary 'fight or flight' reaction is created in the body, forcing to produce the appropriate neuro-chemicals to overcome the oncoming danger: the presence of the known allergen. Tapping at the specific nerve roots will alert the entire nerve pathway, from its origin in the brain to the nerve ending somewhere in the periphery, about the dangerous situation. This will inform the nerve about the adjustment the body is making by releasing appropriate neuro-chemical antidotes such as endorphins to neutralize the threat. During the hyper-chemical state, the allergen is once again totally ignored. At a later time, whenever that particular allergen comes into contact with the body, the body will automatically go into a hyper-chemical state by releasing the particular chemical and will no longer react adversely to the allergen. The same allergen can trigger different individual reactions in people depending upon the number of energy pathways affected by the allergen's invasion.

The pathology can then be clearly demonstrated initially as a kinetic weakness observable through standard muscle response testing techniques, borrowed from applied kinesiology. Kinetic weakness, or muscle weakness, makes diagnosis possible. Muscle weakness is the body's way of signaling to the patient and the doctor potential negative reactions to allergens. Since a simple and effective diagnostic tool is now available, it becomes a relatively simple matter of good detective work to identify all of the substances that may be responsible for the presenting symptoms.

This brings us to a concept that is totally revolutionary to most people. Allergic reactions are the result of messages received and acted upon by the central nervous system and are not the result of the inherent properties of the substances we come in contact with. The central nervous system must be reprogrammed to sense allergens differently than before treatment. Is this possible? Can NAET offer a solution? The answer is a resounding YES.

The answer to this question was discovered quite by accident in 1983. I was being treated by acupuncture for the relief of a severe allergy to raw carrots. During the treatment, I fell asleep with the carrots still on my body. After the treatment (and a restful nap during the needling period), I woke up and experienced a unique feeling. I had never felt quite that way following other similar acupuncture treatments in the past. I realized that I had been lying on some of the carrot. A piece was still in my hand. I knew that some of the needles were supposed to help circulate the electrical energy and balance the body. If there is any energy blockage, the balancing process is supposed to help clear it during the treatment and bring the body to a balanced state.

I asked my husband who was assisting me in the treatment process to test me for carrots again. The carrot's energy field had interacted with my own energy field, and my brain had accepted this once deadly poison as a harmless item. The two energy fields no longer clashed. This was an amazing NEW DISCOVERY. Subsequent tests for carrots by MRT confirmed that something phenomenal had happened indeed. What followed was a series of experiments treating my own allergies and those of my family. I cured most of my allergies in a year's time. The method was extended to my practice. In every case, allergies were 'cleared out,' never to return. After treating thousands of patients for a wide variety of allergens, the procedure is no longer experimental or of questionable value. It is a proven treatment method and the premise of NAET methodology.

Physical contact with the allergen during and after a treatment(which consists of stimulating certain specific points on the acupuncture meridians, thus stimulating the central nervous system0 produces the necessary immune mediators or antidotes to neutralize the adverse reaction coming from the allergen held in the hand. This produces a totally new, permanent and irreversible response to the allergen. It is possible, through stimulation of the appropriate points of the acupuncture meridians, which have direct correspondence with the brain, to reprogram the brain.

The success of the NAET procedure confirms that a major portion of the illnesses we observe result from allergies. Yes, the prognosis is bright. The evidence suggests a convincing argument can be made that a significant number of patients suffering from latent, undiagnosed allergies, normally treated by traditional western medical practitioners for temporary relief, are going to experience a cure from holistic health practitioners. Freedom from allergies is becoming a fact for many patients formerly presenting a wide range of symptoms, from chemical dependency and stroke to eczema and asthma. [153]

Another researcher of the relationship of food sensitivities to illnesses, Jeffrey Zavik, came to the same conclusion as Nambudripad in regards to the need for eliminating allergies. Rather than using the word allergies, which includes all types of sensitivities in addition to food, Zavik confined his research to foods only and used the words Toxic Food Syndrome to describe the condition. He reached the conclusion that 95 percent of the population suffers from Toxic Food Syndrome.

Zavik conducted research into methods for testing for adverse reactions to foods. He developed a technique which proved to be very successful in identifying food sensitivities, which led to his forming a company, Immuno Laboratories. The testing procedure involves the use of food extracts given to patients whose blood cells are observed with the

---

[153] Dr. Devi Nambumripad. *Say Good-Bye To Illness*. Buena Park, CA: Delta Publishing, 1999, pp. 130-138.

use of a microscope. Zavik describes what his company does as follows: "Today, my laboratory enjoys a reputation for being the finest toxic food-testing laboratory in the world. We have performed over 250,000 tests through a network of physicians in more than 24 different countries.

Unlike Nambudripad whose method called NAET, actually eliminates allergies to specific allergens, Zavik identifies the food allergens through his testing procedure and then provides guidance on how to relieve reactions by the avoidance of the identified allergens and by the use of rotation diets to obtain relief from the specific food allergen." [154]

Both methods provide substantial benefits to people with allergies by identifying the allergens they are sensitive to. It is estimated that 95 percent of the population have allergies with symptoms that cause chronic ailments. People are treated with medication to relieve the symptoms when all they have to do is avoid the food which they are allergic to or make use of the treatments mentioned above.

Reiki

Reiki is a powerful healing method that makes use of the healing energies of the universe which was discovered by a Japanese monk by the name of Usui. An insight into how Usui became aware of this healing power is furnished in the following excerpt from the book, *The Healing Power of Light:*

"Usui, the Japanese founder of Reiki experienced the power of light after an extended 21-day meditation and fast. There was an awareness of a white light striking him at the brow chakra, the Third Eye, with many rainbow bubble particles of light in front of him and, on what felt like a white screen, the symbols from the Sanskrit scriptures blazed in Gold. He felt charged with energy to start new healing and teaching work. The light was inside him and working within him." [155]

The following information about the power of Reiki to heal the body and mind is based on the book *The Reiki Magic Guide to Self-Attunement* by Brett Bevell.

Reiki is a form of hands-on energy healing that comes from the Divine. It is an intelligent healing energy that flows through anyone who

---

[154] Jeffrey Zavik. *Toxic Food Syndrome.* Fort Lauderdale, FL: Fun Publishing, 2007.
[155] Cooper, op. cit., pp. 110-111.

has received a Reiki initiation, which is called an attunement. Once a person is attuned to Reiki, he or she has the ability to use this energy for healing themselves or others; an ability that remains for an entire lifetime….Thus, Reiki has intelligence as well as compassion and a healing quality much greater than that of any individual human being. It is as limitless as the Divine source from which it comes.

During Reiki sessions it always seems to know where to go and what to do, unlike psychic energy, which needs to be consciously directed. The beautiful thing about Reiki is that it does not require you to be psychic or intuitive or have any special abilities. Once you are attuned to this sacred energy, all you have to do is desire it to run through your own hands into whomever or whatever you intend to heal."

There are three degrees in Reiki. In First Degree Reiki, the energy flows out of your hands. In Second Degree, you learn Reiki symbols for empowering the flow of Reiki, so you can send it across time and space, or direct it to heal mental and emotional issues. Third Degree Reiki is the Master Level, where you are empowered with more symbols which allow you to perform the sacred attunement ceremony.

….Learning Reiki is something that requires an initiation ceremony, called an attunement. You cannot access Reiki simply through intellectual or meditative means. There are attunements for each level of Reiki that open the hands and crown chakra to the energy of Reiki at each level (For those unfamiliar with the term, Chakras are sacred energy wheels that exist in seven places in our energetic body, starting at the bottom of the torso and moving upward. The crown chakra, which is at the very top of the skullcap, both influences and is influenced by our spiritual awareness and connection to the Divine.) Traditionally these attunements are performed in person by a Reiki master. The unique thing about this book is that it reveals a new method of attunement that allows easy access for all to be attuned to Reiki without going to a Reiki Master. The intention is to provide all of humanity with the capacity to use Reiki in their lives every day for health and spiritual growth….All humans do need Reiki, for their own health, for the sake of elevating the entire vibration of the human race, and for the sake of the planet as a whole. [156]

---

[156] Brett Bevell. *The Magic Guide to Self-Attunement.* Berkley, CA: Crossing Press, 2007, pp. 1-7.

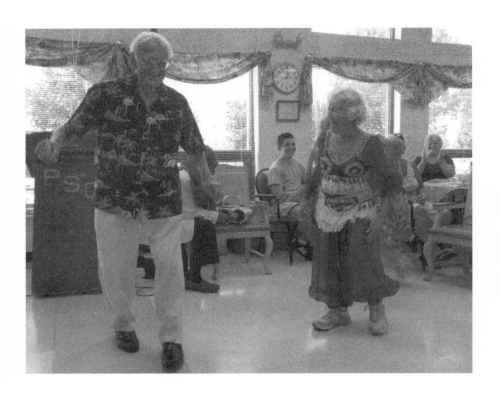

CHAPTER TEN

BREATHING FOR HEALTH

Pranayama

A powerful method of increasing total well-being is deep breathing. There is a substantial body of knowledge about the benefits and techniques of deep breathing, dating back to the ancient art of Pranayama, which is an Indian practice that includes a variety of breathing techniques. Besides its basic functions of bringing in oxygen and exhaling carbon dioxide, breathing affects our state of mind. It can make us excited or calm, tense or relaxed. It can make our thinking confused or clear.

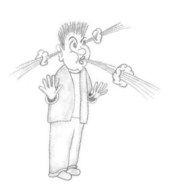

In the yogic tradition, air is the primary source of prana or life force that provides vital energy throughout the universe. Pranayama is a term that includes the control of breathing for the purpose of maximizing the benefits of prana. It is a separate part of yoga used to help clear the body and mind in preparation for meditation. Full Yogic breathing is done during meditation and some of the techniques involved are described in sections of this book on meditation and on yoga.

Basically, pranayama is practiced while sitting in the lotus position which consists of sitting on the floor or on a mat with both legs crossed over another. It is easier to sit on a cushion which is about two to four inches thick. Since most people are unaccustomed to sitting with their legs crossed, it is very uncomfortable to sit this way for any length of time. The problem gradually goes away by itself. The common cross-legged posture consists of bending both knees in front of you and drawing them close to the torso; then place one leg over the other, resting in the crease of the bent leg or as far above the knee as you can, while the other leg remains flat on the floor. If your legs become numb while sitting, uncross them and relax. It also helps to change the leg which is in the lifted position to the other leg from time to time. Sitting cross-legged restricts the normal blood flow and the body needs time to adjust to the new position. It is easier to sit with both legs crossed with both feet resting flat on the floor without pulling one leg higher than the other. In either sitting position, your hands should be held close to your abdomen, one on top of the other, with the tips of the thumbs touching. This position helps you feel your breathing as you expand your abdomen while inhaling and will develop deeper breathing.

Posture is very important. Do not slouch or lean forward or backward. Sit upright, looking straight ahead. To help maintain the proper position, think of your head being pulled up by a string hanging from above like a puppet. Relax completely and focus your attention on your breath or on a single object in front of you. The object is to control your mind so it is clear of all extraneous thoughts.

There are many different breathing exercises involved, all of which include holding your hands and fingers in various positions. The overall purpose is to develop your ability to breathe more deeply, thus bringing in more prana, and at the same time obtaining the benefits of keeping your mind free of its usual clutter. The various techniques used in the practice of pranayama can be found in most books on yoga. Space does not allow for them to be included here. Some of the many benefits of Pranayama breathing are listed below:

1. It releases chronic and acute muscular tensions around the heart and digestive organs.
2. It helps sufferers of respiratory illnesses such as asthma and emphysema to overcome shortness of breath. It actually increases lung capacity.

3. It encourages proper nerve stimulus to the cardio-vascular system.
4. Dramatically reduces emotional and nervous anxiety.
5. It improves detoxification through exchange of carbon dioxide and oxygen.
6. It amplifies the autoimmune system by increased distribution of energy to the endocrine system.
7. It calms the mind and integrates the mental physical balance.
8. It contributes to both vitality and relaxation.

In the Chinese tradition, the vital energy in the air that we breathe is called Qi. Chi Gong makes use of deep breathing techniques similar to Pranayama but places more emphasis on various ways of directing the Qi energy to different parts of the body. The section on Chi Gong and the one on Meditation in this book present some of these techniques.

Rebirthing

Another method of increasing our total well-being by deep breathing is known as a technique used in the Rebirthing process. The theory behind this method is based upon the traumatic experiences of a newborn infant during childbirth. In addition to emotional problems that may be transmitted to the newborn during delivery, a lack of oxygen entering the newborn infant usually occurs during the interval after the umbilical cord is cut and the infant begins to breathe on its own. We are familiar with the usual scene of a newborn being held upside down and being slapped on the back in order to start the breathing process. When the newborn starts to cry it is a good sign that the breathing process has begun. A result of this experience is that the newborn, while gasping for its first breath of air, is only able to bring in a small portion of the air needed to fill the lungs' capacity. The outcome is that a pattern of shallow breathing remains with each person throughout life unless a deep breathing pattern is established to replace the pattern of shallow breathing. A special method of bringing about this change of breathing came to be known as the *twenty-five breaths* which is an essential part of the Rebirthing Process. When deep breathing is established by this method there is a marked improvement in one's health and sense of well-being. I know from personal experience that it really works. The technique consists of the following steps:

While lying on your back, preferably when you lie down to sleep, start counting up to five as you breathe in. Then count to five as you breathe out. It should be a slow steady count, about one second for each count without any pause between the in and out phase. Each sequence of inhaling and exhaling counts as one breath. You repeat the sequence 25 times. That is all there is to it. If you have difficulty breathing in and out to the count of five, it is alright to count to just three or four at first and then gradually increase the count as your lung capacity increases. Another thing you can do to improve the effectiveness of this breathing exercise is to hold your hands over your abdomen while breathing in and feel the hands being pushed up as the air enters the lower part of the lungs. Then notice how your hands drop as you breathe out. Focusing on your breath in this way will encourage you to breathe as deeply as possible. Do not strain; your lung capacity will increase slowly over a period of time. The benefits will be obvious. Among other things, you will find that you fall to sleep more quickly and more soundly. If you awaken during the night, do the twenty-five breaths and you will be able to fall back to sleep more quickly.

Do not strain to breathe in more deeply than you can handle comfortably as it is possible to get too much oxygen and then hyper-ventilate. This situation can be handled by breathing out into a paper bag held over your nose. By inhaling the carbon dioxide that you exhaled into the bag, you will compensate for the excess oxygen. Do this a few times until you get over the dizzy feeling brought on by hyperventilating.

CHAPTER ELEVEN

LAUGHTER & MUSIC

Not enough can be said about the health-promoting effects of a playful attitude, a sense of humor, and the ability to have fun. Bob Hope and George Burns, both famous comedians, each lived for 100 years by cultivating light-hearted attitudes. They pursued lives of fun and laughter while they tried to make others laugh. And well-known author, Norman Cousins cured himself of a painful life-threatening disease with laughter and vitamin C. Humor and a light-hearted attitude can add years to your life, and they are powerful stimulants for your healing system.

Benefits of Laughter

A happy disposition raises the spirit and enhances well being. Laughter can actually prevent and even cure serious diseases. One of the best examples of the healing power of laughter is that of the famous Norman Cousins experience.

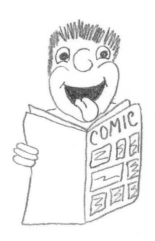

Norman Cousins was the highly respected and well-known editor of the _Saturday Review_, a weekly magazine section of the

New York Times that featured articles about the entertainers and entertainment in New York City.

Back in 1964, he came down with a rare spinal disease, *ankylosing spondylitis,* for which there was no known cure. The condition was so serious that he had to be placed in a hospital and confined to a special bed that was designed to keep him as comfortable as possible since he could not walk and his every movement brought on excruciating pain.

After a few weeks of this constant suffering, Cousins decided that he was going to try to ease his suffering by watching his favorite comical movies with such outstanding comics as Charlie Chaplin, etc. He also encouraged entertainers who came to visit him to perform for him. A group of entertainers came on a regular basis each week performing comical routines and also musicians played his favorite music.

This went on for several months during which time Cousins started to slowly get better. He needed less and less medication to ease his pains. He started to get out of bed and walk a little. Over a period of six months he steadily improved to the point where he no longer needed painkillers and the spinal disease went into remission. At that time, he was discharged from the hospital and was able to resume his job at the *Saturday Review.*

In 1979, he wrote a book about his experiences, *Anatomy of an Illness,* which became a best-seller and introduced the health benefits of laughter to a wide audience. On the basis of Cousins' experience a number of research studies were conducted to determine the association of laughter and health. The results of these studies confirmed the value of laughter as indicated in the following article which appeared in the March, 2008 issue of *Energy Times:*

> Today, laughter is known to have a wide array of healthcare applications. And it has become more apparent why so many comedians who have had troubled and sometimes tragic upbringings, from Charlie Chaplin to Rodney Dangerfield and Carol Burnett, were so drawn to their line of work.
>
> A study by the University of Maryland School of Medicine showed the positive effects of laughter on the functioning of blood vessels and on overall cardiovascular health.

Healthy volunteers watched two movies shown at the extreme ends of the emotional scale: the furiously violent opening scene of *Saving Private Ryan* and a segment of the comedy *Kingpin*. Laughter caused by the second clip appeared to cause the endothelium, or inner lining of the participants' blood vessels to expand in order to increase blood flow. In contrast, the stress response from watching the first clip triggered *vasoconstriction,* or reduced blood flow, within the blood vessels. Overall, average blood flow increased 22% during laughter and decreased 35% during stress—even among those who had already previously seen *Ryan* and knew what to expect.

'The act of laughing out loud vigorously has benefits similar to a workout,' says Kelly McGonigal, PhD, a health psychologist at Stanford University. 'It increases heart rate and stimulates breathing'…A growing number of proponents of laughter as medicine are embracing the idea that harnessing self-driven laughter can yield tremendous therapeutic benefits.

Laughter enthusiasts trace the movement to Madame Kataria, MD, himself inspired by Cousins. Kataria started a playful form of laughter yoga in Mumbai, India in 1995. Steve Wilson, a psychologist, met Kataria three years later and picked up the torch, creating a training program (www.worldlaughtertour.com) through which therapists become Certified Laughter Leaders who direct sessions and laughter clubs.

Some 5000 laughter Clubs are organized in 40 countries, according to Kataria's website, www.yogalaff.com. Certified Laughter Leaders have been dispatched to help families of military who have shipped out to Iraq or returned home with permanent injuries. They've also trained teachers to introduce laughter into the classroom, hoping to develop more receptive students.

At the laughter therapy session at the Philadelphia cancer hospital, patients, their family members and hospital staff appeared to shift from the artificial laughter into heartfelt giggles and sincere laughs very quickly. Laughter therapy is but one tool in the Cancer Treatment Centers of America Psycho-neuroimmunology Program, which includes naturo-pathic medicine and Reiki.

Citing a study of laughter's sonic structure, Brain notes that laughter can trigger "ha-ha-ha" or 'ho-ho-ho sounds, but never a hybrid of the two. That observation underscores the artifice of the "hee hee, ha ha, ho ho" stew of chants practiced at the laughter therapy session at the Philadelphia cancer hospital and among other laughter groups. [157]

Another outcome was the widespread formation of laughing classes in different localities. I had the personal experience of attending a number of laughing classes near my home in N.J. The classes definitely improved my feelings of happiness and left me feeling light-hearted and energized with a feeling of reduced stress as well. The leader of the class, Yvette Halpin, made the following comments when she was interviewed for a featured article in the local newspaper, The Courier News on May 8, 2009:

"The economy still resembles a sink-hole, or maybe you're out of work, or maybe you're dealing with a chronic disease or cancer. In any of these situations I know exactly when laughter is needed, said Yvette Halpin, certified laughter leader and yoga teacher.

I like to start a Laugh Out Loud session near World Laughter Day, which is celebrated the first Sunday in May, Halpin said. She said the first World Laughter Day was celebrated Jan. 11, 1998, in Mumbai, India. The holiday was created by Dr. Madan Kataria, founder of the World Laughter Yoga movement.

Halpin's course teaches new and return laughers to connect with their positive energy. Each week's interactive class uses props to take the class on an excursion, for example to be a pirate, or go on a train trip, or attend a graduation or carnival

'The idea is for the participants to become completely involved and engrossed in the present, to divorce oneself from what's going on in one's life. First-time participants are not used to laughing heartily for no reason,' said Halpin, who added that a good laugh also improves circulation and breathing, relaxes muscles and reduces stress. As the course progresses, Halpin will introduce the philosophy of

---

[157] *Energy Times, March, 2008.*

good hearted living,' which suggests that concentrating on a particular good-hearted goal each day of the week promotes physical peace—a kind of laughter for the mind. Laughter classes similar to Halpin's have been covered by Oprah WINFREY and on TV Newscasts, Halpin said." [158]

Music, Singing, and Dancing

The value of listening to uplifting music, plus the associated activities of singing and dancing, all contribute to our health and wellbeing. Studies have been made of the effects of different kinds of music on the mind. It was determined that children who listened to classical music, such as baroque music, by composers such as, Bach and Vivaldi, actually scored higher on intelligence tests than children who did not listen to such music. On the other hand children who listened frequently to "Rap" 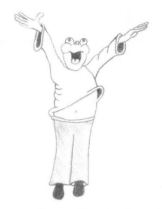 music had lower IQs. Other researchers such as Don Campbell and Alfred Tomatis found that the music of Mozart had the greatest beneficial effect on the mental and physical development of humans as compared to all other kinds of music. The many benefits of listening to music such as Mozart's are presented in great detail by Campbell in his book, *The Mozart Effect for Children: Awakening Your Child's Mind, Health, and Creativity with Music.* Excerpts from this book follow below:

"A recent study found that visual tracking eye-hand coordination, and other positive behaviors developed more rapidly in babies whose mothers participated in a pilot program of prenatal exposure to music. Another study found that remedial first graders who were given seven months of music instruction and visual arts training soon caught up in all subjects with an average group of children not exposed to the arts, and actually surpassed them in math.

It has been proven time and time again that music is a powerful implement for stimulating a child's brain, nourishing his spirit, and

---

[158] Yvette Halpin. *Benefits of Laughter.* Somerset, NJ: Courier News, May 8, 2009, pp. B1-B2.

strengthening his body, even prior to birth. Music is the perfect tool to improve children's language, movement, and emotional skills at home, play, and school.

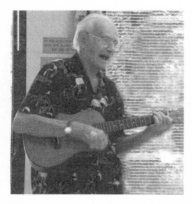

There is more to listening to music - something that seems to bestow a group serenity or transcendence and banish all fear and anxiety, if only for a moment. Most of us have experienced this feeling during a concert or when singing hymns at church." [159]

Don Campbell, cites research studies which confirm the benefits of listening to the music of Mozart: "The researcher reported that the subjects who listened to Mozart reduced their theta brain waves in exact rhythm to the underlying beat of the music, and displayed improved focus, mood control, and social skills. Seventy percent of the subjects who improved maintained that improvement for at least six months afterward....Another music researcher, Alfred Tomatis, found that listening to quality music such as Mozart's gradually retrains the ear, easing the symptoms of ADD as well as certain emotional problems and physical challenges. He states, 'Mozart is an ideal transition from a world of noise to an orderly and organized thinking process." [160]

Music therapists obtain good results, especially in the improving of the quality of sleep, by various methods as described below:

"RESPONDENT CONDITIONING – Follow these steps:

Listen to different selections of music until you find one that seems most restful to you.

After turning out the light, turn on the music you selected. Listen to it over and over until you fall asleep.

Listen to this same selection each night when you are ready to sleep, but don't listen to it at any other time. Eventually the music will stimulate a 'time to sleep', response and you will drift off be-

---

[159] Don Campbell. *The Mozart Effect for Children: Awakening Your Child's Mind, Health, and Creativity with Music.* New York: William Morrow, 2000.
[160] Ibid, pp.181-182.

fore it has hardly begun.

Calming Disquieting Thoughts.

Turn on the light; fix something soothing to drink.

Get comfortable, turn on music that makes you feel good, close your eyes a moment and listen. The music provides a focal point to help you feel in control.

Write down in a notebook whatever thoughts the music suggests, no matter how little sense they seem to make. Keep listening and writing until you feel sleepy.

The next day, read what you wrote and share it with a counselor or friend.

Tonal Massage-By visualizing tones, and by massaging our bodies, we relax muscles and promote inner harmony. The more harmonious we feel, the more easily we fall asleep. Follow the steps below:

1. Turn on the music and concentrate on the sounds while clearing your mind of regrets and worries.

2. Imagine that the tones, starting at your feet are moving up your legs and into your abdomen like the fingers of a masseur or masseuse.

3. Imagine how your heart looks, then imagine how your lungs look. Visualize the tones relaxing these organs, slowing down and regulating their rhythms.

4. Visualize the tonal fingers working on your neck and shoulders, then on your jaws, eyeballs and temples.

5. Visualize the tones entering and tuning your glandular system, especially the lymph nodes, pancreas and liver. Imagine the glands working together at an appropriate pace.

6. Visualize your muscles, organs and glands as a complex machine with all the parts interacting in harmony. Your increasingly slow, even breathing lets you know that you are about to fall asleep.

Breathing away muscle tension - Try breathing and listening to music to get rid of tension.

1. Put on some appropriate relaxing music.

2. Think of nothing except your breathing. Say to yourself something like this: I am relaxing, breathing slowly and easily. With each breath I feel more and more relaxed.

3. Breath in and out several times as you focus on successive groups of muscles. Start with your toes and ankles, move to your legs, then to your buttocks and lower back, your abdomen, your hands and wrists, your chest, your shoulder and neck, your face and scalp and your jaw. Feel each muscle group feel heavy and relaxed.

4. Picture in succession three numbers appearing on a blackboard. Take a deep breath as you conjure up each number. For example, the number three is your symbol for complete body relaxation. The number two is your symbol for complete mental relaxation. The number one is your symbol for oneness of mind and body.

5. Drift with the music for a few moments longer until you fall asleep." [161]

---

[161] *Everyday Health Tips.* Prevention Magazine, 1998. Rodale Press.

CHAPTER TWELVE

COLORS & LIGHT

As we know, rainbows are formed when the sun shines through moisture in the air causing ordinary light to break apart into seven beautiful colors. This also occurs when sunlight shines through prisms or crystals. Looking at these colors gives us a joyful, uplifting feeling.

Light Therapy

Dr. W. Brugh Joy, in his book, *Joy's Way,* describes from a scientific viewpoint how light and colors can be used as a way to heal the body and mind:

> In modern physics, one current theory holds that all matter—and, thus, all energy—is actually trapped light. I find this suggestion intriguing, because many mystical and cosmic experiences report light of various colors emanating from all objects. This light appears to be intrinsic to an object, rather than being reflected from the object; that is, the object itself emits the light and can be seen in total darkness. Without considering the nature of intrinsic light, with all our sophistication, we do not even know what ordinary light is.
>
> Light and sound are accepted in conventional medicine as energy forces capable of healing. Light, in the many frequencies that we know as colors, has been shown to be effective in influencing certain abnormalities of the body. For example, blue light is used to treat jaundiced infants, and the mechanism is clearly known; the frequency of blue light is capable of

breaking up the chemical bonding of the bilirubin molecule and thus converting it into a substance less toxic to the central nervous system. For another example, ultraviolet light is used to treat certain skin disorders and, in sterilization techniques, to kill bacteria and influence virus replication. Sun tanning and sunburn are both produced by light beyond visible frequencies, and when light is produced in a single frequency-as a laser beam-it can make incisions into the body and, outside of medicine, it can cut metal, fabrics and other materials.

Sound is used in orthodox medicine in the form of ultrasonic sound frequencies far above the range audible to humans. These frequencies are used to vaporize liquids in inhalation therapy for respiratory patients, in diagnostic equipment which bounces sound waves through the body to produce so-called echograms, and in direct application to the body to promote the healing of injured tissue. Down in the ordinary listening ranges, sound in the form of music is used to soothe or calm supermarket shoppers, operating room personnel, and office and factory workers. Sonar uses sound waves in the sea in a way analogous to the diagnostic equipment that makes echograms. And I will share some further insights about sound-in the form of music played at high volume-as a tool in precipitating expanded experiences in awareness.

Does this information begin to pique your curiosity as to what we really are? Doesn't it begin to shift your attitude about what is real and what is only apparent? If you can see that a body is an energy interaction, can you see that a disease must be an energy interaction, too? Isn't it conceivable then, that there are unexplored combinations of energy interaction that may alter a disease-energy interaction? Could energy fields produced by human thought be among these therapeutic configurations? Could essential thought even originate matter-create it, and its counterpart, energy-or at least organize it into forms and structures? What cures is not penicillin or other medicine in tablet or liquid form; what cures is actually a combination of energy forces that is capable of influencing other energy forces. There are many such energy configurations, as yet unknown-or denied by science that can influence the fields of energy that are manifested as the apparent physical form.

I hope, for the average reader to feel tilted out of his or her comfortable belief structure about reality and to begin to enter into dimensions of awareness that are based on scientific probing and personal observation as well as the mystical, spiritual and holistic experiences of reality. I feel that if more information from many belief systems is presented to a developing human consciousness there will be less fantasizing and greater application of our potential as conscious beings. [162]

Another researcher into the healing power of light and colors, Dr. Jacob Liberman, in his book, *LIGHT: Medicine of the Future,* reviews the latest findings in this field, excerpts of which follow below:

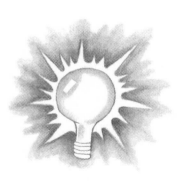

The studies of many researchers have clearly shown that cool-white fluorescent lighting, which is used in most classrooms, creates bodily stress and thus interferes with learning ability. A series of experiments were conducted to evaluate the effects of light and color in a school setting. The subjects were children with severe handicaps including blind and sighted children. Physiology and behavior were monitored and measured before and after full-spectrum lighting was installed and classrooms were painted with selected shades of warm colors. The decision to repaint the walls was based on the work of Ertel, who found that the use of bright warm colors such as yellow and orange improved the intelligence quotient (IQ) and academic achievement of school-age children.

The results were *highly significant.* In the newly painted rooms with full-spectrum lighting, systolic blood pressure dropped an average of 20 points per child, and behavior (es-

---

[162] W. Brugh Joy, M.D. *Joy's Way.* Pp. 31-33.

pecially the reduction of aggression) improved dramatically. However, when the full-spectrum lighting was changed back to the original cool-white fluorescent tubes, blood pressure increased and the children once again became disorderly. Another very interesting finding was that the *blind subjects were as affected as the sighted ones.*

Color Therapy

Dr. H. Wohlfard, one of the world's leading color researchers, designed a follow-up study in which four different schools with different lighting and colors in each school were compared for the effects over a complete school year. He substituted warm shades of light yellow and light blue for the original orange, white, beige and brown wall paints, and replaced the cool-white fluorescent lights with full-spectrum ones.

The best results were consistently found in school number two where both lighting and wall color were changed. The worst results were in school number one where, neither lighting nor colors were changed. In school number two, students were less stressed, quieter, less moody, showed the greatest improvement on combined academic and IQ test scores, and were absent due to illness only one-third as often as the children in school number one. With such impressive results, one wonders why all children's classrooms are not designed with such warm colors and full-spectrum lighting.

A well-known educator, author, and lecturer, Barbara Meister Vitale has used color in her work since 1970. She wrote the following list of effects of colors:

"Placing appropriately colored pieces of felt within the visual work space of a child frequently reduces hyperactivity, increases attention span and improves the speed and accuracy of completing assignments. In most cases, the color red seems to be the most effective for reducing activity levels.

Behavioral changes are sometimes noticed in children when they wear different colored clothing.

By writing with different colored markers or putting words on different colored paper, some children and adults experience an increase in reading fluency, fewer punctuation errors, and improved comprehension. They also experience an increase in long-time recall when notes are taken in their favorite color.

Some adults and children respond very well to reading or working under a blue light.

Adults and children who have difficulty with letter and word reversals, frequent loss of place and or words appearing to float above the page, respond very well to having a specific colored transparency placed over their reading material This alone can drastically change their reading levels.

Nonreaders, when asked to visualize their favorite color, can frequently begin reading at the level of instruction they have been exposed to.

The value of color seems to be individual specific. In most cases, the color that works most effectively is either the person's favorite color or the color that is opposite on the color wheel.

If light and color can significantly improve learning and behavior of normal children and adults, what might be its effects on individuals with leaning difficulties? The effects of color on learning ability received wide publicity as a result of the work of Helen Irlen, a California psychologist. Using different colors she was able to transform nonreading learning disabled individuals into fluid readers. Irlen described her newly discovered form of 'visual dyslexia,' Scoptic Sensitivity Syndrome, and explained that this condition is caused by light that, when received by the eyes, actually distorts what the eyes see. Individuals suffering from this condition respond inappropriately to specific wavelengths of light; they feel overwhelmed in the presence of those wavelengths, almost as if they are allergic to them. Irlen's technique basically involves using colored transparencies and lenses to modify the light entering the eyes, thus eliminating the distortions perceived. Irlen's lenses selectively reduce or eliminate those wavelengths that the eyes cannot handle and transmit those wavelengths that the eyes can handle." [163]

In the book, *The Healing Power of Light,* Primrose Cooper offers an overview of healing theories of light, from the pioneering work of Rudolf Steiner, to the full spectrum light treatment developed by Dr. Norman Rosenthal. Based on her research she states:

"Light is - and has been - a healing agent for various disorders ranging from depression to cancer. Exposure to light is extremely important for your overall health." She points out the importance of being exposed to sunlight as did Dr. Liberman: "Doctors have long known that sunlight is a nutrient and a healer particularly useful for tuberculosis and deep skin wounds. It is also helpful for those with osteoporosis, depleted immune systems and the winter depression. In the 1920s and 30s, Dr. A. Rollier pioneered the building of special sanatoria high in the Swiss Alps and introduced 'sun baths' at his own clinic at Leysin.

It was only with the coming of penicillin in 1938 and the growth of the drug industry that doctors prescribe pills rather than free healing sunlight. Now with the reemergence of tuberculosis in the Western world, the benefits of sunlight are being rediscovered.

Another practitioner who recognized the healing properties of sunlight was Dr. Bates, an oculist working in New York at the beginning of the twentieth century to improve natural vision. He developed a set of exercises to enable his patients to take in as much sunlight as possible. These included periods of 'sunning', looking at the sun through closed lids, 'palming, placing the palms of the hands over the eyes to rest them in an enveloping blackness, blinking, swaying and shifting. He trained his patients to focus with and through the centre of sight in the eyes, the *fovea centralis.* He believed that with this and the supporting exercises it should be possible to do without glasses.

---

[163] Jacob Liberman, O.D., *LIGHT: Medicine of the Future.* New York: Bear & Co. Publishing, 2006, pp. 101-105

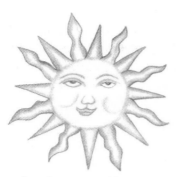 As we have seen, we live by sunlight. This reaches our brain through the eyes and is monitored by a very important gland—the pineal, which is really a light meter. The gland controls puberty and influences our sleep patterns. It secretes a hormone called melatonin, which induces sleep and hibernation. With limited sunlight levels of melatonin are high by day as well as at night. Sunlight, however, suppresses melatonin. We are, after all, programmed to be active in the daylight and to sleep at night. Sunlight suppresses melatonin, but so does light from a light box. Bright light therapy, as it is called, can lift moods, and has also been found helpful to those suffering from eating disorders and those undergoing detoxification from drugs and alcohol.

Most of our domestic lighting is deficient at the green/blue end of the spectrum. It is concentrated on the orange/red end for a 'cozy' effect. That is our choice, of course, but for public areas of work and leisure such as schools, hospitals, prisons, offices, and recreational spaces, it is important to have full spectrum lighting. Research has shown that hyperactivity in children and their levels of dental decay have been linked with poor classroom lighting and have improved with full-spectrum lighting. " [164]

Cooper provides us with an overview of how light is used therapeutically to heal the body; a few excerpts follow below:

Light can be delivered to the body, an area or a point. In ocular light therapy it is delivered to the eye. The treatment was developed by D. John Downing in the course of 20 years in the neurosensory field. It increases the ability to absorb light energy so that the brain and body can function more efficiently. This leads to improved mental emotional and physical well-being and performance. The treatment is particularly valuable for those with learning difficulties, dyslexia,

---

[164] Primrose Cooper. *Healing Power of Light.* York Beach, Maine: Weiser, 2001, pp. 16-23.

hyperactivity, cerebral palsy and autism, Anorexia, bulimia, and ME or chronic fatigue syndrome. SAD and depression may also be helped.

Research demonstrated that light travels to the brain and stimulates and improves its performance. An increasing amount of light can be delivered by the Lumatron. The treatment consists of listening to music and looking at wavebands of light in colors indicated by assessment to be beneficial. Physical and psychological improvements in well-being are often immediate, while for some further courses may be indicated. Light wave stimulation can be used with auditory integration training (AIG) with excellent results. Dr. Downing quotes a case in which he treated a woman of 30 suffering from severe depression, chronic pain and no sense of smell. After nine session of violet light her depression cleared completely and although she still had pain, her sense of smell-lost for years—returned. [165]

The medical profession has researched light for decades. In the USA in 1972, Dr. Thomas Dougherty used light and photofrin, a light sensitive chemical, in cancer treatment at Roswell Park Institute. He discovered that the photofrin gathered in the area of the malignancy, where it luminesced in response to violet or ultra-violet. If Dougherty then focused a red laser beam on the tumor within 10 minutes it would begin to self-destruct. Dr. Kira Samoilova, a world authority on lasers, reported that blood could be cleaned by irradiating it with ultraviolet light. It has proved a highly successful procedure which has cleaned the blood of viruses, cancer and other chronic conditions. One to two percent of a patient's blood is taken, irradiated and reintroduced into the patient's system. [166]

---

[165] Ibid, pp. 81-82
[166] Ibid, pp. 83-84.

APPENDIX A

OAHSPE

Oahspe was channeled by angelic beings through a physician, John Ballou Newbrough circa 1881. The first edition was published in 1882. Newbrough describes in his own words how it happened, as follows:

Briefly, then, *Oahspe* was mechanically written through my hands by some other intelligence than my own. Many spiritualists are acquainted with this automatic movement of the hands, independent of one's volition. There are thousands and thousands of persons who have this quality. It can also be educated, or rather; the susceptibility to external power can be increased. In my own case I discovered, many years ago, in sitting in circles to obtain spiritual manifestations that my hands could not lay on the table without flying off into these "tantrums." Often they would write messages, left or right, backward or forward, nor could I control them in any other way than by withdrawing from the table. Sometimes the power thus baffled would attack my tongue, or my eyes, or my ears, and I talked and saw and heard differently from my normal state. Then I went to work in earnest to investigate spiritualism, and I investigated over two hundred mediums, travelling hundreds and hundreds of miles for this purpose.

Often I took them to my own house and experimented with them to my heart's content. I found that nearly all of them were subject to this involuntary movement of the hands, or to entrancement. They told me it was angels controlling them. In course of time, about ten or fifteen years, I began to believe in spiritualism. But I was not satisfied with the communications; I was craving for the light of heaven. I did not desire communications from friends or relatives, or information about earthly things; I wished to learn something about the spirit-world; what the angels did, how they travelled, and the general plan of the universe. So, after awhile I took it into my head that wise and exalted angels would commune better with us if we purified ourselves physically and spiritually. Then I gave up eating flesh and fish, milk and butter, and took to rising before day, bathing twice a day, and occupying a small room alone, where I sat every morning half-an-hour before sunrise, recounting daily to my Creator my shortcomings in governing myself in thought and deed. In six years' training I reduced myself from two hundred and fifty pounds down to one hundred and eighty; my rheumatism was all gone, and I had no more headaches. I became limber and sprightly. A new lease of life came to me.

Then a new condition of control came upon my hands; instead of the angels holding my hands as formerly, they held their hands over my head (and they were clothed with sufficient materiality for me to see them) and a light fell upon my hands as they lay on the table. In the meantime I had attained to hear audible angel voices near me. I was directed to get a typewriter, which writes by keys, like a piano. This I did, and I applied myself industriously to learn 'it, but with only indifferent success. For two years more the angels propounded to me questions relative to heaven and earth, which no mortal could answer very intelligently. I always look back on those two years as an enigma.

Perhaps it was to show me that man is but an ignoramus at best; perhaps I was waiting for constitutional growth to be good. Well, one morning the light struck both my hands on the back, and they went for the typewriter, for some fifteen minutes, very vigorously. I was told not to read what was printed, and I had worked myself into such a religious fear of losing this new power that I obeyed reverently. The next morning, also before sunrise, the same power came and wrote (or printed rather) again. Again I laid the matter away very religiously, saying little about it to anybody. One morning I accidentally (seemed accidental to me) looked out of the window and beheld the line of light that rested on my hands extending heavenward like a. telegraph wire towards the sky. Over my head were three pairs of hands, fully materialized; behind me stood another angel, with her hands on my shoulders. My looking did not disturb the scene; my hands kept right on, printing . . . printing.

For fifty weeks this continued, every morning half-an-hour or so before sunrise, and then it ceased, and I was told to read and publish the book *Oahspe*. The peculiar drawings in *Oahspe* were made with pencil in the same way. A few of the drawings I was told to copy from other books, such as Saturn, the Egyptian ceremonies, etc.

Now during all the while I have pursued my vocation (dentistry) nor has neither this matter nor my diet (vegetables, fruit and farinaceous food) detracted any from my health or strength, although I have continued this discipline for upwards of ten or more years. I am firmly convinced that there are numberless persons who might attain to marvelous development if they would thus train themselves. A strict integrity to one's highest light is essential to development. Self-abnegation and purity should be the motto and discipline of everyone capable of angel communion. The fact that the plates are all bound together at the end of the volume. Almost at the same time there appeared the first English edition (also at a low price) issued New-brough immediately printed and published the manuscript, the first edition of the work, a folio, being issued in New York and London in 1882. A second edition, a quarto, and cheaper in price, was published in Boston and London in 1891. This contained in addition, a series of reproductions of paintings of great spiritual teachers made by the author when in the trance state. They were not, however, an integral part of the original work.

Half a century later in 1936 the Kosmon Press in California acquired a number of sheets of this imprint (including two important pages which for some reason were not included therein) and issued a new edition, which is now obtainable in America and England.

The first cheap edition was one which was printed privately in England in 1912, but which is now no longer in circulation. It may be identified through by the Kosmon Press in London. A revised edition was published in London, Sydney and Melbourne in 1926.

As to the original manuscript of Oahpse, from which all these editions ultimately take their authority, for some time after New-brough's death this was kept in the basement of a house in El Paso, Texas, until it was ultimately destroyed by a flood. Although this happening may appear to be unfortunate from the point of view of the scholar and the archaeologist it is clear also that there was thereby avoided all danger that authority should come to be vested in a historical document rather than in that interior light of the soul in which Oahpse itself teaches man to place his trust.

It appears, however, that the destruction) of the manuscript took place only when its correspondence with the printed version had already been carefully established. In the Preface to the second edition it is stated that although certain errors had crept into the first edition they had been thoroughly eliminated by existence. As Newbrough died the same year in April it is just possible that he himself was able to undertake the task before he passed over.

With regard to the contents of this extraordinary book, it will suffice here to say that it contains detailed teachings regarding the Creator and His relation to Man and the Universe; the history of the earth and its heavens for the past 24,000 years; the principles of cosmogony and cosmology embracing a completely revolutionary conception of physics; the nature of the angelic worlds and their relation to the earth; the origin of man and his path onwards and upwards during life and after death towards spiritual emancipation; the principles of an enlightened morality; the lost keys to all the different religious doctrines and symbols in the world; the history of the great teachers who have been sent to humanity in different cycles; the character of the civilization which will supersede that in which we are at present living; and a mass of remarkable teachings regarding metaphysics, rites and ceremonies, magic, prophecy and the like. It may profitably be read on every level. The simple may find set forth therein that which they need to know, while the philosopher, the mystic and the esotericist will never exhaust the profundity of its more recondite pages.

APPENDIX B

THE ORIGINS OF THE URANTIA BOOK

Years of experience have demonstrated that the first thing people wish to know about *The URANTIA Book* is its authorship and origin. It does little good to tell them that the book should be judged by its content, not by claims of authorship or events associated with its publication. This is a natural reaction as we have been conditioned by our culture to depend on sources and authority in evaluating publications of all kinds. Religious literature, in particular, is appraised in this way.

The authenticity of persons or literature which are classified by religious groups as having revelatory authority or which make claim to such status is always open to question. Hopefully, we have left behind those days of cultural naivete when claim or authority has any meaning as criterion of truth. There are only two sources through which this question can be approached with any credibility. The one is personal judgment based on the evidence of the quality of the material being evaluated. The other is the testimony of the judgment of society through years of historical experience. Social tradition is an especially powerful influence. Even when Biblical scholars like Rudolf Bultmann declare that our reliable historical knowledge of Jesus is so meager, "We can know almost nothing concerning the life and personality of Jesus," few people are troubled by such statements. Our historical experience has socially validated the quality of the New Testament.

At present there are obviously no traditions associated with *The URANTIA Book*. It must be analyzed and judged on the basis of the quality of its content. Although, technically, they have little relevance in determining the quality of *The URANTIA Book*, there are two sources of information regarding its origin.

THE AUTHORS' ACCOUNT

First is the account you will find in the book itself. We are told the URANTIA papers were authorized by high deity authorities and written by numerous supermortal personalities. These papers are designated as the fifth epochal revelation to our planet, Urantia.The authors acknowledge the difficulty of attempting to portray the realities of eternity in the language of time. We are told there are severe limitations placed on the knowledge they are allowed to share with man. They even admit that all time-space revelation is partial and incomplete needing to be upstepped in the process of planetary development.

In general terms the authors discuss the problems associated with bridging communication between the spiritual levels of the universe and material mortals on our planet. They speak of necessary preparations such as making contact with the Thought Adjuster (indwelling spirit of God) of a human being on our world but hasten to assure us they are not involved in phenomena related to "spiritualism "or "mediumship." Specific details are not discussed. The book simply states the URANTIA papers were materialized in the English language in 1934 and 1935.

THE HUMAN STORY

The second source of information related to the origin of *The URANTIA Book* is the human side of the story. Following my discovery of the book in December of 1955 and after introducing it to some of my clerical friends, we spent years researching the human side of the origin of the book. While space does not allow reporting in detail, the following is a summary of our findings.

We quickly discovered the papers were received by a small

group of people in Chicago and that the leader of this group was Dr. William S. Sadler. As you may know, Dr. Sadler was a highly respected psychiatrist who is sometimes referred to as the father of American psychiatry. For many years he taught at the Post-graduate School of Medicine at Chicago University and for almost thirty years he was a lecturer in Pastoral Counseling at McCormick Theological Seminary.

Discussions with Dr. Sadler revealed that in the mid 1920's a group of people from all walks of life were meeting at the Sadler residence as a psychological-medical discussion group. It was known as the Forum. This group was in communication with the revelators and eventually members of the Forum assumed responsibility for forming the URANTIA Foundation and publishing *The URANTIA Book.*

Dr. Sadler candidly discussed any questions we asked him but he would not talk about two things the name of the individual who was used in some way in the materialization of the URANTIA papers and details associated with this materialization. He said they were asked to take vows of secrecy regarding two things. When I asked him why these restrictions were imposed on them, he gave me the following reasons:

The main reason for not revealing the identity of the contact personality is that the revelators do not want any human being – any human name –ever to be associated with *The URANTIA Book.*

They want this revelation to stand on its own   declarations and teachings. They are determined that future generations shall have the book wholly free from all mortal   connections they do not want a St. Peter, St. Paul, Luther, Calvin, or Westly. The book does not even bear the imprint of the printer who brought the book into being.

2. There is much connected with the appearance of the URANTIA papers which no human being fully understands. No one really knows just how this phenomenon was executed. There are numerous missing links in the story of how this revelation came to appear in written English. If anyone should tell all he really knows about this technique and methods employed throughout the years of getting this revelation, such a narration would satisfy no one   there are too many missing links."

Our group of ministers found in the appendix of Sadler's book

The Mind at Mischief written in 1929 statements which appear to refer to this individual. He says:

"Eighteen years of study and careful investigation have failed to reveal the psychic origin of these messages. I find myself at the present time just where I was when I started. Psychoanalysis, hypnotism, intensive comparison, fail to show that the written or spoken messages of this individual have origin in his own mind. Much of the material secured through this subject is quite contrary to his habit of thought, to the way in which he has been taught, and to his entire philosophy. In fact, of much that we have secured, we have failed to find anything of its nature in existence. Its philosophic content is quite new, and we are unable to find where very much of it has ever been found in human expression." p.383

During Dr. Sadler's investigation of this phenomenon he consulted with men like Howard Thurston, the renowned sleight of hand artist who devoted considerable time to exposing fraudulent mediums and psychics, and Sir Hubert Wilkens, the noted scientist and explorer who was interested in investigating psychic phenomena. All of them agreed that the phenomena connected with this individual could not be classified with other types of psychic phenomena such as automatic writing, telepathy, clairvoyance, trances, spirit mediumship, or split personality.

On May 7, 1958 our group of ministers had an appointment with Dr.Sadler to discuss phenomena associated with the origin of *The URANTIA Book*. When we arrived he had prepared a paper for us listing every imaginable form of subconscious mind or psychic activity at the bottom of the outline he had a note saying, "The technique of the reception of *The URANTIA Book* in English in no way parallels or impinges upon any of the above phenomena of the marginal consciousness." He went on to tell us that so nearly as he could determine, the appearance of the URANTIA papers was associated with some form of superconscious mind activity.

On numerous occasions Dr. Sadler told me that he really did not know how the materialization was accomplished and that just about everything known about the origin of *The URANTIA Book* is found in various places in the book.

In 1939 the revealators requested the leaders of the Forum ask for volunteers who would meet each Wednesday evening to seriously and systematically study the URANTIA papers. Seventy persons volunteered and they became known as "The Seventy." The Seventy were trained by directives from the revelators and their own leadership up to the time of the publication of *The URANTIA Book*. Special emphasis was placed on the evolutionary nature of the acceptance of new truth and the danger of using broadcast, indiscriminate, or revolutionary methods in presenting the message of The URANTIA Book.

After many years of study and discipline, they were given permission to publish the book. They were told the book did not belong to the era in which they were living but would slowly take root in our society in the years to come. An early publication of the book was given, they were told, so that leaders and teachers may be trained and so that men of means may be found to provide for translations into other languages. The cost of the first printing was $75,000, all of which was raised by voluntary contributions of those who had been members of the Forum.

URANTIA Foundation was established as a non-profit, educational organization in 1950 and they published *The URANTIA Book* under international copyright on October 12, 1955. URANTIA Brotherhood was also organized in 1955 as an ecumenical fellowship of people interested in studying and dissemination the teachings of *The URANTIA Book*. Both organizations have offices at 533 Diversey Parkway, Chicago, Illinois 60614.

JUDGE BY CONTENT

This brief account of events associated with the origin of *The URANTIA Book*, as we mentioned earlier, has nothing to do with the truth or spiritual quality of the book. This must be judged by the reader on the basis of the content of the book. The message of *The URANTIA Book* has amazing self-authentication and historical-philosophical truth consistency. The indwelling spirit in man is, in the final analysis, the only ground of being which can reject or affirm the truth of its message. **Meredith J. Sprunger, PhD (4-6-79)**

APPENDIX C

A COURSE IN MIRACLES

There is a set of three books titled *A Course in Miracles* that adds further confirmation to the reality of on-going revelations being transmitted to humans from higher sources. The manner by which the Course came into being plus the deep insights contained in the contents attests to superhuman influences being involved.

The channel through whom the Course was transmitted was Dr. Helen Schucman, a professor of psychology at Columbia University School of Physicians and Surgeons. She was assisted in compiling the material by the head of the department, Dr. William Thetford, who was then Director of the Psychology Department of Presbyterian Hospital. An excellent summary of what took place was described in the book *Double Vision* by Judith Skutch who assisted the professors in bringing about the publication of the Course. Judith and her husband Douglas were invited to meet the professors at the Medical Center on May 29, 1975. The professors told them the following story about the origin of the Course: They told me they had worked together for six years, surviving the vicissitudes of academia, their personal relationship worn but intact. Both of them wondered how they had maintained their willingness to continue, as it was getting more and more difficult to weather their private storms.

One June day in 1965, after a particularly trying staff meeting, Bill and Helen returned to their office. Bill said he felt acutely frustrated by the stress-reflecting attitudes by themselves and associates, and even more resentful at the way in which they interacted with each other. At this point in their story, Helen chimed in to describe the confrontation. 'Bill wanted to say something which he evidently felt hard to talk about. He drew a deep breath, grew slightly red-faced, and actually delivered a speech. Based on the past, he hardly expected a favorable response from me. But he said he had been thinking things over and had concluded that our approach to relating to others was wrong. He said vehemently 'There *must* be another way, and I am determined to find it.' The new way Bill suggested was cooperation rather than competition. He was going to look for the constructive side in all his relationships and not let negative feelings prevail. Somehow Bill's gravity and sincerity struck a chord deep within me and I knew he was right. Though he obviously expected ridicule, I jumped up and told Bill with conviction that I would join with him in the new approach, whatever it might be.'

Helen and Bill told Douglas and me that this joining represented a real commitment that was unprecedented in their relationship. It seemed to be the signal for the beginning of a series of remarkable events that occurred during the summer of 1965. Helen had begun to have both sleeping and waking dreams (or visions) which were three-dimensional and in color. She told us this was not an unfamiliar occurrence, as she had many times in the past caught flashes of inner pictures which she likened to black-and-white stills. These new pictures were heightened by color, and she was included in the action. ...

After three months of what seemed like 'cosmic' preparation, Helen had told Bill she was about to do something very unusual. She did not know what this would be, but the thought of it discomforted her greatly. One evening while she was sitting in her bedroom, an inner voice with which she had become familiar began to give her definite instructions. Afraid, she telephoned Bill. "It keeps saying 'This is a course in miracles. Please take notes.'" In a kindly and supportive manner Bill suggested that Helen, with her excellent shorthand, might just as well sit still and let the inspiration flow. He promised to meet her in their office before the staff arrived and listen to what she had taken down. Still dubious, Helen assented. She settled herself in an attentive position and listened. That first night Helen was given the introduction to *A Course in Miracles*. As Bill had suggested, she brought it into her office the next morning whereupon Bill agreed to type it as he was the better typist, while Helen read her notes out loud.

Douglas and I listened, fascinated, as they continued their narrative, reliving the days when Helen acted as a scribe to the inner voice with Bill as her collaborator. The material they transcribed, through a process Helen called 'inner dictation' eventually comprised three volumes and was revealed to them in the form of a self-study course in spiritual psychotherapy. The purpose of the course was to heal relationships and bring about inner peace.

As they told us of its emphasis on forgiveness as the process to remember one' true identity in God, I felt a force begin to stir in me that I had unknowingly long suppressed. An ancient call so very familiar was resounding in my mind, almost drowning out the details Helen and Bill were sharing. I heard them say the *Course* consisted of a text, a workbook for students and a teacher's manual, and that it had taken them almost ten years to complete the project. I listened to the stories of its origin and its message, which certainly were gripping. (pp.123-126)

Judith was given a copy of the manuscript to read. She became so impressed with the inspirational and practical knowledge contained in the *Course* that she decided to give up working for her doctorate at Columbia University which she had almost completed and to devote her full time to studying the *Course*. She eventually became the most helpful person involved with getting the *Course* published and promoted. She formed a non-profit organization called The Foundation for Inner Peace that became the publisher of the *Course*.

A little booklet published in 1977 by the Foundation contains an excellent summary of what the *Course* is about. An excerpt from the booklet follows below:

"Nothing real can be threatened.
Nothing unreal exists.
Herein lies the peace of God."

This is how *A COURSE IN MIRACLES* begins. It makes a fundamental distinction between the real and the unreal; between knowledge and perception. Knowledge is truth, under one law, the law of love or God. Truth is unalterable, eternal and unambiguous. It can be recognized, but it cannot be changed. It applies to everything God created, and only what he created is real. It is beyond learning because it is beyond time and process. It has no opposite; no beginning and no end. It merely is.

The world of perception, on the other hand, is the world of time, of change of beginnings and endings. It is based on interpretation, not on facts. It is the world of birth and death, founded on the belief in scarcity, loss, separation and death. It is learned rather than given, selective in its perceptual emphases, unstable in its functioning, and inaccurate in its interpretations.

From knowledge and perception respectively, two distinct thought systems arise which are opposite in every respect. In the realm of knowledge no thoughts exist apart from God, because God and His Creation share one Will. The world of perception, however, is made by the belief in opposites and separate wills, in perpetual conflict with each other and with God. What perception sees and hears appears to be real because it permits awareness only what conforms to the wishes of the perceiver. This leads to a world of illusions, a world which needs constant defense precisely *because* it is not real.

Once an individual has been caught in the world of perception he is caught in a dream. He cannot escape without help, because everything his senses show him merely witnesses to the reality of the dream. God has provided the Answer, the only Way out, the true Helper. It is the function of His Voice, His Holy Spirit, to mediate between the two worlds. He can do this because, while on the one hand He knows the truth, on the other He also recognizes our illusions but without believing in them. It is the Holy Spirit's goal to help us escape from the dream world by teaching us how to reverse our thinking and unlearn our mistakes. Forgiveness is the Holy Spirit's great learning aid in bringing this thought reversal about. However, the Course has its own definition of what forgiveness really is, just as it defines the world in its own way.

The world we see merely reflects our own internal frame of reference; the dominant ideas, wishes and emotions in our minds. "Projection makes perception." We look inside first, decide the kind of world we want to see, and then project that world outside, making it the truth *as we see it*. We make it true by our interpretations of what it is we are seeing. If we are using perception to justify our own mistakes, -our anger, our impulses to attack, our lack of love in whatever form it may take, -we will see a world of evil, destruction, malice, envy and despair. All this we must learn to forgive; not because we are being "good" and "charitable," but because what we are seeing is not true. We have distorted the world by our twisted defenses, and are therefore seeing what is not there. As we learn to recognize our perceptual errors, we also learn to look past them or "forgive" them. At the same time we are forgiving ourselves, looking past our distorted self concepts to the Self that God created in us and as us.

Sin is defined as "lack of love." Since love is all there is, sin in the sight of the Holy Spirit is a mistake to be corrected, rather than an evil to be punished. Our sense of inadequacy, weakness and incompletion comes from the strong investment in the "scarcity principle" that governs the whole world of illusions. From that point of view, each individual seeks in others what he feels is wanting in himself. He "loves" another in order to get something from him. That, in fact, is what passes for love in the dream world. There can be no greater mistake than that, for love is incapable of asking for anything.

Only minds can really join, and whom "God has joined no man *can* put asunder." It is, however, only at the level of the Christ Mind that true union is possible, and has, in fact, never been lost. The "little I" seeks to enhance itself by external approval, external possessions and external "love." The Self that God created needs nothing. It is forever complete, safe, loved and loving. It seeks to share rather than to get; to extend rather than project. It has no needs and wants to join with others out of their mutual awareness of abundance.

The special relationships of the world are destructive, selfish and childishly egocentric. Yet, if given to the Holy Spirit, these relationships can become the holiest things on earth; the miracles that point the way to the return to Heaven. The world uses its special relationships as a final weapon of exclusion and a demonstration of separateness. The Holy Spirit transforms them into perfect lessons in forgiveness and in awakening from the dream. Each one is an opportunity to let perceptions be healed and errors corrected. Each one is another chance to forgive oneself by forgiving the other. And each one becomes still another invitation to the Holy Spirit and to the remembrance of God.

Perception is a function of the body, and therefore represents a limit on awareness. Perception sees through the body's eyes and hears through the body's ears. It evokes the limited responses which the body makes. The body appears to be largely self-motivated and independent, yet it actually responds only to the intentions of the mind. If the mind wants to use it for attack in any form, it becomes prey to sickness, age and decay. If the mind accepts the Holy Spirit's purpose for it instead, it becomes a useful way of communicating with others, invulnerable as long as it is needed, and to be gently laid by when its use is over. Of itself it is neutral, as is everything in the world of perception. Whether it is used for the goals of the ego or the Holy Spirit depends entirely on what the mind wants to use it *for*.

… God-like vision is the Holy Spirit's gift; God's alternative to the illusion of separation and to the belief in the reality of sin, guilt and death. It is the one correction for all errors of perception; the reconciliation of the seeming opposites on which this world is based. Its kindly light shows all things from another point of view, reflecting the thought system that arises from knowledge and making return to God not only possible but inevitable. What was regarded as injustices done to one by someone else now becomes a call for help and for union. Sin, sickness and attack are seen as misperceptions calling for remedy through gentleness and love. Defenses are laid down because where there is no attack there is no need for them. Our brother's needs become our own, because they are taking the journey with us as we go to God. Without us they would lose their way. Without them we could never find our own.

Forgiveness is unknown in Heaven, where the need for it would be inconceivable. However, in this world forgiveness is a necessary correction for all the mistakes that we have made. To offer forgiveness is the only way for us to have it, for it reflects the law of Heaven that giving and receiving are the same. Heaven is the natural state of all the Sons of God as He created them. Such is their reality forever. It has not changed because it has been forgotten.

Forgiveness is the means by which we will remember. Through forgiveness the thinking of the world is reversed. The forgiven world becomes the gate to Heaven, because by its mercy we can at last forgive ourselves. Holding no one prisoner to guilt, we become free.

APPENDIX D

RESOURCES

Some of the alternative health care treatments and supplements mentioned in this book may require the services of professionals. This list of resources is provided to assist the reader in finding them plus sources of various products. This does not constitute an endorsement on the part of the author or publisher for any particular product or service.

For additional up-to-date resources visit us on the web at: www.BernardSinger.com and www.ImproveWithAge.org

Organic Foods

Whole Foods Store - This is a national chain of stores that carry a very large selection of natural food products including an excellent selection of fresh fruits and vegetables, many of which are organic.

Farmer Markets - Many local communities throughout the country have locations called 'The Farmers Market' where local farmers bring their produce including fruits and vegetables, many of which are organic.

County Agriculture Agents - Government agriculture agents are listed in phone directories and on the Web. They are knowledgeable in how to grow vegetables and fruits organically that are suitable for the geographic area where you live. They help individuals and groups with technical knowledge on how to grow crops organically. Some assist in locating fields that are available for community gardening for individuals to grow their own vegetables.

The Organic Network by Jean Winter is a directory of Organic growers. For more information call 517-456-4288.

Chiropractic Physicians

Holistic chiropractors are those who offer more than just spinal adjustments. They may provide many additional services such as NAET allergy testing and relief from allergies, massage, and nutritional consultation. Some of them carry the natural, organic supplements manufactured by the Standard Process Co. My own personal holistic chiropractor who has contributed to my good health for the past thirty years is:

Dr. Harry Schick, D.C., Highland Park, NJ, (732) 819-7890.

Alternative Health Care Physicians

Doctors who offer alternative treatments such as chelation therapy, nutritional consultations, acupuncture, laser therapy, massage, etc. for most illnesses including fibromyalgia, cancer, Lupus, MS, and Parkinson's Disease.

Dr. Carlos Manuel Garcia, M.D., Utopia Wellness Center, Clearwater, Florida. phone (727) 799-9060 or www.utopiaawaits.com.

Neurologic Health Centers - www.nrc.md

Wellness Professionals - wellnessspeakers.org

Natural Vitamins and Supplements

Standard Process Co. - Manufactures natural supplements made for the most part from organically grown foods and herbs. Holistic chiropractors are the best way to obtain these products as they know which items are best suited for individual patient's needs. Call 800-848-5061 to locate chiropractors in your area.

Swanson Health Products - The largest and least expensive mail order supplier of natural vitamins and supplements. Call for free catalog 800-437-4148.

Holistic Health Centers and Spas

Omega Institute for Holistic Studies - located at Rhinebeck, NY is one of the largest and best staffed organizations where people can come to be rejuvenated and learn how to maintain their health and longevity. Call 800-944-1000 and/or visit www.eOmega.org.

The Ann Wigmore Foundation - located in San Fidel, New Mexico offers a 10 day Living Foods Lifestyle Retreat based on the diet and philosophy of Ann Wigmore. Phone (505) 552-0595.

SELECTED BIBLIOGRAPHY

Alternative Health Care

Bottom Line Editors. *The 50 Lifesaving Secrets of the World's Greatest Doctors.* Stamford, CT: Boardroom, 2007.
More Ultimate Healing. Stamford, CT: Boardroom, 2007.

Buhner, Stephen. *Herbal Antibiotics.* Pownal, VT: Storey Books, 1999.

Fitzgerald, Randall. *The Hundred-Year Lie.* NY: Dutton, 2006.

Hickey, Dr. Steve & Dr. Hilary Roberts. *Ascorbate: The Science of Vitamin C.* Manchester, England: Lulu Press, 2004.

Kallet, Arthur and F. Schlink. *100,000,000 Guinea Pigs.* New York: Vanguard Press, 1933.

Loes, Michael, M.D. and David Steinman. *The Aspirin Alternative: Escape the Toxicity of NSAIDs.* Topango, CA: Freedom Press, 1999.

Mason, Roger. *The Natural Prostate Cure.* Sheffield, MA: Safe Goods, 2000.

Mertz, Dr. CJ and Co-Authors. *The World's Best Kept Health Secret Revealed.* Minnesota, USA: Chiropractic Press, 2003.

Norden, Michael, M.D. *Beyond Prozac.* NY: Harper-Collins,1995.

Richards, Byron J. *Fight for Your Health.* Wellness Resources, 2006.

Stengler, Mark, Dr. *Supplement to Natural Healing.* Stamford, CT: Boardroom,2007.

Schwartz-Nobel, Loretta. *Poisoned Nation.* New York: St. Martins Press, 2007.

Trudeau, Kevin. *Natural Cures 'They Don't Want You to Know About.'* Elk Grove *Village, IL:* Alliance Publishing, 2004.
More Natural 'Cures' Revealed. IL: Alliance Pub., 2006.

West, Bruce, Dr. *Health Alert* (Monthly *Newsletter).* Monterey, CA: Self Published, 2005-2008.

Wickenden, Leonard. *Our Daily Poison.* NY: Devin-Adair Co., 1956.

Acid and Alkaline Balance (PH)

Aihara, Herman. *Acid and Alkaline.* Oroville, CA: George Ohsawa
    Macrobiotic Foundation, 1985.
Boutenko, Victoria. *Green for Life.* Raw Family Publishing,2005.
    (www.rawfamily.com)
Brown, Dr. Susan, and Larry Trivieri, Jr.The Acid Alkaline Food
    Guide. Garden City, NY: Square One Publishers,2006.
Kliment, Felicia Drury. *The Acid Alkaline Balance Diet.* Chicago:
    Contemporary Books, 2002.
Smith, Esther l. Good Foods That Go *Together.* New Canaan, Conn:
    Keats Publishing, 1975.
Vasey, Christopher, N.D. *The Acid-Alkaline Diet.* Rochester,
    Vermont: Healing Arts Press, 1999.

Acupressure and Acupuncture

Blate, Michael. *The Natural Healer's Acupressure Handbook*
    New York: Holt, Rinehart and Winston, 1977.
Kunz, Kevin and Barbara. *Hand and Foot Reflexology: A Self-*
    Help Guide. New York: Simon & Schuster, 1984.
Porkert, Manfred. *The Theoretical* Foundations of Chinese
    Medicine. Phainon Edition, 1997.
Wright, Janet. *Reflexology and Acupressure.* Summertown, TN:
    Crcs Book Publishing Co., 2000.

ADD and ADHD

Feingold, Ben, M.D. *Why Your Child Is Hyperactive.* New York:
    Random House, 1975.
    The Feingold Cookbook for Hyperactive Children. NY:
    Random House, 1979.

Allergies

Nambumripad, Devi S. *Say Good-Bye to Illness.* Buena Park, CA:
    Delta Publishing, 1999.
    Say Good-Bye to Allergy-Related Autism. Buena Park, CA:
    Delta Publishing, 1997.
Zavik, Jeffrey S. with Jim Thompson. *Toxic Food Syndrome.* Fort

Lauderdale, FL: Fun Publishing, 2007.

Chiropractic Care

Mertz, Dr. CJ and Co-Authors. *The World's Best Kept Health Revealed.* Minnesota: Chiropractic Press, 2000.

Cancer

Henderson, Bill. *Cancer-Free: Your Guide to Gentle, Non-Toxic Healing. Internet:* Booklocker.com, 2007.

Hickey, Dr. Steve & Dr. Hilary Roberts. (op. cit.)

Bricklin, Mark. *The Practical Encyclopedia of Natural Healing.* Emmaus, PA: Rodale Press, 1983.

Campbell, T. Colin and Thomas M. Campbell. *The China Study.* Dallas Texas: Benbella Books, 2006.

Fischer, William L. *How to Fight Cancer and Win.* Baltimore: Agora South, 2000.

Second Edition. Baltimore: Agora Health Books, 2001.

Fitzgerald, Randall. *The Hundred-Year Lie.* (Op.Cit.)

Levy, Thomas, M.D. *Curing the Incurable.* Henderson, NV: LivOnBooks. com, 2002.

Rodale, J.I. & Staff. *Cancer: Facts and Fallacies.* Emmaus, PA: Rodale Books, 1969.

Thomas, Richard. *The Essiac Report.* Los Angeles, CA: Alternative Treatment Information Network, 1993.

Wigmore, Ann. *You are the Light of the World.* Massachusetts: Self published, 1990.

Rebuild Your Health. Puerto Rico: Quality Printers, 1991.

Colors and Healing

Cooper, Primrose. The Healing Power of *Light.* York Beach, Maine: Weiser, 2001.

Dinshah, Darius. *Let There Be Light.* Vineland, NJ: Dinshah Health Society, 1990.

Gimbel, Theo. *The Healing Energies of Color.* NY: Sterling, 2005.

Lieberman, Jacob, O.D., Ph.D. *LIGHT: Medicine of the Future.* New York: Bear & Co. Publishing, 1990.

Detoxing the Body – Weight Loss

Atkins, Dr. Robert C. *Dr.Atkins' New Diet Revolution.* New York: Avon Books, 1999.

Haas, Elson, M.D. *The Detox Diet.* Berkley, CA: Celestial Arts Publishing, 1996.

Harris, Ben Charles. *Eat The Weeds.* Connecticut: Keats Publishing, 1973.

Junger, Alejandro, M.D. *CLEAN: The Revolutinary Program to Restore the Body's Natural Ability to Heal Itself.* New York: Harper-Collins, 2009.

Kloss, Jethro. *Back to Eden.* Loma Linda, CA: Back to Eden Publishing Co., 1988.

Ross, Julia, MA. *The Diet Cure.* New York: Penguin Books, 1999.

Slaga, Thomas, Ph.D. *The Detox Revolution.* New York: McGraw Hill, 2003.

Exercise

Frantzis, Bruce. *Tai Chi: Health for Life.* Berkley, CA: Blue Snakes Books, 2006.

Greene, Bob and Oprah Winfrey. *Make the Connection: Ten Steps to a Better Body-And a Better Life.* New York: Hyperion, 1996.

Loupos, John. Exploring Tat Chi: *Contemporary Views on an Ancient Art.* Boston: YMAA Publication Center, 2003.

Pawlett, Raymond. *Tai Chi.* San Diego: Thunder Bay Press, 1999.

Qingshaan Liu. *Chinese Fitness: A Mind/Body Approach* Jamaica Plain, MA: YMAA Publication Center, 1997.

Yang, Dr. Jwwing-Ming. *QIGONG for HEALTH and MARTIAL ARTS.* Boston, MA: YMAA Publication Center, 1998.
The Root of Chinese Qigong. Boston, MA: YMAA Publication Center, 1989.
Muscle/Tendon Changing and Marrow/Brain Washing Chi Kung: The Secret of Youth. Boston: YMAA Publication Center, 1998.

Heart Disease

Hickey, Dr. Steve & Dr. Roberts. *Ascorbate The Science of Vitamin C.* Manchester, England: Lulu Press, 2004.

Junger, op. cit. under Detox.

(Also look at books by Kevin Trudeau, Bricklin and Colin Campbell)

Kinesiology

Diamond, John. *Behavioral Kinesiology.* New York: Harper & Row, 1979.

Goodheart, G. *Applied Kinesiology*, 12th *Edition.* Detroit: Privately Published, 1976.

Hawkins, David R. M.D.. Ph.D. *Power vs Force: An Anatomy of Consciousness.* Sedona, AZ: Veritas Publishing, 2004.

Longevity

Balch. James F. *Is It Possible To Fight Off Every Sign of Aging. Henderson, NY:* Journal of Health and Longevity, Vol.3 July, 2008. pp. 1-4.

Clement G. Martin, M.D. *How To Live To Be 100* New York: Frederick Fell Book Publishers, 1961.

Editors of Prevention. *Healing With Vitamins.* Emmaus, PA: Rodale Press, 1996.

Null, Gary, Ph.D. *Gary Null's Power Aging.* New York: New American Library, Division of Penguin Group, 2003.

Rowe, John W., M.D. and Robert Kahn, Ph.D. *Successful Aging.* New York: Pantheon Books, 1998.

Sears, Barry, Ph. D. *The Anti-Aging Zone.* New York: Harper Collins, 1999.

Meditation

Bloomfield, Harold, M.D. and Robert Kory. *HAPPINESS: The TM Program.* New York: Dawn Press, 1976.

Bloomfield Harold, M.D., Michael Cain and Dennis Jaffe. *TM: Discovering Inner Energy and Overcoming Stress.*

New York: Delacorte Press, 1975.

Denniston, Denise and Peter McWilliams. *The Transcendental Meditation TM BOOK*. Allen Park, Michigan: Versemonger Press, 1975.

Forem, Jack. *Transcendental Meditation: Maharhishi Mahesh Yogi and the Science of Creative Intelligence*. New York: E.P.Dutton and Co., 1973.

Music and Sounds for Healing

Campbell, Don. *The Mozart Effect for Children: Awakening Your Child's Mind, Health, and Creativity with Music*. New York: William Morrow, 2000.

Gaynor, Mitchell, M.D. *Sounds of Healing: A Physician Reveals the Therapeutic Power of Sound, Voice, and Music*. New York: Broadway Books, 1999.

Watson, Andrew & Nevill Drury. *Healing Music*. New York: Avery Publishing Group, 1987.

Nutrition

Campbell, T. Colin & T.Campbell. *The* China Study. (op. cit.)

Rodale Editors. *Healthy Living*. Emmaus, PA: Rodale Press, 1996.

Cousens, Gabriel. *Spiritual Nutrition*. Berkley, CA: North Atlantic Books, 2005.

Diamond, Harvey & Marilyn. *Fit For Life*. NY: Warner Books, 1987.

Editors of FC&A. *Super life, Super Health*. Peachtree City, GA: FC&A Medical Publishing, 1997.

Feingold, Ben, M.D. and Helene Feingold. *The Feingold Cookbook for Hyperactive Children*. NY: Random House, 1979.

Jarvis, Wm. M.D. *Folk Medicine*. Greenwich, Conn: Fawcett Publishing Co., 1958.

Price, Weston A. *Nutrition and Physical Degeneration*. NY:

Taub, Edward A, M.D. *Balance Your Body, Balance Your Life*. Westchester, PA: Kensington Press, 1999.

West, Dr. Bruce. *The Elusive Vitamin K2*. Monteray, CA: Health Alert, September, 2008.

Organic Foods and Health

Balfour, E.B. *The Living Soil*. London: Faber and Faber, 1944.

Banik, Dr. Allen and Renee Taylor. Long Beach, CA: Whitehorn Pub. Co.,1995.

Boutenko, Victoria. *Green for Life*. www.rawfamily .com: Raw Family Publishing, 2005.

Howard, Sir Albert. *An Agricultural Testament.* London: Oxford University Press, 1949.
The Soil and Health. New York: Devin Adair, 1956.

McCarrison, Sir Robert. *Nutrition and* National Health. London: Faber and Faber, 1944.

Mons, Barbara. *High Road to Hunza*. London: Faber and Faber, 1958.

Rodale, J.I. *The Organic Front.* Emmaus, PA: Rodale Press, 1948.
The Healthy Hunzas; Emmaus, PA: Rodale Press, 1949.
Organic Gardening. Emmaus, PA: Rodale Press, 1955.

Cooper, Robert K., Ph.D. *Healthy Living* .Emmaus, PA: Rodale Press, 1996.

Jarvis, Wm. M.D. *Folk Medicine.* Greenwich, Conn: Fawcett Publishing Co., 1958.

Taub, Edward A, M.D. *Balance Your Body,* Balance Your Life.

Power of Beliefs and Thoughts

Ardagh, Arjuna. *Awakening Into ONENESS: The Power of Blessing in the Evolution of Consciousness*. Boulder, Colorado: Sounds True Inc., 2007.
The Magic Guide to Self-Attunement. Berkley, CA: Crossing Press. 2007.

Byrne, Rhonda. *The Secret.* New York: Atria Books, 2006.

Daniel, Alma, et al. *Ask Your Angels.* NY: Ballantine Books, 1992.

Eker, T. Harv. *Secrets of the Millionaire Mind.* New York: Harper Collins, 2005.

Germain, Saint.(Channeled)*The 'I Am' Discourses*. Schaumburg, IL: Saint Germain Foundation, 1940.

Chimenti, Sandra Agazzi. *The Real Me: Awakening Your True Self, Positive Affirmations for Empowering Your Life*. Rochester Hills, MI: Creative Books, 2007.

Chopra, Deepak. *The Spontaneous Fulfillment of Desire,* New York: Harmony Books, 2003. *The Book of Secrets.* New York: Harmony Books, 2004.

Cousins, Norman. *Anatomy of an Illness*. NY: Bantam Books, 1981.

Dwoskin, Hale. *The Sedona Method*. Phoenix, AZ: Sedona Press, 2003.

Dyer, Dr .Wayne W. *The Power of Intention*. Carlsbad, CA: Hay House, 2004.

Goldsmith, Joel. *Realization of Oneness*. New York: Citadel Press, 1965.
Conscious Union with God. NY: Citadel Press, 1962.
Beyond Words and Thoughts. NY: Citadel Press, 1963.
Leave Your Nets. New York: Citadel Press,1964.

Hanh, Thich Nhat. *Nothing to Do Nowhere to Go*. Berkeley, CA: Parallax Press, 2007.

Hill, Napoleon. *Think and Grow Rich*. Los Angeles: Highlands Media, 2004.

Huber, Cheri. *That Which You Are Seeking Is Causing You To Seek*. Mountain View, CA: Zen Center, 1990.

Joy, W. Brugh, M.D. *Joy's Way*. Los Angeless: J.P. Tarcher, 1979.

Losier, Michael J. Law of Attraction: *The Science of Attracting more of what you want and less of what you don't want*. New York: Wellness Central, 2007.

Maharshi, Ramana. *The Spiritual Teaching of Ramana Maharshi*. Boston: Shambala Publications, 1988.

Marvelly, Paula. *The Teachers of ONE*. London: Watkins Publishing, 1988.

Masaru, Emoto. *The Hidden Messages in Water*. NY: Atria Books, 2000.

Modi, Shakuntala, M.D. *Remarkable Healings*. Charlottesville, VA: Hamptom Roads Publishing Company, 1997.

Myss, Caroline, Ph.D. *Anatomy of the Spirit*. New York: Harmony Books, 1996.

Schick, Dr. Harry. *What Else Can I Do?* www.xlibris.com, 2009

Singer, Bernard *Life Beyond Earth: The Evidence and its Implications.* Piscataway, NJ: Eloist Press, 2001.

Tsu, Lao. *TAO TE CHING.* New York: Vantage Books, 1989.

Weil, Andrew, M.D. *Spontaneous Healing.* New York: Ballantine Books, 1995.

Healthy Aging. New York: Alfred Knopf, 2005.

Relaxation Response and Stress

Benson, Herbert, M.D. and Eileen M. Stuart. *The Wellness Book.* N.Y.: Fireside, 1992.

Norden, Michael J., M.D. *Beyond Prozac.* N.Y.: Harper Collins Publishers, 1995.

JOURNALS

AARP *The Magazine.* Washington, DC.

Cutler, Dr. Michael. *Natural Health Answers.* Warrior, Alabama.

Douglass, William Campbell II, M.D. *The Douglass Report.* Baltimore, MD.

Laux, Dr. Marcus. *Naturally Well Today.* Lancaster, PA

Life Extension Foundation. *Life Extension Magazine.* Ft. Lauderdale, FL: LE Publications.

Mayo Clinic. *Health Letter.* Rochester, MN: Mayo Foundation.

Shallenenberger, Dr. Frank M.D. *Real Cures.* Soundview Publishing

West, Dr. Bruce. *Health Alert.* Monteray, CA: Health Alert.

Whitaker, Dr. Julian, M.D. *Health & Healing.* Potomac, MD: Healthy Directions.

Williams, Dr. David. *Alternatives.* Potomac, MD: Health Directions.

Wright, Dr. Jonathan. *Nutrition & Healing.* Renton WA: Healthier News.

INDEX

Chondroiton 265
Cilantro 199, 212, 247, 265
Coenzyme Q10 197
Cocaine 27, 162, 164, 168
Coconut Oil 224-225
Cod Liver Oil 188, 208, 258
Coincidences 7, 80
Cola Drinks 212-213
Colds 4, 217, 255, 259
Colitis 17, 38, 273, 278-279
Color Therapy 318
Consciousness 72, 86-91,
    100-104, 112, 119, 122-
    125, 289, 295, 317, 330
Constipation 45, 157, 246,
    278-280
Corn Syrup 205, 212, 269
Cortisol 37, 40-41, 217, 219
Course in Miracles 68, 95-
    99, 109, 333-338
Cranberries 212
Crestor 197-200
Crohn's Disease 278
Curcumin 220, 230, 263,
    272
DDT 151, 154, 264
Dementia 197-198, 221-228
Depression 27, 30, 38, 128,
    135, 163, 181, 185, 205,
    211, 218, 226, 258, 266,
    276, 320-322
DHEA 35, 40
Diabetes 2, 21-23, 33-34,
    150-154, 172, 179, 190,
    197-198, 205, 224-226,
    231, 233, 242, 253-255,
    264, 268-270
Dianetics 68-70

DNA 33, 207, 211, 231,
    260
Dualism 119-122
Dyer, Wayne, 112-113
Echinacea 259
EDTA 252, 282, 284-285
Ego 4, 86-88, 119-125, 338
Emotion 90, 281, 295
Emotional Freedom-EFT
    281
Emphysema 35, 263, 304
Encephalitis 38
Endurance 41, 51-52, 55,
    62-63, 225
Engrams 69-70
Enzymes 16, 47, 190, 207,
    216, 244, 262
Epilepsy 202, 225
Essiac 236-239
Estrogen 35, 44, 65, 151,
    197, 278
Eucalyptus 259
Exercise 49-66, 145,161,
    200, 215, 219, 242, 248,
    250, 253-254, 264-266,
    268-269, 291, 293, 306
Fasting 242
Fat 23-25, 54, 152, 200,
    203, 208-210, 224-226,
    240-241, 265, 268-271
Feingold Diet 170-172
Fenugreek 254
Fiber 14, 23-24, 28, 32, 43,
    200, 215, 219, 248, 255,
    265, 266
Fibromyalgia 205, 210,
    256-258

Water 44-46
Water Crystals 102-107
Watercress 43
Watermelon 263
Weight Loss 13, 24-28, 35,
  46, 210, 270,
Weil, Dr. Andrew, 74, 248
Wheat Germ Oil 41
Wheat Grass 242-243
Wigmore, Ann 242-243

Yin and Yang 55, 88, 123,
  145
Yoga 65-66
Yogurt 190, 200, 212, 265
Zinc 197, 241, 244, 248,
  260
Zoloft 181